NURSES' GUIDE TO

UNDERSTANDING LABORATORY AND DIAGNOSTIC TESTS

Acquisition Editor: Susan Keneally
Production Editor: Jahmae Harris
Senior Production Manager: Helen Ewan
Production Coordinator: Patricia McCloskey
Designer: Doug Smock

Library of Congress Cataloging in Publication Data

Wilson, Denise D.
    Nurses' guide to understanding laboratory and diagnostic tests /
Denise D. Wilson.
        p.   cm.
    Includes bibliographical references and index.
    ISBN 0–7817–1834–1
    1. Diagnosis, Laboratory—Handbooks, manuals, etc.   2. Nursing-
-Handbooks, manuals, etc.   I. Title.
    [DNLM: 1. Laboratory Techniques and Procedures nurses'
instruction.   2. Diagnostic Tests, Routine nurses' instruction.   QY
4 W747n   1998]
    RB38.2.W54   1998
    616.07′56—dc21
    DNLM/DLC
    for Library of Congress   98–3764
                                                                CIP

Care has been taken to confirm the accuracy of the information presented and to describe generally accepted practices. However, the authors, editors, and publisher are not responsible for errors or omissions or for any consequences from application of the information in this book and make no warranty, express or implied, with respect to the contents of the publication.

The authors, editors and publisher have exerted every effort to ensure that drug selection and dosage set forth in this text are in accordance with current recommendations and practice at the time of publication. However, in view of ongoing research, changes in government regulations, and the constant flow of information relating to drug therapy and drug reactions, the reader is urged to check the package insert for each drug for any change in indications and dosage and for added warnings and precautions. This is particularly important when the recommended agent is a new or infrequently employed drug.

Some drugs and medical devices presented in this publication have Food and Drug Administration (FDA) clearance for limited use in restricted research settings. It is the responsibility of the health care provider to ascertain the FDA status of each drug or device planned for use in their clinical practice.

9   8   7   6   5   4   3   2   1

NURSES' GUIDE TO

UNDERSTANDING LABORATORY AND DIAGNOSTIC TESTS

Denise D. Wilson, PhD, RN, CS, FNP

Associate Professor
Mennonite College of Nursing
Bloomington, Illinois
Family Nurse Practitioner
Medical Hills Internist
Bloomington, Illinois

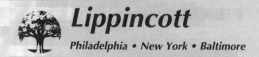

Lippincott

Philadelphia • New York • Baltimore

I dedicate this book with love to four very special people . . .

. . . to my husband, Gary, whose never-ending love,
support, and encouragement made this dream a reality

. . . to Cole and Lauren . . . I could never ask
for more wonderful and loving children

. . . to my mother, Ida Williams,
who has always been there for me.

Preface

··

The *Nurses' Guide to Understanding Laboratory and Diagnostic Tests* is designed to assist those caring for patients to quickly understand and interpret the diagnostic procedures most commonly ordered in health care today.

The tests are arranged alphabetically according to the most current name used for the test. However, it is recognized that many health care providers are more familiar with terminology previously used for some tests. To meet this need, each test lists other names commonly used for the test. The index is complete with all of the test names, both old and new, so that anyone can find the test they need quickly and without frustration.

The following format is used for each test.

Name of the Test

The primary test name is given in large bold print. Other commonly used names are listed in bold print under the primary name.

Description of the Test

Information is provided to assist the reader in understanding the test. Information is included regarding relevant anatomy and physiology, indications for the test, the theoretical basis for the test, and other information specific to the test.

Normal Values

The normal values listed are intended to serve as general guidelines, or reference values. They are not meant to replace test norms provided by each laboratory. Most of the values contained in this text are those published by the *New England Journal of Medicine.*

When available, values are given in both conventional and SI units. Conventional units, such as milligram and liter, are those which have been used historically in health care in the United States. In an attempt to standardize the measurements worldwide, a system of international (SI) units has been developed. Although the change is occurring slowly, many laboratories are now reporting values in both systems.

Abnormal Values

For a few of the tests there are abnormal values listed. This is done when there are "degrees" of abnormality, such as "borderline," and with some tests involving titer determination.

Possible Meanings of Abnormal Values

This section provides a compilation of conditions that *may* account for an abnormal result for the test. The lists are presented alphabetically to assist the reader in quickly locating the desired information.

Contributing Factors to Abnormal Values

This section provides information regarding patient conditions, equipment or procedural peculiarities, foods, and drugs that may affect test results. Drugs are listed either as individual generic names, or, when an entire group of drugs is applicable, as a broad classification.

Please refer to Appendix A for a drug name reference guide and to Appendix B for a broad classification reference. The reader may wish to add additional drug names used in a particular practice to supplement those chosen for inclusion here.

Contraindications

This section lists the primary types of patients on whom a particular test should *not* be performed. In addition, the health care provider must always assess the individual patient to determine the presence of other factors that may cause the test to be contraindicated for that particular patient.

Pre-Test Nursing Care

This section includes areas of patient teaching to be completed prior to the test and other aspects of patient preparation for the test, such as dietary restrictions and obtaining informed consent.

Procedure

This section includes the steps carried out during the actual procedure. Some institutions may use different colored tubes for collecting blood samples than those used at other facilities. Thus, the *type* of collection tube, such as one containing heparin, is listed, rather than indicating a tube top *color*.

Although the nurse may not be present during the procedure, this information is important for patient teaching purposes. Most procedures involve potential contact with the patient's body fluids. *The institution's infection control policy regarding collection and handling of specimens should be reviewed and carefully followed. This includes compliance with the universal precautions developed by the Centers for Disease Control and Prevention (CDC).*

The proper collection and handling of a specimen is essential, not only for obtaining accurate results, but also for the safety of the health care worker. If the registered nurse (RN) delegates the collection of a specimen to another individual, such as a certified nursing assistant (CNA), it is the responsibility of the RN to ensure that the CNA understands and follows the proper procedure.

Post-Test Nursing Care

This section lists first, in bold print, the complications that may be experienced by the patient. It also lists assessment, intervention, and patient teaching aspects of care following completion of the test.

In addition to the drug references found in Appendix A and Appendix B, which were discussed previously, this text includes a list of common test groupings in Appendix C that should be helpful in understanding relationships among the various tests. The appendices are followed by a bibliography of sources used for this text, and a comprehensive index listing of all test names and abbreviations used in the text.

It is my hope that you, the reader, find this a helpful guide for use in your nursing practice.

Denise Wilson

Acknowledgments

I would like to acknowledge and thank those individuals who have, in some way, played a part in the completion of this text. Thank you to: Lisa Stead, Editor, Nursing and Allied Health Publishing for Lippincott Williams & Wilkins, for believing in me. Susan M. Keneally, Associate Editor, for her guidance and encouragement throughout the production of this book. My colleagues at Mennonite College of Nursing, for their encouragement, sharing of knowledge, and friendship throughout the years. My graduate students, Linda Ahrens, RN, BSN; Yvonne M. Campbell, RN, BSN; Cindy Chaffin, RN, MSN, FNP; Phyllis Coulter, RN, BSN; Penny S. Kilhoffer, RN, MSN, FNP; M. Elizabeth Koglin, RN, MS; Katherine A. Krall, RN, MSN, FNP, ONC; Nancy Machens, RN, MS, FNP; Karen M. Manson, RN, MSN, FNP; Sue S. McGinnes, RN, MSN, FNP; Sue S. Mendez, RN, C, MSN, FNP; Patricia A. Thompson, RN, MSN, FNP, CCRN; Sue A. Valentine, RN, MSN, FNP; Keli Wagner, RN, MSN, FNP; and Nancy S. White, RN, MSN, FNP, who made me realize that both generic name *and* trade names of drugs were needed in this text and who worked diligently to compile the drug lists found in the Appendix. The Reviewers of the text for their careful review and thoughtful comments. My family and friends who were always there to offer support. Cole and Lauren Wilson, who helped me while I developed the lengthy list of what tests would be included in the text. A very special thank you to Gary Wilson, my husband, for always believing in me and for taking over many of my responsibilities at home as the manuscript deadlines quickly approached.

Contents

List of Figures

List of Tables

Table

Abdominal Aorta Sonogram
(Ultrasonography of the Abdominal Aorta)

Ultrasonography is a noninvasive method of diagnostic testing in which ultrasound waves are sent into the body with a small transducer pressed against the skin. The transducer not only sends the sound waves into the body but also receives any returning sound waves, which are deflected back as they bounce off various structures. The transducer converts the returning sound waves into electric signals that are then transformed with a computer into a visual display on a monitor.

In this particular type of ultrasonography, the transducer is passed over the area from the xiphoid process to the umbilicus. The purpose is to detect and measure a suspected abdominal aortic aneurysm. The lumen of the abdominal aorta is normally less than 4 cm in diameter. It is considered to be aneurysmal if it is greater than 4 cm and at high risk of rupture if it is greater than 7 cm. This test can also be used as a follow-up evaluation after surgery for repair of an aneurysm.

Normal Values

Negative for presence of aneurysm
Abdominal aorta lumen diameter < 4 cm

Possible Meanings of Abnormal Values

Abdominal aortic aneurysm

Contributing Factors to Abnormal Values

- The transducer must be in good contact with the skin as it is being moved. A lubricant, such as mineral oil, glycerin, or a water-based jelly, is used to ensure good contact with the skin.
- Clear imaging can be hampered by the presence of retained gas or barium in the intestine, obesity, and patient movement.

Pre-Test Nursing Care

- Explain to the patient the purpose of the test. Provide any written teaching materials available on the subject. Note that there is no discomfort involved with this test.
- No fasting is required before the test.

Procedure

- The patient is assisted to a supine position on the ultrasonography table.
- A coupling agent, such as a water-based gel, is applied to the area to be evaluated.
- A transducer is placed on the skin and moved as needed to provide good visualization of the structures.
- The sound waves are transformed into a visual display on the monitor. Printed copies of this display are made.

Post-Test Nursing Care

- Cleanse the patient's skin of remaining coupling agent.
- Report abnormal findings to the primary care provider.

Acetylcholine Receptor Antibodies
(AChR, Anti-ACh Antibodies)

Acetylcholine (ACh) and the catecholamines epinephrine and norepinephrine are the main neurotransmitters of the autonomic nervous system. In normal contraction of the muscles, ACh is released from the terminal end of the nerve into the neuromuscular junction. ACh then binds with receptor sites on the muscle membrane, resulting in the opening of sodium channels. This allows sodium ions to enter and depolarize the cell. This begins an action potential that passes along the entire muscle fiber, resulting in muscle contraction.

Myasthenia gravis (MG) is an autoimmune disease that affects neuromuscular transmission. In this disease, antibodies form that interfere with the binding of ACh to the receptor sites on the muscle membrane. This prevents muscle contraction from occurring. These antibodies are present in more than 85% of the patients with MG. Thus, this test is used for diagnosis of MG and for the monitoring of patient response to immunosuppressive therapy for the disease.

Normal Values

Negative or ≤ 0.03 nmol/L

Possible Meanings of Abnormal Values

Increased

Myasthenia gravis

Contributing Factors to Abnormal Values

- *False-positive* results may occur in patients with amyotrophic lateral sclerosis (ALS).
- Drugs that may *decrease* ACh receptor antibodies titers: immunosuppressive drugs.

Pre-Test Nursing Care

- Explain to the patient the purpose of the test and the need for a blood sample to be drawn.
- No fasting is required before the test.

Procedure

- A 7-mL blood sample is drawn in a collection tube containing no additives.
- Gloves are worn throughout the procedure.

Post-Test Nursing Care

- Apply pressure at venipuncture site. Apply dressing, periodically assessing for continued bleeding.
- Label the specimen and transport it to the laboratory.
- Report abnormal findings to the primary care provider.

• • • • • • • • • • • • • • • •

Acid-Fast Bacilli
(AFB)

The acid-fast method is a special staining technique that is particularly useful when identifying mycobacteria in sputum specimens, which often contain a variety of organisms. Examples of mycobacteria are those causing leprosy, tuberculosis, and respiratory infection in patients with acquired immune deficiency syndrome (AIDS). Mycobacteria retain stain coloring even after treatment with a decolorizing acid-alcohol solution. Once bacilli are determined to be acid-fast, a culture is done to differentiate the type of mycobacteria, along with sensitivity testing to determine appropriate pharmacologic treatment.

Normal Values

Negative for bacilli

Possible Meanings of Abnormal Values

Positive

Acquired immune deficiency syndrome (AIDS)
Leprosy
Tuberculosis

Contributing Factors to Abnormal Values

- Collection of saliva, rather than sputum, will provide inaccurate test results.

Pre-Test Nursing Care

- The sputum should be collected before antimicrobial therapy is begun.
- Explain to the patient the purpose of the test and the need for a sputum specimen.
- Explain the procedure to the patient:
  - An early morning specimen is best, because sputum is most concentrated at that time.
  - The patient should brush the teeth and rinse the mouth with water before collecting the sputum to reduce contamination of the sample.
  - The sputum must be from the bronchial tree. The patient must understand this is different from saliva in the mouth.
  - The sample is collected in a sterile sputum container.
- If tuberculosis is suggested, three consecutive morning specimens may be ordered. This increases the chance of isolating the microbes.
- If the sputum is very thick, it can be thinned by inhaling nebulized saline or water or by increasing fluid intake the evening before sample collection. Postural drainage and chest physiotherapy may also prove helpful.

Procedure

- The patient should take several deep breaths and then cough deeply to obtain the specimen. At least 1 teaspoon of sputum is needed.
- Other ways to collect sputum include endotracheal suctioning and fiberoptic bronchoscopy.

- After collection of the sputum, the sample is sent to the laboratory for a Gram stain. This is used to differentiate between true sputum and saliva, which contains many epithelial cells. Decolorizing solution is used to determine acid-fastness of the bacilli.
- The sputum is then placed on the appropriate culture medium and allowed to incubate. Final reports for tuberculosis (AFB culture) may take 1 to 6 weeks.
- Gloves are worn throughout the procedure.

Post-Test Nursing Care

- Label the specimen container and transport it to the laboratory as soon as possible. Note any current antimicrobial therapy on the label.
- Report abnormal findings to the primary care provider.

• • • • • • • • • • • • • • • •

Acid Phosphatase
(Prostatic Acid Phosphatase [PAP])

Acid phosphatase, also known as prostatic acid phosphatase (PAP), is an enzyme found primarily in the prostate gland, with high concentrations found in the seminal fluid. It is found in smaller concentrations in the kidneys, liver, spleen, bone marrow, erythrocytes, and platelets. Acid phosphatase is used to diagnose advanced metastatic cancer of the prostate and to monitor the patient's response to therapy for prostate cancer. This test has been considered a tumor marker for prostatic cancer. However, with the advent of the prostate-specific antigen (PSA) test, monitoring of the acid phosphatase is decreasing in popularity. An additional use of acid phosphatase testing is testing for its presence in vaginal secretions during the investigation of cases of alleged rape.

Normal Values

2.2–10.5 IU/L (37–175 nkat/L SI units)

Possible Meanings of Abnormal Values

Increased

Acute renal impairment
Bone metastases
Breast cancer
Cancer of the prostate
Cirrhosis
Eclampsia
Gaucher's disease
Hemolytic anemia
Hepatitis
Hyperparathyroidism
Liver tumor

Multiple myeloma
Obstructive jaundice
Paget's disease

Contributing Factors to Abnormal Values

- Hemolysis of the blood sample may alter test results.
- Any manipulation of the prostate gland, including rectal examination or cystoscopy, should be avoided for 2 days before the test.
- Acid phosphatase levels vary during the day. Multiple tests of acid phosphatase should be drawn at the same time each day.
- Drugs that may *increase* acid phosphatase: anabolic steroids, androgens, clofibrate.
- Drugs that may *decrease* acid phosphatase: alcohol, fluorides, oxalates, phosphates.

Pre-Test Nursing Care

- Explain to the patient the purpose of the test and the need for a blood sample to be drawn.
- No fasting is required before the test.

Procedure

- A 7-mL blood sample is drawn in a collection tube containing a silicone gel. The tube should be kept on ice.
- Gloves are worn throughout the procedure.

Post-Test Nursing Care

- Apply pressure at venipuncture site. Apply dressing, periodically assessing for continued bleeding.
- Label the specimen and transport it to the laboratory immediately.
- Report abnormal findings to the primary care provider.

• • • • • • • • • • • • • • • • •

Adrenal Function Tests

Adrenal Cortex:

Glucocorticoids

See:
Adrenocorticotropic Hormone
Adrenocorticotropic Hormone Stimulation Test
Cortisol, Blood
Cortisol, Urine
Dexamethasone Suppression Test
17-Hydroxycorticosteroids

Mineralocorticoids

See:
Aldosterone
Renin Activity, Plasma

Sex Hormones
See:
Pregnanetriol
17-Ketosteroids

Adrenal Medulla:
See:
Vanillylmandelic Acid and Catecholamines

• • • • • • • • • • • • • • • • •

Adrenocorticotropic Hormone
(ACTH, Corticotropin)

In response to a stimulus such as stress, the hypothalamus secretes corticotropin-releasing hormone. This hormone stimulates the secretion of adrenocorticotropic hormone (ACTH) by the anterior pituitary gland. ACTH, in turn, causes the adrenal cortex to release the glucocorticoid hormone cortisol. As levels of cortisol in the blood rise, the pituitary gland is stimulated to decrease ACTH production via a negative feedback mechanism. See Figure 1.

Diurnal variations in ACTH level occur, with peak levels occurring between 6 and 8 AM and trough levels occurring between 6 and 11 PM. Trough levels are approximately one-half to two-thirds the peak levels.

Assessment of ACTH levels is used in conjunction with knowledge of cortisol levels to evaluate adrenal cortical dysfunction. For example, consider the patient with Addison's disease in which the adrenal cortex is hypoactive, thus producing abnormally low levels of cortisol in the

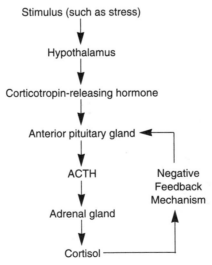

Figure 1 Cortisol production.

blood. The anterior pituitary gland senses the low serum cortisol levels and, as a result, increases its release of ACTH. This is an attempt to stimulate the adrenal gland to increase its production of cortisol. Thus, the combination of high ACTH and low cortisol levels indicates adrenocortical hypoactivity. Correlation of ACTH and cortisol levels with the underlying cause is summarized in Table 1. "Primary" type problems, such as primary adrenal insufficiency, deal with abnormalities of the target organ (adrenal gland) itself, whereas "secondary" problems deal with abnormalities of the pituitary gland. See Table 1.

Normal Values

6.0–76.0 pg/mL (1.3–16.7 pmol/L SI units)

Possible Meanings of Abnormal Values

Increased	Decreased
Addison's disease	Cushing's syndrome
Ectopic ACTH syndrome	Hypopituitarism
Pituitary adenoma	Primary adrenocortical hyperfunction (tumor)
Pituitary Cushing's disease	Secondary hypoadrenalism
Primary adrenal insufficiency	
Stress	

Contributing Factors to Abnormal Values

- Levels of ACTH may vary with exercise, sleep, and stress.
- Testing for ACTH should be scheduled no sooner than 1 week after any diagnostic tests using radioactive materials.
- Drugs that may *decrease* ACTH levels: amphetamines, calcium gluconate, corticosteroids, estrogens, ethanol, lithium carbonate, spironolactone.

Pre-Test Nursing Care

- Explain to the patient the purpose of the test and the need for a blood sample to be drawn. Usually one morning sample is drawn, but when ACTH hypersecretion is suggested, a second sample is drawn in the evening.
- The patient should consume a low-carbohydrate diet for 48 hours before the test.
- Fasting and limited physical activity for 10 to 12 hours is required before the test.

TABLE 1
Correlation of ACTH and Cortisol Levels

ACTH Level	Cortisol Level	Indication
High	Low	Adrenocortical hypoactivity (Addison's disease)
Low	High	Adrenocortical hyperactivity (Cushing's syndrome). Probable adrenal tumor.
High	High	Adrenocortical hyperfunction due to excessive ACTH production (due to pituitary tumor or nonendocrine ACTH-producing tumor)

Procedure

- A 7-mL blood sample is drawn in either a plastic tube (because ACTH may adhere to glass), a collection tube containing heparin, or a collection tube containing EDTA.
- Gloves are worn throughout the procedure.

Post-Test Nursing Care

- Apply pressure at venipuncture site. Apply dressing, periodically assessing for continued bleeding.
- The sample is to be placed on ice, labeled, and taken to the laboratory immediately.
- Report abnormal findings to the primary care provider.

• • • • • • • • • • • • • • • • •

Adrenocorticotropic Hormone Stimulation Test

(ACTH Stimulation Test, Corticotropin Stimulation, Cortisol Stimulation Test, Cortrosyn Stimulation Test, Cosyntropin Test) [See also: Adrenocorticotropic Hormone]

The hypothalamus secretes corticotropic-releasing hormone. This hormone stimulates the secretion of adrenocorticotropic hormone (ACTH) by the anterior pituitary gland. ACTH, in turn, causes the adrenal cortex to release the glucocorticoid hormone cortisol. Problems occurring in the adrenal cortex are considered "primary" disorders, whereas those occurring in the anterior pituitary gland are known as "secondary" disorders. It is important to determine whether a patient's problem is of a primary or a secondary nature.

Various tests may be used to evaluate adrenal hypofunction through stimulation of the adrenal glands. The most common is the rapid ACTH test, for which cosyntropin (Cortrosyn) is administered. ACTH stimulation testing is especially valuable in the diagnosis of Addison's disease. If plasma cortisol levels increase after administration of ACTH, the adrenal gland has the ability to function when stimulated and the cause of the adrenal insufficiency would be due to a problem in the pituitary gland. If, however, the plasma cortisol levels do not rise or increase only minimally, the problem lies with the adrenal gland.

Normal Values

Rise of at least 7 µg/dL above baseline level

Possible Meanings of Abnormal Values

Lack of or Minimal Increase

Addison's disease
Adrenal insufficiency
Adrenocortical tumor

Contributing Factors to Abnormal Values

- Levels of ACTH may vary with exercise, sleep, and stress.
- Drugs that may alter the test results: amphetamines, calcium gluconate, corticosteroids, estrogens, ethanol, lithium carbonate, spironolactone.

Pre-Test Nursing Care

- Explain to the patient the purpose of the test and the need for multiple blood samples to be drawn.
- Fasting and limited activity for 10 to 12 hours is required before the test.

Procedure

- A 5 mL blood sample is drawn in a collection tube containing heparin for a baseline plasma cortisol level, labeled, and sent to the laboratory.
- Within 30 minutes of drawing the baseline cortisol level, cosyntropin (Cortrosyn) is administered either intravenously (preferable) or intramuscularly.
- Plasma cortisol levels are drawn at 30 and 60 minutes after cosyntropin administration.
- Gloves are worn throughout the procedure.

Post-Test Nursing Care

- Apply pressure at venipuncture site. Apply dressing, periodically assessing for continued bleeding.
- Each blood sample must be carefully labeled as to the time it was drawn, including whether it was baseline, 30 minutes after the cosyntropin administration, or 60 minutes after the cosyntropin administration.
- Transport the specimens to the laboratory.
- Report abnormal findings to the primary care provider.

• • • • • • • • • • • • • • • •

Alanine Aminotransferase
(ALT, Formerly SGPT: Serum Glutamic-Pyruvic Transaminase)

Alanine aminotransferase (ALT) is an enzyme found in the kidneys, heart, and skeletal muscle tissue but primarily in liver tissue. It functions as a catalyst in the reaction needed for amino acid production. The test is used mainly in the diagnosis of liver disease and to monitor the effects of hepatotoxic drugs.

ALT is assessed along with asparate aminotransferase (AST) in monitoring liver damage. These two values normally exist in an approximately 1:1 ratio. The AST is greater than the ALT in alcohol-induced hepatitis, cirrhosis, and metastatic cancer of the liver. ALT is greater than AST in the case of viral or drug-induced hepatitis and hepatic obstruction due to causes other than malignancy.

The degree of increase of these enzymes may provide a clue as to the source of the problem. A twofold increase is suggestive of an obstructive problem, often requiring surgical intervention. A 10-fold increase of ALT and AST indicates a probable medical problem such as hepatitis.

Normal Values

Female:　7–30 U/L　(0.12–0.50 μkat/L SI units)
Male:　　10–55 U/L　(0.17–0.91 μkat/L SI units)

Possible Meanings of Abnormal Values

Increased

Biliary obstruction
Bone metastases
Cholestasis
Cirrhosis
Congestive heart failure
Eclampsia
Hepatic ischemia
Hepatic necrosis
Hepatitis
Infectious mononucleosis
Liver cancer
Muscle inflammation
Obesity
Pancreatitis
Pulmonary infarction
Reye's syndrome
Shock
Trauma

Contributing Factors to Abnormal Values

- Hemolysis of the blood sample may alter test results.
- Drugs that may *increase* ALT levels: acetaminophen, allopurinol, ampicillin, ascorbic acid, azathioprine, barbiturates, bromocriptine mesylate, captopril, carbamazepine, cephalosporins, chlordiazepoxide, chlorpromazine, chlorpropamide, cholinergics, clofibrate, cloxacillin sodium, codeine, dicumerol, erythromycin, griseofulvin, guanethidine analogs, heparin, hydralazine hydrochloride, indomethacin, isoniazid, meperidine hydrochloride, methotrexate, methyldopa, morphine, nafcillin sodium, nalidixic acid, nitrofurantoin, oral contraceptives, oxacillin sodium, para-aminosalicylic acid, phenothiazines, phenylbutazone, phenytoin, diphenylhydantoin, procainamide hydrochloride, propoxyphene hydrochloride, propranolol hydrochloride, quinidine, salicylates, tetracycline, verapamil hydrochloride.

Pre-Test Nursing Care

- Explain to the patient the purpose of the test and the need for a blood sample to be drawn.
- No fasting is required before the test.

Procedure

- A 7-mL blood sample is drawn in a collection tube containing a silicone gel.
- Gloves are worn throughout the procedure.

Post-Test Nursing Care
(Possible complication: With liver dysfunction, patient may have prolonged clotting time.)

- Apply pressure for 3 to 5 minutes at venipuncture site. Apply dressing, periodically assessing for continued bleeding.
- Teach the patient to monitor the site. If the site begins to bleed, the patient should apply direct pressure and, if unable to control the bleeding, return to the laboratory or notify the nurse.
- Label the specimen and transport it to the laboratory.
- Report abnormal findings to the primary care provider.

• • • • • • • • • • • • • • • • •

Aldolase

Aldolase is a glycolytic enzyme that is present in all body cells. The highest concentrations of aldolase are found in the cells of skeletal muscles, the heart, and liver tissue, although the test is considered most specific for muscle tissue destruction. When damage to muscle tissue occurs, cells are destroyed, resulting in the release of aldolase into the blood. Thus, testing for aldolase is useful in monitoring the progress of muscle damage in such disorders as muscular dystrophy.

Normal Values
Adult:	0–7 U/L (0–117 nkat/L SI units)
Child:	two times adult norms
Newborn:	four times adult norms

Possible Meanings of Abnormal Values

Increased	Decreased
Burns	Late muscular dystrophy
Cancer of the prostate	
Dermatomyositis	
Gangrene	
Hepatitis	
Liver cancer	
Muscle inflammation	
Muscle necrosis	
Muscle trauma	
Myocardial infarction	
Myositis	
Polymyositis	
Progressive muscular dystrophy	
Pulmonary infarction	

Contributing Factors to Abnormal Values

- Hemolysis of the blood sample falsely increases the test results.
- Drugs that may *increase* aldolase levels: corticotropin, cortisone acetate, hepatotoxic drugs.
- Drugs that may *decrease* aldolase levels: phenothiazines.

Pre-Test Nursing Care

- Explain to the patient the purpose of the test and the need for a blood sample to be drawn.
- Although fasting is not required before the test, some institutions require a short fasting period to improve the accuracy of the test results.

Procedure

- A 5-mL blood sample is drawn in a collection tube containing a silicone gel.
- Gloves are worn throughout the procedure.

Post-Test Nursing Care

- Apply pressure at venipuncture site. Apply dressing, periodically assessing for continued bleeding.
- Label the specimen and transport it to the laboratory.
- Report abnormal findings to the primary care provider.

• • • • • • • • • • • • • • • •

Aldosterone

Aldosterone is a mineralocorticoid secreted by the adrenal cortex. Its effects occur in the renal distal tubule, where it causes increased reabsorption of sodium and chloride and increased excretion of potassium and hydrogen ions. The result of these actions is an increase in the extracellular fluid. The ultimate effect of changes in aldosterone level is regulation of blood pressure.

The release of aldosterone is controlled primarily by the renin-angiotensin-aldosterone system. The sequence of events is shown in Figure 2.

Measurement of aldosterone level is performed on both the plasma and the urine. This information assists in the diagnosis of primary aldosteronism , caused by an abnormality of the adrenal cortex, and of secondary aldosteronism, which may result from overstimulation of the adrenal cortex by a substance such as angiotensin or ACTH.

Normal Values

Plasma, standing:	4–31 ng/dL (111–860 pmol/L SI units)
Plasma, recumbent:	< 16 ng/dL (< 444 pmol/L SI units)
Urinary excretion:	6–25 µg/d (17–69 nmol/day SI units)

Possible Meanings of Abnormal Values

Increased	Decreased
Adrenal cortical hyperplasia	Addison's disease
Aldosterone-producing adenoma	High-sodium diet
Aldosteronism	Hypernatremia
Cirrhosis of liver with ascites	Hypokalemia
Congestive heart failure	Salt-losing syndrome
Hemorrhage	Septicemia
Hyperkalemia	Stress

Increased	Decreased
Hyponatremia	Toxemia of pregnancy
Hypovolemia	
Low-sodium diet	
Malignant hypertension	
Nephrosis	
Nephrotic syndrome	
Potassium loading	
Pregnancy	
Primary hyperaldosteronism (Conn's syndrome)	
Stress	

Contributing Factors to Abnormal Values

- Test results may be altered by diet, exercise, licorice ingestion, and posture.
- Drugs that may *increase* aldosterone levels: corticotropin, diazoxide, diuretics, fludrocortisone acetate, hydralazine hydrochloride, nitroprusside sodium, oral contraceptives, potassium, steroids.
- Drugs that may *decrease* aldosterone levels: fludrocortisone acetate, methyldopa, propranolol hydrochloride.

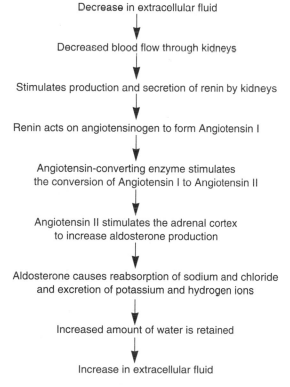

Decrease in extracellular fluid

↓

Decreased blood flow through kidneys

↓

Stimulates production and secretion of renin by kidneys

↓

Renin acts on angiotensinogen to form Angiotensin I

↓

Angiotensin-converting enzyme stimulates
the conversion of Angiotensin I to Angiotensin II

↓

Angiotensin II stimulates the adrenal cortex
to increase aldosterone production

↓

Aldosterone causes reabsorption of sodium and chloride
and excretion of potassium and hydrogen ions

↓

Increased amount of water is retained

↓

Increase in extracellular fluid

Figure 2 Renin-Angiotensin-Aldosterone system.

Pre-Test Nursing Care

- Explain to the patient the purpose of the test and the need for a blood sample to be drawn. Explain the effect of the upright position on the test results.
- No fasting is required before the test.
- Unless otherwise ordered, instruct the patient to follow a 3-g sodium diet for at least 2 weeks before the test. Explain to the patient that this is considered "normal" sodium intake.
- Explain 24-hour urine collection procedure to the patient.
- Stress the importance of saving *all* urine in the 24-hour period. Instruct the patient to avoid contaminating the urine with toilet paper or feces.
- Inform the patient of the presence of a preservative in the collection bottle.
- If possible, drugs that may affect test results should be withheld for at least 2 weeks before the test.

Procedure
Blood Sampling

- A 7-mL blood sample is drawn in a collection tube containing no additives. The sample should be drawn while the patient is in a supine position before arising in the morning.
- If a second specimen is ordered, it is drawn 4 hours later with the patient in an upright position and after ambulation.
- Gloves are worn throughout the procedure.

Urine Collection

- Obtain the proper container containing the appropriate preservative from the laboratory.
- Begin the testing period in the morning after the patient's first voiding, which is discarded.
- Timing of the 24-hour period begins at the time the first voiding is discarded.
- *All* urine for the next 24 hours is collected in the container, which is to be kept refrigerated or on ice.
- If any urine is accidentally discarded during the 24-hour period, the test must be discontinued and a new test begun.
- The ending time of the 24-hour collection period should be posted in the patient's room.
- Gloves are to be worn whenever dealing with the specimen collection.

Post-Test Nursing Care

- Apply pressure at venipuncture site. Apply dressing, periodically assessing for continued bleeding.
- Label the specimen and transport it to the laboratory.
- At the end of the 24-hour collection period, label and send the urine container on ice to the laboratory as soon as possible.
- Resume medications as taken before the testing period.
- Report abnormal findings to the primary care provider.

Alkaline Phosphatase
(ALP)

Alkaline phosphatase (ALP) is an enzyme found in the liver, bone, placenta, intestine, and kidneys but primarily in the cells lining the biliary tract and in the osteoblasts involved in the formation of new bone. ALP is normally excreted from the liver in the bile. Increased ALP levels are found most commonly during periods of bone growth, such as in children, in various types of liver disease, and in biliary obstruction. ALP is also considered a tumor marker that increases in the case of osteogenic sarcoma and in breast or prostate cancer that has metastasized to the bone.

Normal Values

Female:	30–100 U/L (0.5–1.67 µkat/L SI units)
Male:	45–115 U/L (0.75–1.92 µkat/L SI units)
Elderly:	Slightly higher norms
Children:	One to three times adult norms
Puberty:	Six to seven times adult norms

Possible Meanings of Abnormal Values

Increased	Decreased
Biliary obstruction	Celiac disease
Bone metastases	Chronic nephritis
Calcium deficiency	Cystic fibrosis
Cancer of head of pancreas	Excessive vitamin D intake
Cirrhosis	Genetic defect
Eclampsia	Hypophosphatemia
Healing fracture	Hypothyroidism
Hepatitis	Lack of normal bone formation
High-fat intake	Malnutrition
Hyperparathyroidism	Milk-alkali syndrome
Infectious mononucleosis	Pernicious anemia
Leukemia	Placental insufficiency
Liver cancer	Scurvy
Osteogenic sarcoma	
Osteomalacia	
Paget's disease	
Pancreatitis	
Pregnancy	
Rheumatoid arthritis	
Rickets	
Vitamin D deficiency	

Contributing Factors to Abnormal Values

- Hemolysis of the blood sample may alter test results.
- Drugs that may *increase* ALP levels: acetohexamide, albumin, allopurinol, amitriptyline, anabolic steroids, androgens, antibiotics, asparaginase, aspirin, azathioprine, barbiturates, bromocriptine mesylate, carbamazepine, carmustine, chlordiazepoxide, chlorpromazine, chlorpropamide, cholestyramine, cimetidine, clonazepam, colchicine, estrogens, floxuridine, flurazepam hydrochloride, imipramine hydrochloride, indomethacin, isoniazid, methyldopa, metoprolol tartrate, naproxen, niacin, nifedipine, nitrofurantoin, oral contraceptives, papaverine hydrochloride, phenobarbital, phenothiazines, phenylbutazone, phenytoin, probenecid, procainamide hydrochloride, propranolol hydrochloride, propylthiouracil, rifampin, salicylates, sulfamethoxazole, tolbutamide, tolmetin, valproic acid, vitamin D.
- Drugs that may *decrease* ALP levels: arsenicals, cyanides, clofibrate, fluorides, nitrofurantoin, oxalates, phosphates, propranolol hydrochloride, zinc salts.

Pre-Test Nursing Care

- Explain to the patient the purpose of the test and the need for a blood sample to be drawn.
- Fasting of 10 to 12 hours is usually required before the test.

Procedure

- A 7-mL blood sample is drawn in a collection tube containing a silicone gel.
- Gloves are worn throughout the procedure.

Post-Test Nursing Care

Possible complication: With liver dysfunction, patient may have prolonged clotting time.

- Apply pressure 3 to 5 minutes at venipuncture site. Apply dressing, periodically assessing for continued bleeding.
- Teach the patient to monitor the site. If the site begins to bleed, the patient should apply direct pressure and, if unable to control the bleeding, return to the laboratory or notify the nurse.
- Label the specimen and transport it to the laboratory.
- Report abnormal findings to the primary care provider.

• • • • • • • • • • • • • • • • • •

Allergen-Specific IgE Antibody
(RAST Test, Radioallergosorbent Test, Allergy Screen)

The protein of the blood is composed of albumin and globulins. One type of globulin is the group of gamma globulins, also called immunoglobulins or antibodies. Gamma globulins are produced by certain white blood cells known as B lymphocytes in response to stimulation by antigens. There are five types of immunoglobulins: IgA, IgD, IgE, IgG, and IgM. IgE is the antibody of allergies.

Testing for allergies to various substances has typically involved skin testing, which can be quite uncomfortable for the patient and carries the risk of causing an allergic reaction, because allergens are actually introduced into the body. Another way to now test for such allergies is the allergen-specific IgE antibody test. This test is also called the radioallergosorbent test, or RAST test, because it involves the use of radioimmunoassay to identify the specific allergens that are affecting the person. The specific antigens, or allergens, are bound to a carrier substance. If the person is allergic to a particular allergen, a specific IgE antibody in the person's blood sample will react with the allergen.

Normal Values

Negative, 0:   No IgE detected

Abnormal Values

1:                      Borderline
Positive, 2–4:   Increasing levels of IgE

Possible Meanings of Abnormal Values

Increased

Positive allergy to tested substance

Contributing Factors to Abnormal Values

- Testing with radioactive dyes within 1 week before the test will alter test results.
- Test results are affected by the type of allergen, length of exposure to the allergen, and any previous hyposensitization therapy.

Pre-Test Nursing Care

- Explain to the patient the purpose of the test and the need for a blood sample to be drawn.
- No fasting is required before the test.

Procedure

- A 20-mL blood sample is drawn in a collection tube containing no additives.
- Gloves are to be worn throughout the procedure.

Post-Test Nursing Care

- Apply pressure at venipuncture site. Apply dressing, periodically assessing for continued bleeding.
- Label the specimen and transport it to the laboratory.
- Report abnormal findings to the primary care provider.

• • • • • • • • • • • • • • • •

Alpha₁-Antitrypsin Test
(AAT)

Alpha₁-antitrypsin (AAT) is a protein produced by the liver. It has a protective function, in that it prevents the release of proteolytic enzymes that can damage tissues such as that of the lung. AAT deficiency is an inherited disease most often noted in individuals of European descent. This deficiency occurs in young children with liver disease. It is also associated with pulmonary emphysema. In cases of infection, inflammation, and necrosis, AAT levels are elevated.

Normal Values

85–213 mg/dL (0.85–2.13 g/L SI units)

Possible Meanings of Abnormal Values

Increased	Decreased
Acute inflammatory disorders	AAT deficiency
Cancer	Chronic liver disease
Chronic inflammatory disorders	Emphysema
Chronic liver disease	Malnutrition
Hepatitis	Nephrotic syndrome
Pregnancy	Severe hepatic damage
Stress	
Systemic lupus erythematosus	
Thyroid infection	

Contributing Factors to Abnormal Values

- Drugs that may *increase* AAT levels: estrogens, oral contraceptives, steroids.

Pre-Test Nursing Care

- Explain to the patient the purpose of the test and the need for a blood sample to be drawn.
- No fasting is required before the test unless the patient has hypercholesterolemia or hyperlipidemia. If so, the patient should fast for 8 to 10 hours before the test.

Procedure

- A 10-mL blood sample is drawn in a collection tube containing a silicone gel.
- Gloves are worn throughout the procedure.

Post-Test Nursing Care

- Apply pressure at venipuncture site. Apply dressing, periodically assessing for continued bleeding.
- Label the specimen and transport it to the laboratory.
- Report abnormal findings to the primary care provider.
- Teach patients who are AAT deficient to avoid smoking and employment in occupations in which air pollutants are common.

Alpha-Fetoprotein
(AFP, Maternal Serum Alpha-Fetoprotein [MSAFP], Triple Marker)

Alpha-fetoprotein (AFP) is a globulin protein formed in the yolk sac and liver of the fetus. As the fetus develops, the level of AFP found in the mother's serum increases. Only minute amounts of AFP remain in the bloodstream after birth.

This test is used primarily to screen for the presence of neural tube defects in the fetus, such as spina bifida and anencephaly. The test, done between 15 and 20 weeks of pregnancy, does not absolutely diagnose a birth defect. However, if the AFP is found to be abnormally high, additional testing, including ultrasonography and testing of the amniotic fluid for AFP, is needed.

In many institutions, the test for alpha-fetoprotein is now combined with measurement of estriol (uE$_3$) and human chorionic gonadotropin (hCG). This combination testing is known by various names, including "triple marker." The measurement of these three substances provides screening for neural tube defects, trisomy 18, and trisomy 21 (Down syndrome). An accurate fetal gestational age is essential for accurate test results, because the levels of the substances all vary with gestational age. The most accurate method of assessing gestational age is ultrasonography; if unavailable, gestational age by last menstrual period is used. This testing is a screening tool; negative results do not guarantee a normal baby.

Normal Values

Pregnant female:	
First trimester:	< 130 ng/mL (< 130 µg/L SI units)
Second trimester:	< 300 ng/mL (< 300 µg/L SI units)
Third trimester:	< 400 ng/mL (< 400 µg/L SI units)
Nonpregnant female:	< 10 ng/mL (< 10 µg/L SI units)
Male:	< 10 ng/mL (< 10 µg/L SI units)

Possible Meanings of Abnormal Values

Increased	Decreased
Biliary cirrhosis	Down syndrome
Fetal death	
Fetal distress	
Fetal neural tube defect	
Gastric cancer	
Hepatic cancer	
Hepatitis	
Lung cancer	
Multiple fetuses	
Testicular cancer	
Tyrosinemia	
Ulcerative colitis	

Contributing Factors to Abnormal Values

• Hemolysis of the blood sample may alter test results.

Pre-Test Nursing Care

- Explain to the patient the purpose of the test and the need for a blood sample to be drawn.
- No fasting is required before the test.

Procedure

- A 7-mL blood sample is drawn in a collection tube containing no additives. (*Note:* Some laboratories use a collection tube containing EDTA for the triple marker screening test.)
- Gloves are worn throughout the procedure.

Post-Test Nursing Care

- Apply pressure at venipuncture site. Apply dressing, periodically assessing for continued bleeding.
- Label the specimen and transport it to the laboratory.
- Report abnormal findings to the primary care provider.

• • • • • • • • • • • • • • • • •

Ambulatory Electrocardiography
(Ambulatory Monitoring, Event Monitoring, Holter Monitoring)

Ambulatory electrocardiography involves the monitoring of the electrical activity of the heart as the patient carries out normal life activities. By continuously monitoring the patient's heart, ambulatory electrocardiography is able to detect dysrhythmias that occur only sporadically and are easily missed during periodic electrocardiographic assessments.

Holter monitoring is performed by attaching several chest electrodes to a small recorder that is carried with the patient. The monitoring is conducted for a 24 to 48 hour period. The patient maintains a diary of activities and any symptoms experienced during the testing period.

Event monitoring, which is conducted for a 30-day period, is used for those patients whose symptoms occur infrequently. This monitor consists of two electrodes that can be removed for bathing and reapplied by the patient and a small recorder. When symptoms such as fluttering or discomfort are experienced, the patient presses the "Record" button. A recording is then made of the heart's electrical activity for the 15 seconds before the "Record" button being pushed and for 1 minute afterward. The patient maintains a diary of the symptoms experienced.

Normal Values

Normal rate, rhythm, and waveforms

Possible Meanings of Abnormal Values

Cardiac arrhythmias

Contributing Factors to Abnormal Values

- Interferences to the recording of the electrocardiogram are shown on the recording as artifacts. This may occur due to equipment failure, electrode adherence problems, or electromagnetic interference.

- The adequacy of the testing is dependent on the patient maintaining normal daily activities during the testing period and keeping a detailed diary of activities and symptoms.

Pre-Test Nursing Care

- Explain to the patient the purpose of the test and the need for electrodes to be attached to the chest. Note that the test causes no discomfort but does require wearing a small tape recorder for 24 to 48 hours for Holter monitoring and 30 days for event monitoring.
- Instruct the patient to maintain a diary of activities and situations, such as emotional stress, that occur during the test period. Included in the diary should be any symptoms experienced and the time at which they occur. The symptoms will then be able to be correlated with the electrocardiographic pattern occurring at that time.
- No fasting is required before the test.

Procedure

- The skin is cleansed with an alcohol swab and then abraded until slightly reddened.
- The electrodes are securely applied to the skin.
- The monitor and case are positioned; then the electrode cable is attached to the monitor.
- The recorder is turned on.
- The patient is provided with the recording diary and with a telephone number of the cardiology technician who may be called with questions or problems.

Post-Test Nursing Care

- At the end of the testing period, remove the electrodes and cleanse the skin of any residual gel or adhesive.
- Label the recording tape and send the tape and diary to the cardiologist for interpretation.
- Inform the patient that interpretation of the electrocardiographic tape and diary by the physician will take several days.
- Report abnormal findings to the primary care provider.

• • • • • • • • • • • • • • • • •

Aminolevulinic Acid
(ALA, Delta-Aminolevulinic Acid, Delta-ALA)

Aminolevulinic acid (ALA), a urine pigment, is the precursor to porphobilinogen in the formation of heme of hemoglobin. The pathway of heme synthesis is shown in Figure 3. If a problem occurs during heme formation, the ALA accumulates and is excreted in the urine. ALA is normally absent from urine. The presence of ALA in the urine usually indicates lead poisoning. The test can be used as a screening device for detection of excessive absorption of lead before the appearance of symptoms.

Normal Values

Random specimen:	0.1–0.6 mg/dL (7.6–45.8 µmol/L SI units)
24-Hour urine:	1.5–7.5 mg/dL/24 hr (11.15–57.2 µmol/24 hrs SI units)

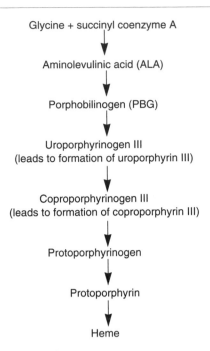

Glycine + succinyl coenzyme A

Aminolevulinic acid (ALA)

Porphobilinogen (PBG)

Uroporphyrinogen III
(leads to formation of uroporphyrin III)

Coproporphyrinogen III
(leads to formation of coproporphyrin III)

Protoporphyrinogen

Protoporphyrin

Heme

Figure 3   Pathway of Heme synthesis.

Possible Meanings of Abnormal Values

Increased

Lead exposure
Lead poisoning
Porphyria hepatica
Hepatitis
Hepatic carcinoma

Contributing Factors to Abnormal Values

- Failure to protect the urine from light may alter test results.
- Drugs which may *increase* ALA levels: barbiturates, griseofulvin, penicillin, rifampin.

Pre-Test Nursing Care

- Explain 24-hour urine collection procedure to the patient.
- Stress the importance of saving *all* urine in the 24-hour period. Instruct the patient to avoid contaminating the urine with toilet paper or feces.
- Inform the patient of the presence of a preservative in the collection bottle.

Procedure

- Obtain the proper container containing the appropriate preservative from the laboratory.
- Begin the testing period in the morning after the patient's first voiding, which is discarded.
- Timing of the 24-hour period begins at the time the first voiding is discarded.

- *All* urine for the next 24 hours is collected in the container, which is to be kept refrigerated or on ice and protected from light. This is accomplished with either a dark container or a container covered with aluminum foil.
- If any urine is accidentally discarded during the 24-hour period, the test must be discontinued and a new test begun.
- The ending time of the 24-hour collection period should be posted in the patient's room.
- Gloves are to be worn when dealing with the specimen collection.

Post-Test Nursing Care

- Label and send the container on ice to the laboratory as soon as possible after the end of the 24-hour collection period.
- Report abnormal findings to the primary care provider.

• • • • • • • • • • • • • • • •

Ammonia, Blood

A mmonia is a waste product that forms as a result of nitrogen breakdown during intestinal protein metabolism and from digestion of blood from such areas as leaking esophageal varices. Normally, it is converted into urea by the liver and then excreted by the kidneys. If a physical disorder prevents this conversion from occurring, the ammonia accumulates in the bloodstream. Another major source of ammonia is from the synthesis and conversion of glutamine by the renal tubules. In the kidneys, ammonia serves as an important renal buffer. Toxic levels of ammonia in the blood lead to a problem known as *hepatic encephalopathy*, in which brain function is affected by the high ammonia levels.

Normal Values

Adult:	35–65 µg/dL (25–46 µmol/L SI units)
Child:	45–80 µg/dL (32–57 µmol/L SI units)
Newborn:	90–150 µg/dL (64–107 µmol/L SI units)

Possible Meanings of Abnormal Values

Increased	Decreased
Acute bronchitis	Essential hypertension
Azotemia	Malignant hypertension
Cirrhosis	Renal failure
Cor pulmonale	
Heart failure	
Hemolytic disease of the newborn	
Hepatic encephalopathy	
Hepatic failure	
Leukemia	
Pericarditis	
Pulmonary emphysema	
Renal failure	
Reye's syndrome	

Contributing Factors to Abnormal Values

- Drugs that may *increase* serum ammonia levels: acetazolamide, alcohol, ammonium salts, asparaginase, barbiturates, chlorothiazide, furosemide, heparin, methicillin sodium, thiazide diuretics.
- Drugs that may *decrease* serum ammonia levels: kanamycin, lactulose, neomycin sulfate, potassium salts.

Pre-Test Nursing Care

- Explain to the patient the purpose of the test and the need for a blood sample to be drawn.
- Fasting for 8 to 10 hours is required before the test. Water is permitted.

Procedure

- A 7-mL blood sample is drawn in a collection tube containing either sodium heparin or lithium heparin, *not* ammonium heparin. The tube should be kept on ice.
- Gloves are worn throughout the procedure.

Post-Test Nursing Care

- Apply pressure at venipuncture site. Apply dressing, periodically assessing for continued bleeding.
- The sample is labeled, placed in ice water, and transported to the laboratory immediately.
- Report abnormal findings to the primary care provider.

• • • • • • • • • • • • • • • • • •

Amniocentesis
(Amniotic Fluid Analysis)

Amniocentesis involves the transabdominal needle aspiration of amniotic fluid. A 10 to 20 mL sample of the amniotic fluid is withdrawn for analysis. This test is useful in detecting birth defects such as Down syndrome and spina bifida, in determining fetal maturity, and in detecting hemolytic disease of the newborn. It can also be used for determining gender and detecting chromosomal abnormalities. The timing of the procedure is based on the reason the procedure is being done. If it is to determine fetal defects, it is performed during the 14th to 16th weeks of gestation. This allows time after the test results are received 2 weeks later for an abortion to be performed, if indicated. If the procedure is being done to determine fetal maturity, it is more likely to be performed after the 35th week of gestation.

The amniotic fluid is analyzed for the following: acetylcholinesterase, alpha-fetoprotein, bacteria, bilirubin, chromosomal karyotype, color, creatinine, glucose, lecithin-to-sphingomyelin (L/S) ratio, meconium, and phosphatidylglycerol. Hemolytic disease of the newborn is indicated by high levels of bilirubin in the fluid. Meconium staining indicates possible fetal distress. Fetal pulmonary immaturity is demonstrated by a low L/S ratio and the absence of phosphatidylglycerol. A decreased creatinine level may also indicate fetal immaturity. Neural tube defects are suspected with increased levels of alpha-fetoprotein and acetylcholinesterase.

Normal Values

Acetylcholinesterase:	absent
Alpha-fetoprotein:	varies with gestational age (peaks at 13–14 weeks)
Bacteria:	absent
Bilirubin:	absent at term
Chromosomes:	normal karyotype
Color:	colorless or light straw
Creatinine:	> 2 mg/dL when mature
Glucose:	< 45 mg/dL
L/S ratio:	> 2 indicates pulmonary maturity
Meconium	absent
Phosphatidylglycerol:	present with pulmonary maturity

Possible Meanings of Abnormal Values

Chromosomal abnormalities (e.g., Down syndrome)
Fetal distress
Genetic aberrations (e.g., galactosemia)
Hereditary metabolic disorders (e.g., cystic fibrosis)
Neural tube defects (e.g., spina bifida)
Pulmonary immaturity
Rh isoimmunization
Sex-linked disorders (e.g., hemophilia)
Sickle cell anemia
Thalassemia

Contributing Factors to Abnormal Values

- Alpha-fetoprotein and acetylcholinesterase may be falsely elevated if the sample is contaminated with fetal blood.
- Bilirubin may be falsely elevated if the sample is contaminated with maternal hemoglobin or if meconium is present in the sample.
- Bilirubin may be falsely low if the sample is exposed to light.

CONTRAINDICATIONS

- Patients with abruptio placentae, incompetent cervix, placenta previa
- Patients with a history of premature labor

Pre-Test Nursing Care

- Explain to the patient the purpose of the test and procedure to be followed.
- No fasting is required before the test.
- Obtain a signed informed consent.
- If an ultrasonography is to be performed just before the amniocentesis, the patient needs to be well hydrated and have a full bladder. The bladder must then be emptied before the amniocentesis to avoid accidental puncture.

Procedure

- The patient is assisted to a supine position.
- The skin of the lower abdomen is cleansed with an antiseptic solution and draped.
- The skin overlying the chosen site is anesthetized with 1% lidocaine.
- A 20-gauge spinal needle is inserted into the amniotic cavity and the stylet is withdrawn. A 10-mL syringe is then attached to the needle.
- The fluid sample is aspirated and placed in an amber or foil-covered test tube. This will protect the sample from light and avoid breakdown of bilirubin in the sample.
- The needle is withdrawn, and a dressing is applied over the site.
- Gloves are worn throughout the procedure.

Post-Test Nursing Care

Possible Complications:
Amniotic fluid embolism
Fetal injury
Hemorrhage
Infection
Premature labor
Rh sensitization (fetal bleeding into maternal circulation)
Spontaneous abortion

- Monitor fetal heart rate and maternal vital signs every 15 minutes until stable.
- If the patient complains of nausea or feeling faint, assist her to lie on her left side. This will relieve uterine pressure on the vena cava.
- Observe the puncture site for drainage.
- Instruct the patient to notify the physician immediately if any of the following occur: abdominal pain, cramping, chills, fever, vaginal bleeding, fetal hyperactivity, or unusual fetal lethargy.
- Protect the specimen from light, label it, and transport it to the laboratory immediately.
- Inform the patient that up to 3 weeks is required for results.
- Report abnormal findings to the primary care provider.

• • • • • • • • • • • • • • • •

Amnioscopy

Amnioscopy is the direct visualization of amniotic fluid by means of an amnioscope inserted into the cervical canal. This procedure is used to assess for the presence of meconium staining of the amniotic fluid. When meconium staining is present, it can be an indication of fetal distress. During the procedure, if fetal distress is suspected, blood samples can be obtained through the amnioscope from the scalp of the fetus for determination of fetal blood pH and oxygen, carbon dioxide, and bicarbonate levels.

Normal Values

Normal amniotic fluid with no meconium staining present

Possible Meanings of Abnormal Values

Fetal death

Fetal distress

 CONTRAINDICATIONS

- Patients in labor
- Patients with ruptured membranes
- Patients with active cervical infection or sexually transmitted disease (e.g., gonorrhea)

Pre-Test Nursing Care

- Explain to the patient the purpose of the test. Note that some discomfort will be felt during dilation of the cervix.
- No fasting is required before the test.
- Obtain a signed written consent.

Procedure

- The patient is placed in the lithotomy position with her legs supported in the stirrups. Privacy is maintained with proper draping.
- The external genitalia are cleansed and a vaginal speculum is inserted.
- The cervix is dilated to 2 cm. The amnioscope is then inserted into the cervical canal.
- The lighted amnioscope allows for visualization of the amniotic fluid through the intact amniotic sac.
- No amniotic fluid is obtained. If a fetal blood sample is needed, it can be obtained at this time.
- Gloves are worn throughout the procedure.

Post-Test Nursing Care

Possible complication: ruptured membranes

- Inform the patient that mild cramping and vaginal discomfort may occur after the procedure. Instruct the patient to report immediately any excessive pain or ruptured membranes.
- Report abnormal findings to the primary care provider.

• • • • • • • • • • • • • • • • •

Amylase, Serum

Amylase is an enzyme found primarily in the pancreas and salivary glands and in minor amounts in the liver and fallopian tubes. Its function is to assist in the digestion of complex carbohydrates into simple sugars. Measurement of serum amylase is often performed to differentiate abdominal pain due to acute pancreatitis from other causes of abdominal pain that may require surgical treatment. The serum amylase begins to rise 3 to 6 hours after the onset of acute pancreatitis and peaks in approximately 24 hours. The values return to normal within 2 to 3 days after onset.

Normal Values

    Adult: 53–123 U/L (0.88–2.05 nkat/L SI units)
    Elderly: slightly higher norms

Possible Meanings of Abnormal Values

Increased	Decreased
Acute pancreatitis	Cirrhosis of liver
Alcoholism	Hepatitis
Biliary obstruction	Pancreatic cancer
Cholelithiasis	Severe burns
Diabetic ketoacidosis	Severe thyrotoxicosis
Hyperlipidemia	
Hyperthyroidism	
Inflammation of salivary glands	
Mumps	
Perforated bowel	
Perforated peptic ulcer	
Pregnancy	
Ruptured tubal pregnancy	

Contributing Factors to Abnormal Values

- Hemolysis of the blood sample will alter test results.
- Contamination of the sample with saliva by talking over an uncovered blood sample may falsely increase test results.
- Drugs that may *increase* serum amylase levels: aminosalicylic acid, asparaginase, aspirin, azathioprine, bethanecol chloride, cholinergics, codeine, corticotropin, cyproheptadine hydrochloride, dexamethasone, ethacrynic acid, ethanol, furosemide, glucocorticoids, iodine-containing diagnostic dyes, meperidine hydrochloride, mercaptopurine, methacholine chloride, methyldopa, morphine, oral contraceptives, phenformin, prednisone, rifampin, sulfasalazine, thiazide diuretics, triamcinolone.
- Drugs that may *decrease* serum amylase levels: citrates, glucose, oxalates.

Pre-Test Nursing Care

- Explain to the patient the purpose of the test and the need for a blood sample to be drawn.
- No fasting is required before the test.

Procedure

- A 7-mL blood sample is drawn in a collection tube containing a silicone gel.
- Gloves are worn throughout the procedure.

Post-Test Nursing Care

- Apply pressure at venipuncture site. Apply dressing, periodically assessing for continued bleeding.
- Label the specimen and transport it to the laboratory.
- Report abnormal findings to the primary care provider.

• • • • • • • • • • • • • • • •

Amylase, Urine
(Amylase Excretion/Clearance)

Amylase is an enzyme found primarily in the pancreas and salivary glands and in minor amounts in the liver and fallopian tubes. Whenever there is an inflammation of the pancreas or salivary glands, more amylase is released into the bloodstream and excreted by the kidneys. Amylase assists in the digestion of complex carbohydrates into simple sugars.

Amylase levels may be measured in the serum and in the urine. Whereas the serum amylase level begins to rise 3 to 6 hours after the onset of acute pancreatitis and returns to normal within 2 to 3 days after onset of acute pancreatitis, the urine amylase level is elevated for 7 to 10 days. Thus, testing for urine amylase is a useful way to demonstrate the presence of acute pancreatitis after serum amylase levels have returned to normal. The test may be conducted with a minimum of a 2-hour urine collection, a 24-hour urine collection, or a variety of other time periods.

Normal Values
0–375 U/L (0–6.25 μkat/L SI units)

Possible Meanings of Abnormal Values

Increased	Decreased
Acute pancreatitis	Cirrhosis of liver
Alcoholism	Hepatitis
Biliary obstruction	Pancreatic cancer
Cholelithiasis	Severe burns
Diabetic ketoacidosis	Severe thyrotoxicosis
Hyperlipidemia	
Hyperthyroidism	
Inflammation of salivary glands	
Mumps	
Perforated bowel	
Perforated peptic ulcer	
Pregnancy	
Ruptured tubal pregnancy	

Contributing Factors to Abnormal Values
- Contamination of the sample with saliva by talking over an uncovered urine specimen may falsely increase test results.
- Drugs that may *increase* urine amylase levels: alcohol, aspirin, bethanechol, codeine, indomethacin, meperidine hydrochloride, morphine, pentazocine, thiazide diuretics.
- Drugs that may *decrease* urine amylase levels: fluorides, glucose.

Pre-Test Nursing Care

- Explain 24-hour urine collection procedure to the patient.
- *Note:* Shorter urine collection periods, such as 2 hours, may be ordered in place of a 24-hour collection.
- Stress the importance of saving *all* urine in the 24-hour period. Instruct the patient to avoid contaminating the urine with toilet paper or feces.

Procedure

- Obtain the proper container containing no preservative from the laboratory.
- Begin the testing period in the morning after the patient's first voiding, which is discarded.
- Timing of the 24-hour period begins at the time the first voiding is discarded.
- *All* urine for the next 24 hours is collected in the container, which is to be kept refrigerated or on ice.
- If any urine is accidentally discarded during the 24-hour period, the test must be discontinued and a new test begun.
- The ending time of the 24-hour collection period should be posted in the patient's room.
- Gloves are to be worn when dealing with the specimen collection.

Post-Test Nursing Care

- Label and send the container on ice to the laboratory as soon as possible after the end of the 24-hour collection period.
- Report abnormal findings to the primary care provider.

• • • • • • • • • • • • • • • •

Androstenedione

Androstenedione is one of the primary androgens produced in the ovaries and, to a lesser extent, adrenal glands, of women. It is converted to estrone by adipose tissue and the liver. Estrone is a form of estrogen that is of relatively low potency, compared with estradiol. In premenopausal women, estrone levels are relatively small in comparison to estradiol levels. However, in children and postmenopausal women, estrone is a major estrogen source. If, for some reason, androstenedione production is increased, a child may experience premature sexual development. In postmenopausal woman, increased androstenedione production may result in bleeding, endometriosis, ovarian stimulation, and polycystic ovaries. Increased production in obesity may cause menstrual irregularities and, in men, such signs of feminization as gynecomastia. Owing to the results seen with androstenedione overproduction, this test is useful in the diagnosis of menstrual irregularities, premature sexual development, and postmenopausal irregularities.

Normal Values

80–300 ng/dL (3.8–6.6 nmol/L SI units)

Possible Meanings of Abnormal Values

Increased	Decreased
Adrenal tumor	Hypogonadism
Congenital adrenal hyperplasia	
Cushing's syndrome	
Ectopic ACTH-producing tumor	
Hirsutism	
Ovarian tumor	
Stein-Leventhal disease	
Testicular tumor	

Contributing Factors to Abnormal Values

- Radioactive dyes received within 1 week of the test will alter test results.
- Elevated results may be reduced to normal levels through the use of glucocorticoid therapy.

Pre-Test Nursing Care

- Explain to the patient the purpose of the test and the need for a blood sample to be drawn.
- No fasting is required before the test.
- The blood sample is to be drawn 1 week before or after the menstrual period.

Procedure

- A 7-mL blood sample is drawn in a collection tube containing no additives, and an additional 7-mL sample is drawn in a collection tube containing heparin.
- Gloves are worn throughout the procedure.

Post-Test Nursing Care

- Apply pressure at venipuncture site. Apply dressing, periodically assessing for continued bleeding.
- Label the specimens and transport them to the laboratory.
- Report abnormal findings to the primary care provider.

• • • • • • • • • • • • • • • • • •

Angiotensin-Converting Enzyme
(ACE, Serum Angiotensin-Converting Enzyme [SACE])

Angiotensin-converting enzyme (ACE) is an enzyme found primarily in the epithelial cells of the lungs and in smaller concentrations in the blood vessels and kidneys. This enzyme is the responsible for stimulating the conversion of angiotensin I to angiotensin II, a vasoconstricting agent, which, in turn, stimulates the adrenal cortex to produce aldosterone.

There has been found a high correlation between high ACE levels and patients with active sarcoidosis. Thus, this test is used in the diagnosis of sarcoidosis, as well as to monitor patient response to therapy for the disease. It can also be used in the diagnosis of Gaucher's disease, a congenital disorder of lipid metabolism, and leprosy.

Normal Values

Older than age 20:   6.1–21.1 nmol/min/mL (6.1–21.1 U/L SI units)
Younger than age 20:   higher values

Possible Meanings of Abnormal Values

Increased

Diabetic retinopathy
Gaucher's disease
Hyperthyroidism
Leprosy
Liver disease
Sarcoidosis

Contributing Factors to Abnormal Values

• Drugs that may *decrease* ACE levels: prednisone.

Pre-Test Nursing Care

• Explain to the patient the purpose of the test and the need for a blood sample to be drawn.
• Fasting for 12 hours is required before the test.

Procedure

• A 7-mL blood sample is drawn in a collection tube containing either no additives or heparin.
• Gloves are worn throughout the procedure.

Post-Test Nursing Care

• Apply pressure at venipuncture site. Apply dressing, periodically assessing for continued bleeding.
• Label the specimen and transport it to the laboratory.
• Report abnormal findings to the primary care provider.

• • • • • • • • • • • • • • • • •

Anion Gap

When electrolytes are evaluated, the substances being measured include two positive ions, called *cations*, and two negative ions, called *anions*. The cations are sodium (Na^+) and potassium (K^+), and the anions are chloride (Cl^-) and bicarbonate (HCO_3^-). When the total amount of cations and the total amount of anions are compared, there are normally more cations than anions, leading to what is known as the *anion gap*. This is because all of the possible anions are not measured. Those not measured include organic acids, phosphates, and sulfates. The anion gap is calculated as follows:

$$(Na^+ + K^+) - (Cl^- + HCO_3^-) = \text{Anion gap}$$

Measurement of the anion gap assists the health care provider in determining the potential causes of metabolic acidosis. Types of metabolic acidosis that have an increased anion gap include those associated with renal failure, diabetic ketoacidosis, and lactic acidosis.

Normal Values
7–17 mEq/L (7–17 mmol/L SI units)

Possible Meanings of Abnormal Values

Increased	Decreased
Dehydration	Bromide intoxication
Diabetic ketoacidosis	Hypercalcemia
Hyperalbuminemia	Hyperdilution
Hypocalcemia	Hyperkalemia
Hypomagnesemia	Hypermagnesemia
Lactic acidosis	Hypoalbuminemia
Metabolic acidosis	Hyponatremia
Renal failure	Hypophosphatemia
Salicylate toxicity	Multiple myeloma
Uremia	Polyclonal gammopathy
	Waldenström's macroglobulinemia

Contributing Factors to Abnormal Values
- Hemolysis of the sample may alter test results.
- *False decreases* may occur owing to absorption of iodine from povidone-iodine–packed wounds.
- Drugs that may *increase* the anion gap: acetazolamide, ammonium chloride, antihypertensives, carbenicillin, corticosteroids, dextrose 5% in water, dimercaprol, ethacrynic acid, furosemide, methyl alcohol, nitrates, paraldehyde, penicillin, salicylates, sodium bicarbonate, thiazides.
- Drugs that may *decrease* the anion gap: ammonium chloride, antacids containing magnesium, boric acid, chlorpropamide, cholestyramine, cortisone acetate, corticotropin, lithium carbonate, phenylbutazone, polymyxin B, sodium chloride (IV), vasopressin.

Pre-Test Nursing Care
- Explain to the patient the purpose of the test and the need for a blood sample to be drawn.
- No fasting is required before the test.

Procedure
- A 10-mL blood sample is drawn in a collection tube containing a silicone gel.
- Gloves are worn throughout the procedure.

Post-Test Nursing Care
- Apply pressure at venipuncture site. Apply dressing, periodically assessing for continued bleeding.
- Label the specimen and transport it to the laboratory.
- Report abnormal findings to the primary care provider.

• • • • • • • • • • • • • • • • •

Anticentromere Antibody Test

CREST syndrome is a variant of scleroderma characterized by calcinosis, Raynaud's phenomenon, esophageal dysfunction, sclerodactyly, and telangiectasia. The anticentromere antibody has been found in most patients diagnosed with CREST syndrome.

Normal Values

Negative

Possible Meanings of Abnormal Values

Positive

CREST syndrome

Pre-Test Nursing Care

- Explain to the patient the purpose of the test and the need for a blood sample to be drawn.
- No fasting is required before the test.

Procedure

- A 10-mL blood sample is drawn in a collection tube containing no additives.
- Gloves are worn throughout the procedure.

Post-Test Nursing Care

- Apply pressure at venipuncture site. Apply dressing, periodically assessing for continued bleeding.
- Label the specimen and transport it to the laboratory.
- Report abnormal findings to the primary care provider.

• • • • • • • • • • • • • • •

Antideoxyribonuclease-B Titer
(Anti-DNase B [ADB], Streptodornase)

Deoxyribonuclease B is an antigen produced by group A streptococci. When the body is confronted by this antigen, it produces antibodies against the antigen. The antideoxyribonuclease-B test is designed to detect these antibodies. If the antibodies are present, the person has had a streptococcal infection. The anti-DNase B level increases after the person has recovered from the infection. This test is considered more sensitive than the antistreptolysin-O (ASO) test. When both tests are consistently performed on blood samples, 95% of the streptococcal infections can be identified. The test is particularly useful in the diagnosis of rheumatic fever and post-streptococcal glomerulonephritis, both sequelae of infections involving group-A beta-hemolytic streptococci.

Normal Values

Adult:	< 85 Todd U/mL
Child age 7 and older:	< 170 Todd U/mL
Child younger than age 7:	< 60 Todd U/mL

Possible Meanings of Abnormal Values

Increased

Acute rheumatic fever
Pharyngitis
Poststreptococcal glomerulonephritis
Pyodermic skin infection

Contributing Factors to Abnormal Values

- Hemolysis of the blood sample may alter test results.
- Drugs that may *decrease* results: antibiotics.

Pre-Test Nursing Care

- Explain to the patient the purpose of the test and the need for a blood sample to be drawn.
- No fasting is required before the test.

Procedure

- A 5-mL blood sample is drawn in a collection tube containing no additives.
- Gloves are worn throughout the procedure.

Post-Test Nursing Care

- Apply pressure at venipuncture site. Apply dressing, periodically assessing for continued bleeding.
- Label the specimen and transport it to the laboratory.
- Report abnormal findings to the primary care provider.

• • • • • • • • • • • • • • • • •

Antidiuretic Hormone
(ADH, Vasopressin)

Antidiuretic hormone (ADH), originally known as vasopressin, is a hormone produced by the hypothalamus. It is stored in the posterior pituitary and released when needed as indicated by serum osmolality levels. A high serum osmolality indicates that the serum is concentrated and that the amount of water is limited. When this occurs, ADH is released. ADH increases the permeability of the distal renal tubules and collecting ducts, resulting in water reabsorption. Conversely, a low serum osmolality indicates there is a water excess and that the serum is dilute. In this situation, ADH secretion is reduced, leading to increased excretion of water (diuresis).

Certain conditions can result in an abnormal secretion or lack of secretion of ADH, or in a lack of renal response to ADH secretion. In *diabetes insipidus,* there is either inadequate ADH secretion or the kidneys do not respond appropriately to ADH. Causes of diabetes insipidus include head trauma, brain tumor or inflammation, neurosurgical procedures, or primary renal diseases. In the *syndrome of inappropriate antidiuretic hormone secretion (SIADH),* there is continuing release of ADH in the presence of low plasma osmolality. SIADH may be caused by ectopic ADH-producing tumors of the lung, thymus, pancreas, intestines, and urologic tract; by some pulmonary conditions; or by extreme stress.

Normal Values

1–5 pg/mL (1–5 ng/L SI units)

Possible Meanings of Abnormal Values

Increased	Decreased
Acute porphyria	Central (pituitary)
Addison's disease	diabetes insipidus
Brain tumor	Head trauma
Bronchogenic cancer	Hypervolemia
Circulatory shock	Hypothalamic tumor
Cirrhosis	Metastatic disease
Hemorrhage	Neurosurgical procedures
Hepatitis	Sarcoidosis
Hypothyroidism	Syphilis
Hypovolemia	Viral infection
Nephrogenic diabetes insipidus	
Pneumonia	
Syndrome of inappropriate	
ADH secretion (SIADH)	
Tuberculosis	

Contributing Factors to Abnormal Values

- Test results can be altered by: physical and psychological stress, positive-pressure mechanical ventilation, use of glass tube for blood sample collection.
- Drugs that may *increase* ADH levels: acetaminophen, anesthetics, barbiturates, carbamazepine, chlorothiazide, chlorpropamide, cyclophosphamide, estrogens, lithium, morphine sulfate, nicotine, oxytocin, vincristine sulfate.
- Drugs that may *decrease* ADH levels: alcohol, phenytoin.

Pre-Test Nursing Care

- Explain to the patient the purpose of the test and the need for a blood sample to be drawn.
- Fasting for 10 to 12 hours is required before the test. Physical activity and stress should be avoided during this time.

Procedure

- A 5-mL blood sample is drawn in a collection tube containing either no additives or EDTA and *made of plastic*.
- Gloves are worn throughout the procedure.

Post-Test Nursing Care

- Apply pressure at venipuncture site. Apply dressing, periodically assessing for continued bleeding.
- Label the specimen and transport it to the laboratory immediately. The blood sample must be spun within 10 minutes of collection.
- Report abnormal findings to the primary care provider.

• • • • • • • • • • • • • • • • •

Anti-DNA Antibody Test
(Anti-ds-DNA Antibody)

The anti-DNA antibody test detects the presence of antibodies to native, or double-stranded, DNA. Presence of these antibodies indicates the person has some type of autoimmune disease. These antibodies are particularly prevalent in patients with systemic lupus erythematosus (SLE); thus, this test is useful in monitoring the course of SLE. Progression of the disease is indicated by increasing titers; disease remission is shown by declining titers. A *titer* is the most dilute serum in which the antibody is detected.

Normal Values

Negative at 1:10 dilution

Possible Meanings of Abnormal Values

Increased

Lupus nephritis
Myasthenia gravis
Rheumatoid arthritis
Sclerosis
Sjögren's syndrome
Systemic lupus erythematosus

Contributing Factors to Abnormal Values

- Hemolysis of the blood sample may alter test results.
- Drugs that may *increase* anti-DNA titers: hydralazine hydrochloride, procainamide hydrochloride.

Pre-Test Nursing Care

- Explain to the patient the purpose of the test and the need for a blood sample to be drawn.
- No fasting is required before the test.

Procedure

- A 7-mL blood sample is drawn in a collection tube containing no additives.
- Gloves are worn throughout the procedure.

Post-Test Nursing Care

Possible complication: Infection at venipuncture site due to immunocompromised state.

- Apply pressure at venipuncture site. Apply dressing, periodically assessing for continued bleeding.
- Label the specimen and transport it to the laboratory.
- Teach the patient to monitor the site and to notify the health care provider if signs or symptoms of infection occur, such as drainage, redness, warmth, edema, pain at the site, or fever.
- Report abnormal findings to the primary care provider.

• • • • • • • • • • • • • • • • •

Antiglomerular Basement Membrane Antibody

(AGBM, Glomerular Basement Membrane Antibody)

Goodpasture's syndrome is an autoimmune disease in which antibodies specific for renal structural components, such as the glomerular basement membrane in the kidney, and pulmonary structural components, such as the alveolar basement membrane, are produced. These antibodies then bind to the tissue antigens, resulting in an immune response and the development of such problems as necrotizing glomerulonephritis and hemorrhagic pneumonitis. Because of the renal and pulmonary complications, kidney and lung biopsies may also be performed.

Normal Values

Negative

Possible Meanings of Abnormal Values

Increased

Antiglomerular basement membrane disease
Glomerulonephritis
Goodpasture's syndrome

Contributing Factors to Abnormal Values

- Drugs that may *decrease* test results: antibiotics.

Pre-Test Nursing Care

- Explain to the patient the purpose of the test and the need for a blood sample to be drawn.
- Fasting for 8 hours is required before the test.

Procedure

- A 5-mL blood sample is drawn in a collection tube containing no additives.
- Gloves are worn throughout the procedure.

Post-Test Nursing Care

- Apply pressure at venipuncture site. Apply dressing, periodically assessing for continued bleeding.
- Label the specimen and transport it to the laboratory immediately.
- Report abnormal findings to the primary care provider.

• • • • • • • • • • • • • • • •

Antimicrosomal Antibody Test
(Thyroid Antimicrosomal Antibody)

Microsomes are lipoproteins that are normally present within the epithelial cells of the thyroid. In some types of thyroid disorders, these microsomes escape from their normal locations. Once liberated, these substances appear as antigens to the body. In response, the body produces antibodies against the microsomes, leading to inflammation and destruction of the thyroid gland. Antimicrosomal antibodies are present in the majority of patients diagnosed with Hashimoto's thyroiditis. The most dilute serum in which antimicrosomal antibodies are detected is called the *titer*. This test is usually performed in conjunction with the antithyroglobulin antibody test.

Normal Values

Titer < 1:100

Possible Meanings of Abnormal Values

Increased

Autoimmune hemolytic anemias
Granulomatous thyroiditis
Hashimoto's thyroiditis
Hyperthyroidism
Juvenile lymphocytic thyroiditis
Myasthenia gravis
Myxedema
Nontoxic nodular goiter
Pernicious anemia
Primary hypothyroidism
Rheumatoid arthritis
Sjögren's syndrome
Systemic lupus erythematosus
Thyroid cancer

Contributing Factors to Abnormal Values

- Drugs that may *increase* antimicrosomal antibody titers: oral contraceptives.

Pre-Test Nursing Care

- Explain to the patient the purpose of the test and the need for a blood sample to be drawn.
- No fasting is required before the test.

Procedure

- A 7-mL blood sample is drawn in a collection tube containing no additives.
- Gloves are worn throughout the procedure.

Post-Test Nursing Care

- Apply pressure at venipuncture site. Apply dressing, periodically assessing for continued bleeding.
- Label the specimen and transport it to the laboratory.
- Report abnormal findings to the primary care provider.

• • • • • • • • • • • • • • • • •

Antimitochondrial Antibody Test
(AMA)

The antimitochondrial antibody (AMA) test is used to detect the presence of autoimmune antibodies that have formed against a lipoprotein component of the mitochondrial membrane. These antibodies have a tendency to attack organs that expend a great deal of energy, such as those of the hepatobiliary system. The AMA test is used in the diagnosis of primary biliary cirrhosis. It is usually performed in conjunction with the anti–smooth muscle antibody (ASMA) test.

Normal Values

Negative at 1:20 dilution

Possible Meanings of Abnormal Values

Increased	Decreased/Absent
Autoimmune disease	Drug-induced cholestatic
Chronic active hepatitis	jaundice
Cryptogenic cirrhosis	Extrahepatic obstructive
Drug-induced jaundice	biliary disease
Myasthenia gravis	Sclerosing cholangitis
Primary biliary cirrhosis	Viral hepatitis

Contributing Factors to Abnormal Values

- Hemolysis of the blood sample may alter test results.

Pre-Test Nursing Care

- Explain to the patient the purpose of the test and the need for a blood sample to be drawn.
- No fasting is required before the test.

Procedure

- A 5-mL blood sample is drawn in a collection tube containing no additives.
- Gloves are worn throughout the procedure.

Post-Test Nursing Care

Possible complication: Prolonged bleeding due to vitamin K deficiency secondary to liver dysfunction.

- Apply pressure 3 to 5 minutes at venipuncture site. Apply dressing, periodically assessing for continued bleeding.
- Teach the patient to monitor the site. If the site begins to bleed, the patient should apply direct pressure and, if unable to control the bleeding, return to the laboratory or notify the nurse.
- Label the specimen and transport it to the laboratory.
- Report abnormal findings to the primary care provider.

• • • • • • • • • • • • • • • • • •

Antinuclear Antibody Test
(ANA, FANA, Fluorescent ANA)

A ntinuclear antibodies are antibodies the body produces against nuclear components of its own cells. This results in the development of an autoimmune disease. The antinuclear antibody (ANA) test is commonly used to rule out systemic lupus erythematosus (SLE), because 95% to 99% of SLE patients have positive ANA titers. A *titer* is the most dilute serum in which the ANA is detected. The ANA test uses an indirect immunofluorescent procedure, which results in several staining patterns: homogeneous, nucleolar, peripheral, and speckled patterns. These patterns assist in diagnosing the specific disease process affecting the individual.

Normal Values

Negative at 1:8 dilution or titer < 40

Possible Meanings of Abnormal Values

Positive

Bacterial endocarditis
Chronic autoimmune hepatitis
Cirrhosis
Connective tissue diseases
Dermatomyositis

Positive

Discoid lupus erythematosus
Drug-induced lupus
Human immunodeficiency virus infection
Infectious mononucleosis
Leukemia
Malignancy, especially lymphoma
Mixed connective tissue disease
Myasthenia gravis
Polymyositis
Raynaud's syndrome
Rheumatoid arthritis
Scleroderma
Sjögren's syndrome
Systemic lupus erythematosus
Tuberculosis

Contributing Factors to Abnormal Values

- Hemolysis of the blood sample may alter test results.
- Drugs that may cause a *false-positive* result due to a drug-induced syndrome similar to SLE: acetazolamide, carbidopa, chlorothiazide, chlorpromazine, chlorprothixene, clofibrate, ethosuximide, gold salts, griseofulvin, hydralazine hydrochloride, hydroxytryptophan, isoniazid, lithium, mephenytoin, methyldopa, methysergide, oral contraceptives, para-aminosalicylic acid, penicillin, phenylbutazone, phenytoin, primidone, procainamide hydrochloride, propylthiouracil, quinidine, reserpine, streptomycin, sulfonamides, tetracyclines, thiouracil, trimethadione.

Pre-Test Nursing Care

- Explain to the patient the purpose of the test and the need for a blood sample to be drawn.
- No fasting is required before the test.

Procedure

- A 7-mL blood sample is drawn in a collection tube containing a silicone gel.
- Gloves are worn throughout the procedure.

Post-Test Nursing Care

Possible complication: Infection at venipuncture site due to immunocompromised state.

- Apply pressure at venipuncture site. Apply dressing, periodically assessing for continued bleeding.
- Label the specimen and transport it to the laboratory.
- Teach the patient to monitor the site and to notify the health care provider if signs or symptoms of infection occur, such as drainage, redness, warmth, edema, pain at the site, or fever.
- Report abnormal findings to the primary care provider.

• • • • • • • • • • • • • • • •

Antiscleroderma Antibody
(Scl–70 Antibody, Scleroderma Antibody)

The antiscleroderma antibody is found in individuals with progressive systemic sclerosis (scleroderma) and in individuals with CREST syndrome, which is characterized by calcinosis, Raynaud's phenomenon, esophageal dysfunction, sclerodactyly, and telangiectasia. Positive results with this test are considered highly diagnostic of scleroderma, because the antibody is found only rarely in diseases such as mixed connective tissue disease, rheumatoid arthritis, Sjögren's syndrome, and systemic lupus erythematosus.

Normal Values

Negative

Possible Meanings of Abnormal Values

Increased

CREST syndrome
Scleroderma

Contributing Factors to Abnormal Values

- Drugs that may *increase* antiscleroderma antibody levels: aminosalicylic acid, ethosuximide, isoniazid, methyldopa, penicillin, phenytoin, propylthiouracil, streptomycin, tetracycline, trimethadione.

Pre-Test Nursing Care

- Explain to the patient the purpose of the test and the need for a blood sample to be drawn.
- No fasting is required before the test.

Procedure

- A 5-mL blood sample is drawn in a collection tube containing no additives.
- Gloves are worn throughout the procedure.

Post-Test Nursing Care

- Apply pressure at venipuncture site. Apply dressing, periodically assessing for continued bleeding.
- Label the specimen and transport it to the laboratory.
- Report abnormal findings to the primary care provider.

• • • • • • • • • • • • • • • •

Anti–Smooth Muscle Antibody Test
(ASMA)

The anti-smooth muscle antibody (ASMA) test is used to detect the presence of autoimmune antibodies that have formed against smooth muscle. These antibodies have a tendency to appear in chronic active hepatitis and other diseases in which there is liver damage. The ASMA test is used in the diagnosis of primary biliary cirrhosis and chronic active hepatitis. It is usually performed in conjunction with the antimitochondrial antibody (AMA) test.

Normal Values

Negative at 1:20 dilution

Possible Meanings of Abnormal Values

Increased

Acute viral hepatitis
Chronic active hepatitis
Infectious mononucleosis
Infiltrative tumors
Intrinsic asthma
Malignancies
Primary biliary cirrhosis

Contributing Factors to Abnormal Values

- Hemolysis of the blood sample and the presence of antinuclear antibodies may alter test results.

Pre-Test Nursing Care

- Explain to the patient the purpose of the test and the need for a blood sample to be drawn.
- No fasting is required before the test.

Procedure

- A 5-mL blood sample is drawn in a collection tube containing no additives.
- Gloves are worn throughout the procedure.

Post-Test Nursing Care

Possible complication: Prolonged bleeding due to vitamin K deficiency secondary to liver dysfunction.

- Apply pressure at venipuncture site. Apply dressing, periodically assessing for continued bleeding.
- Teach the patient to monitor the site. If the site begins to bleed, the patient should apply direct pressure and, if unable to control the bleeding, return to the laboratory or notify the nurse.
- Label the specimen and transport it to the laboratory.
- Report abnormal findings to the primary care provider.

• • • • • • • • • • • • • • • •

Antisperm Antibody Test
(Antispermatozoal Antibody)

Antisperm antibodies may form in a male as a result of blocked efferent ducts in the testes. This blockage results in reabsorption of sperm, which can lead to the formation of autoantibodies to the sperm. Antisperm antibodies may also form in a female. Thus, this test may be performed on both males and females as one part of an infertility screening.

Normal Values

Negative

Possible Meanings of Abnormal Values

Increased

Blocked efferent ducts in the testes
Infertility
Vasectomy

Pre-Test Nursing Care

- Explain to the patient the purpose of the test and the specimen samples needed.
- If a semen sample is to be used, the man should avoid ejaculation for 3 days before the test.
- No fasting is required before the test.

Procedure

- The preferred specimen from a male is a semen sample. Provide the appropriate container for the specimen collection.
- A 7-mL blood sample is drawn in a collection tube containing no additives from both the male and female.
- Gloves are worn throughout the procedure.

Post-Test Nursing Care

- Apply pressure at venipuncture site. Apply dressing, periodically assessing for continued bleeding.
- Label all specimens and transport them to the laboratory.
- Semen samples must be transported to the laboratory within 2 hours after collection.
- Report abnormal findings to the primary care provider.

Anti-SS-A (Ro) and Anti-SS-B (La) Antibody

Anti-SS-A (Ro) and anti-SS-B (La) are autoantibodies formed against ribonucleic acid (RNA) protein particles in the body. These antibodies are most often seen in Sjögren's syndrome, a disorder with symptoms similar to those of connective tissue disorders such as rheumatoid arthritis, systemic lupus erythematosus (SLE), or scleroderma. The syndrome is characterized by decreased secretion and eventual destruction of the exocrine glands, resulting in dryness of the mucosa and conjunctiva. The test is used in the differential diagnosis of Sjögren's syndrome, SLE, and mixed connective tissue disease.

Normal Values

Ro: Negative
La: Negative

Possible Meanings of Abnormal Values

Increased

ANA-negative lupus
Neonatal lupus
Scleroderma
Sjögren's syndrome

Pre-Test Nursing Care

- Explain to the patient the purpose of the test and the need for a blood sample to be drawn.
- No fasting is required before the test.

Procedure

- A 7-mL blood sample is drawn in a collection tube containing no additives.
- Gloves are worn throughout the procedure.

Post-Test Nursing Care

Possible complication: Infection at venipuncture site due to immunocompromised state.

- Apply pressure at venipuncture site. Apply dressing, periodically assessing for continued bleeding.
- Label the specimen and transport it to the laboratory.
- Teach the patient to monitor the site and to notify the health care provider if signs or symptoms of infection occur, such as drainage, redness, warmth, edema, pain at the site, or fever.
- Report abnormal findings to the primary care provider.

• • • • • • • • • • • • • • • •

Antistreptolysin-O Titer
(ASO, Streptococcal Antibody Test)

Streptolysin-O is an enzyme produced by group A beta-hemolytic streptococci bacteria. When confronted by this foreign enzyme, the body produces antibodies against it. The antibodies appear 7 to 10 days after the acute streptococcal infection. The antibodies continue to rise for 2 to 4 weeks and remain for up to several months. The antistreptolysin-O (ASO) test is designed to detect these antibodies. If the antibodies are present, the person has had a streptococcal infection. This test is considered less sensitive than the anti-DNase B test. When both tests are consistently performed on blood samples, 95% of the streptococcal infections can be identified. The test is particularly useful in determining whether such conditions as joint pain or glomerulonephritis are the result of a streptococcal infection.

Normal Values

Adult:	< 160 Todd units/mL
Ages 5–12:	< 170–330 Todd units/mL
Ages 2–5:	< 160 Todd units/mL
Ages birth-2:	< 50 Todd units/mL

Possible Meanings of Abnormal Values

Increased

Acute rheumatic fever
Poststreptococcal endocarditis
Poststreptococcal glomerulonephritis
Scarlet fever

Contributing Factors to Abnormal Values
- Hemolysis of the blood sample may alter test results.
- Drugs that may *decrease* ASO titers: antibiotics, corticosteroids.
- False-positive results may occur when blood sample has high lipid content.

Pre-Test Nursing Care
- Explain to the patient the purpose of the test and the need for a blood sample to be drawn.
- No fasting is required before the test.

Procedure
- A 7-mL blood sample is drawn in a collection tube containing no additives.
- Gloves are worn throughout the procedure.

Post-Test Nursing Care

- Apply pressure at venipuncture site. Apply dressing, periodically assessing for continued bleeding.
- Label the specimen and transport it to the laboratory immediately.
- Report abnormal findings to the primary care provider.
- ASO titers are usually repeated in 10 to 14 days for comparison with initial findings.

• • • • • • • • • • • • • • • • • •

Antithrombin III
(AT-III, Heparin Cofactor)

During hemostasis, a substance called thrombin stimulates the formation of fibrin from fibrinogen. This fibrin then forms a stable clot at the site of injury. Any excess amounts of clotting factors which remain following hemostasis are inactivated by fibrin inhibitors which prevent clotting from occurring when it is not needed. One such substance is antithrombin III (AT-III). (See "Coagulation Studies" for a description of the process of hemostasis.)

AT-III is a naturally occurring protein immunoglobulin that is synthesized by the liver. The action of AT-III is catalyzed by heparin. Its role is to inactivate thrombin and other coagulation factors, thus inhibiting the coagulation process. The proper balance between thrombin and AT-III allows for appropriate hemostasis to occur. If, however, this balance is disrupted, problems can arise. For example, if there is a congenital deficiency of AT-III, coagulation will not be inhibited at an adequate level, resulting in a hypercoagulability state with a high risk of thrombosis.

Normal Values

Functional Method

Premature infant:	26%–61%
Full term infant:	44%–76%
After 6 months:	77%–122%

Abnormal Values

Moderate risk for thrombosis:	50%–75%
Significant risk for thrombosis:	< 50%

Possible Meanings of Abnormal Values

Increased	Decreased
Acute hepatitis	Arteriosclerosis
Factor V deficiency	Burns
Factor VII deficiency	Cancer
Inflammation	Cardiovascular disease
Menstruation	Cerebro vascular accident
Renal transplant	Chronic liver failure

Increased	Decreased
Vitamin deficiency	Cirrhosis
	Congenital AT-III deficiency
	Deep vein thrombosis
	Disseminated intravascular coagulation
	Late pregnancy/early postpartum period
	Liver transplant
	Malnutrition
	Nephrotic syndrome
	Postoperative period
	Pulmonary embolism
	Septicemia

Contributing Factors to Abnormal Values

- Hemolysis of the blood sample and presence of lipemia may alter test results.
- Drugs that may *increase* AT-III levels: anabolic steroids, androgens, dicumarol, progesterone-containing oral contraceptives, warfarin sodium.
- Drugs that may *decrease* AT-III levels: estrogen-containing oral contraceptives, fibrinolytics, heparin, L-asparaginase.

Pre-Test Nursing Care

- Explain to the patient the purpose of the test and the need for a blood sample to be drawn.
- No fasting is required before the test.

Procedure

- A 5-mL blood sample is drawn in a collection tube containing sodium citrate and citric acid.
- Gloves are worn throughout the procedure.

Post-Test Nursing Care

- Apply pressure at venipuncture site. Apply dressing, periodically assessing for continued bleeding.
- Label the specimen and transport it to the laboratory.
- Report abnormal findings to the primary care provider.

• • • • • • • • • • • • • • • •

Antithyroglobulin Antibody Test
(Thyroid Antithyroglobulin Antibody)

Thyroglobulin is a thyroid glycoprotein that has a role in the synthesis of triiodothyronine (T_3) and thyroxine (T_4). In some types of thyroid disorders, thyroglobulin may escape from the thyroid gland. Once liberated, these substances appear as antigens to the body. In response, the body produces antibodies against the thyroglobulin, leading to inflammation and destruction of the thyroid gland. Antithyroglobulin antibodies are present in the majority of patients diagnosed with Hashimoto's thyroiditis. The most dilute serum in which antithyroglobulin antibodies are detected is called the *titer*. This test is usually performed in conjunction with the antimicrosomal antibody test.

Normal Values

Titer < 1:100

Possible Meanings of Abnormal Values

Increased

Autoimmune hemolytic anemias
Granulomatous thyroiditis
Hashimoto's thyroiditis
Hyperthyroidism
Juvenile lymphocytic thyroiditis
Myasthenia gravis
Myxedema
Nontoxic nodular goiter
Pernicious anemia
Primary hypothyroidism
Rheumatoid arthritis
Sjögren's syndrome
Systemic lupus erythematosus
Thyroid autoimmune diseases
Thyroid cancer
Thyrotoxicosis

Contributing Factors to Abnormal Values

- Drugs that may *increase* antithyroglobulin antibody titers: oral contraceptives.

Pre-Test Nursing Care

- Explain to the patient the purpose of the test and the need for a blood sample to be drawn.
- No fasting is required before the test.

Procedure

- A 7-mL blood sample is drawn in a collection tube containing no additives.
- Gloves are worn throughout the procedure.

Post-Test Nursing Care

- Apply pressure at venipuncture site. Apply dressing, periodically assessing for continued bleeding.
- Label the specimen and transport it to the laboratory.
- Report abnormal findings to the primary care provider.

• • • • • • • • • • • • • • • • •

Arterial Blood Gas Analysis
(ABGs, Blood Gases)

This section includes discussion regarding the following components:

- pH, blood
- Partial pressure of carbon dioxide (PCO_2)
- Bicarbonate (HCO_3^-)
- Base excess/deficit
- Partial pressure of oxygen (PO_2)
- Oxygen (O_2) content
- Oxygen saturation (SO_2)

Arterial blood gas analysis is performed when information is needed regarding the acid-base status of the patient. The acid-base balance of the body is controlled via three mechanisms: (1) the buffering system, (2) the respiratory system, and (3) the renal system. The buffering system assists with maintaining acid-base balance through the retention or loss of hydrogen ions (H^+). There are also minor buffers in the blood in the form of phosphates and proteins.

The primary buffering system is the *carbonic acid-bicarbonate buffer system*. For the pH of the blood to be within the normal range, these two substances need to be in a 20:1 ratio: 20 parts bicarbonate for every 1 part carbonic acid (H_2CO_3). The breakdown of carbonic acid forms carbon dioxide (CO_2) and water, thus the carbonic acid level can be measured indirectly with the PCO_2 level. The PCO_2 level is controlled by the lungs. The lungs are able to respond relatively quickly to changes in the acid-base balance of the body through the amount of CO_2 retained. The more CO_2 retained, the more carbonic acid in the body, which leads to a state known as *acidosis*. When less CO_2 is retained, the result is less carbonic acid in the body, or *alkalosis*.

Although the lungs are capable of making rapid changes in the acid–base balance of the body, they are only approximately 80% efficient because they must continue to be the site of oxygen exchange. To bring the body into a normal acid–base balance once again, another mechanism must be involved. This mechanism involves the kidneys. The kidneys make changes in the acid–base balance at a slower rate than the lungs, taking several days for their effect to be fully noted. The kidneys regulate the pH of the blood through the excretion or retention of H^+ ions, bicarbonate (HCO_3^-), sodium, potassium, and chloride.

Unlike the lungs, the kidneys are 100% efficient; that is, they will continue to work on the acid–base problem until either the pH of the blood returns to the normal range, a state known as *full compensation*, or the condition worsens. If all of the compensatory mechanisms (buffering system, lungs, and kidneys) are unsuccessful in bringing the acid–base imbalance under control, the problem progresses. Severe acidotic states lead to coma and death, owing to depression of the central nervous system. Alkalotic states stimulate the central nervous system, leading to irritability, tetany, and possibly death. Acidotic states are generally considered more life threatening than alkalotic states.

pH

The pH of the blood is the negative logarithm of the H^+ ion concentration in the blood. For example, if the H^+ ion concentration is 1×10^{-7}, the pH is 7. A blood pH of normal range is needed for many of the chemical reactions in the body to take place. The normal range of pH for arterial blood is 7.35 to 7.45. Blood pH less than 7.35 is considered *acidemia* or *acidosis*. Blood pH greater than 7.45 is considered *alkalemia* or *alkalosis*.

Normal Values

7.35–7.45

Contributing Factors to Abnormal Values

- Drugs that may *increase* the blood pH: sodium bicarbonate.

Partial Pressure of Carbon Dioxide (PCO_2, $PaCO_2$)

The partial pressure of carbon dioxide in the arterial blood, designated as $PaCO_2$, is the amount of pressure exerted by CO_2 dissolved in the blood. It is measured in millimeters of mercury (mm Hg) or torr (1 torr = 1 mm Hg). The normal range for $PaCO_2$ is 35 to 45 mm Hg, but lower values are normal at higher altitudes where the atmospheric pressure is decreased.

When the lungs retain CO_2, the level of CO_2 in the blood increases. This is known as hypercarbia or *hypercapnia,* which is an acidotic state. This problem is exhibited in clinical signs and symptoms of headache, dizziness, and decreasing levels of consciousness. When the lungs expire more CO_2 than normal, the level of CO_2 in the blood decreases, an alkalotic state known as hypocarbia or *hypocapnia.* This results in the patient complaining of tingling of the fingers, muscle twitching, lightheadedness, and dizziness.

Normal Values

35–45 mm Hg (torr)

Contributing Factors to Abnormal Values

- Failure to expel all air from the syringe will result in a falsely low $PaCO_2$ value.
- Drugs that may *increase* $PaCO_2$: aldosterone, ethacrynic acid, hydrocortisone, metolazone, prednisone, sodium bicarbonate, thiazides.
- Drugs that may *decrease* $PaCO_2$: acetazolamide, dimercaprol, methicillin sodium, nitrofurantoin, tetracycline, triamterene.

Bicarbonate (HCO_3^-)

As discussed previously, bicarbonate works with carbonic acid to help regulate the pH of the blood. There are two ways in which bicarbonate may be measured. The first is through direct measurement of the bicarbonate level. The second is an indirect measurement using the values for total CO_2 content and $PaCO_2$ in the following formula:

$$HCO_3^- = \text{Total } CO_2 - (0.03 \times PaCO_2).$$

When the bicarbonate level is less than 22, the value is considered acidotic; if it is greater than 26, it is alkalotic.

Normal Values

22–26 mEq/L (22–26 mmol/L)

Contributing Factors to Abnormal Values

- Drugs that may *increase* bicarbonate: alkaline salts, diuretics.
- Drugs that may *decrease* bicarbonate: acid salts.

Base Excess/Deficit

Determination of the base excess/deficit provides information about the total buffer anions (bicarbonate, hemoglobin, phosphates, and plasma proteins) and whether changes in acid–base balance are respiratory or nonrespiratory (metabolic). Values below −3 mEq/L indicate a base deficit, which correlates to a decrease in bicarbonate level. Values greater than +3 mEq/L indicate a base excess. This information assists in the planning of appropriate treatment for the patient.

Normal Values

−3 to +3 mEq/L

Analysis of Arterial Blood Gases

Following these steps should simplify the analysis of ABG results:

1. Determine whether the pH is acidotic (< 7.35) or alkalotic (> 7.45). (*Note:* If the pH is normal and the PCO_2 and HCO_3^- are abnormal, see step 6.)
2. Determine whether the PCO_2 is acidotic (> 45) or alkalotic (< 35).
3. Determine whether the HCO_3^- is acidotic (< 22) or alkalotic (> 26).
4. Compare the above three values and find the two that "match" in terms of acidity/alkalinity to determine the underlying acid–base imbalance. This step is summarized in Table 2.

TABLE 2
Determining Acid–Base Imbalances

pH	PCO_2 Respiratory Component	HCO_3^- Metabolic Component	Acid–Base Imbalance
Acidotic	Acidotic		Respiratory acidosis
Alkalotic	Alkalotic		Respiratory alkalosis
Acidotic		Acidotic	Metabolic acidosis
Alkalotic		Alkalotic	Metabolic alkalosis

5. If the third value (the one that did not "match" in acidity/alkalinity) is: *normal*, the imbalance is *uncompensated*. If it is *abnormal*, the imbalance is *partially compensated*. For example, if the pH and PCO_2 are both acidotic and the HCO_3^- is alkalotic, the analysis is a "partially compensated respiratory acidosis."
6. If the pH is normal, but the PCO_2 and HCO_3 are abnormal, the imbalance is considered *fully compensated*. To determine the underlying, or initial, imbalance, look at the base excess (shown as BE on a laboratory report). If the base excess is normal when the pH is normal, the underlying problem was *metabolic*. The HCO_3^- value, which is considered the metabolic component, is then referred to in order to determine whether the problem was acidotic or alkalotic.

The previous steps are summarized in Table 3.

TABLE 3
ABG Analysis

pH (7.35–7.45)	Pco₂ (35–45)	HCO₃⁻ (22–26)	Base Excess (–/+ 3)	Acid-Base Imbalance
Acidotic (<7.35)	Acidotic (>45)	Normal		Respiratory acidosis with no compensation
Acidotic (<7.35)	Acidotic (>45)	Alkalotic (>26)		Respiratory acidosis with partial compensation
Normal	Acidotic (>45)	Alkalotic (>26)	Abnormal	Respiratory acidosis with full compensation
Acidotic (<7.35)	Normal	Acidotic (<22)		Metabolic acidosis with no compensation
Acidotic (<7.35)	Alkalotic (<35)	Acidotic (<22)		Metabolic acidosis with partial compensation
Normal	Alkalotic (<35)	Acidotic (<22)	Normal	Metabolic acidosis with partial compensation
Alkalotic (>7.45)	Alkalotic (<35)	Normal		Respiratory alkalosis with no compensation
Alkalotic (>7.45)	Alkalotic (<35)	Acidotic (<22)		Respiratory alkalosis with partial compensation
Normal	Alkalotic (<35)	Acidotic (<22)	Abnormal	Respiratory alkalosis with full compensation
Alkalotic (>7.45)	Normal	Alkalotic (>26)		Metabolic alkalosis with no compensation
Alkalotic (>7.45)	Acidotic (>45)	Alkalotic (>26)		Metabolic alkalosis with partial compensation
Normal	Acidotic (>45)	Alkalotic (>26)	Normal	Metabolic alkalosis with full compensation

Possible Meanings of Abnormal Values

Respiratory Acidosis (increased Pco₂ due to hypoventilation)

Anesthesia/drugs
Asthma
Cardiac arrest
Chronic bronchitis
Congestive heart failure
Emphysema
Head trauma
Neuromuscular depression
Obesity
Pickwickian syndrome
Pneumonia
Pulmonary edema
Respiratory failure

Respiratory Alkalosis (decreased Pco₂ due to hyperventilation)

Adult cystic fibrosis
Anemia
Anxiety
Carbon monoxide poisoning
Cerebral hemorrhage

Fever
Heart failure
Hypoxia
Improperly set ventilator
Myocardial infarction
Pain
Pregnancy (third trimester)
Pulmonary emboli

Metabolic Acidosis (decreased HCO_3^- due to either excess acid production or loss of bicarbonate)

Cardiac arrest (lactic acidosis)
Diabetic ketoacidosis
Diarrhea
Renal failure
Renal tubular acidosis
Starvation (ketoacidosis)

Metabolic Alkalosis (increased HCO_3^- due to either excessive intake of bicarbonate or lactate, or increased loss of chloride, hydrogen, and potassium ions)

Diuretics
Hypochloremia
Hypokalemia
Ingestion of sodium bicarbonate, antacids
Nasogastric suctioning
Sodium bicarbonate infusion
Vomiting

Partial Pressure of Oxygen (PaO_2, PO_2)

The partial pressure of oxygen in the arterial blood, designated as PaO_2, is the amount of pressure exerted by O_2 dissolved in the blood. It is measured in millimeters of mercury (mm Hg) or torr (1 torr = 1 mm Hg). The PaO_2 is used to measure how effective the lungs are in oxygenating the blood. When the value is below normal, the patient is said to be *hypoxic*. The PaO_2 is directly influenced by the amount of oxygen inhaled; thus, it can also be used to assess the effectiveness of oxygen therapy.

Normal Values

75–100 mm Hg (torr)—on room, or ambient air
Elderly: value decreases with age

Possible Meanings of Abnormal Values

Increased	Decreased
High doses of oxygen	Anemia
Polycythemia	Atelectasis
	Cardiac decompensation
	Emphysema

Increased	Decreased
	Hypoventilation
	Insufficient atmospheric oxygen
	Pneumonia
	Pulmonary edema
	Pulmonary embolism

Contributing Factors to Abnormal Values

- Falsely elevated PaO_2 levels may occur owing to failure to expel all air from the syringe.

Oxygen Content (O_2, O_2CT)

The amount of oxygen that the blood can contain is based on the amount of oxygen carried by the hemoglobin and on the amount of oxygen contained in the plasma. One gram of hemoglobin can carry up to 1.34 mL of oxygen. In addition, up to 0.3 mL of oxygen can be carried in 100 mL of blood plasma.

The oxygen content is a measurement of the actual amount of oxygen being carried in the blood. This value is determined through the following formula:

$$O_2 \text{ content} = \frac{SaO_2 \% \times Hgb \times 1.34 + (PaO_2 \times 0.003)}{100\%}$$

Normal Values

Arterial: 15–22 mL/dL of blood (15%–22%)
Venous: 11–16 mL/dL of blood (11%–16%)

Possible Meanings of Abnormal Values

Decreased
Asthma
Chronic bronchitis
Emphysema
Flail chest
Hypoventilation
Kyphoscoliosis
Neuromuscular impairment
Obesity
Postoperative respiratory complications

Oxygen Saturation (SaO_2, SO_2, O_2 sat)

The oxygen saturation value is a comparison of the *actual* amount of oxygen carried by the hemoglobin compared with the amount of oxygen that the hemoglobin is *capable* of carrying. Thus, if the hemoglobin is carrying the amount of oxygen it is capable of carrying, the oxygen saturation is approximately 100%. Oxygen saturation may be measured with arterial blood gases or through pulse oximetry, a noninvasive procedure. (See Oximetry.)

Normal Values

95%–100%

Possible Meanings of Abnormal Values

Increased	Decreased
Adequate oxygen therapy	Carbon monoxide poisoning
	Hypoxia

Contributing Factors to Abnormal Values

- The oxygen saturation is affected by the partial pressure of oxygen in the blood, by the body temperature, by the pH of the blood, and by the structure of the hemoglobin.

ABG Determination

Pre-Test Nursing Care

- Explain to the patient the purpose of the test, noting that the puncture is momentarily painful. (*Note:* Some institutions allow for anesthetizing the area with 1% lidocaine [Xylocaine].)
- Perform the Allen's test to assess for adequate collateral circulation in the ulnar artery. This collateral circulation is important should the radial artery become obstructed by a thrombus after the arterial puncture.
- To perform the Allen's test, apply pressure to both the radial and ulnar pulses of one of the patient's wrists until the pulses are obliterated. The hand will blanch (pale), owing to lack of circulation to the hand. Release the pressure on the ulnar artery. If the hand returns to normal color immediately, the test is considered positive and the arterial puncture may be done in that wrist. If the hand remains pale, the ulnar circulation is inadequate. The test is considered negative, and the other arm should be tested for adequacy. Should both arms be found to be inappropriate sites, the use of the femoral artery may need to be explored.
- No fasting is required before the test.

Procedure

- The area over the radial artery in the wrist is anesthetized with 1% lidocaine, if allowed per institutional policy.
- An airtight syringe containing 0.2 mL of heparin is used to draw a 3 to 5-mL arterial blood sample. (*Note:* Venous blood can be used if arterial blood is unaccessible; however, venous blood is useful only for evaluating pH, $PaCO_2$, and base excess.)
- All air bubbles are expelled from the syringe. The syringe is capped to prevent loss of gases from the sample.
- The syringe is labeled, placed in ice, and taken to the laboratory immediately for analysis.
- Gloves are worn throughout the procedure.

Post-Test Nursing Care

Possible complication: Circulatory impairment

- Apply continuous pressure on the radial site for at least 5 minutes, 10 minutes if the femoral site was used.

- Apply dressing, periodically assessing for continued bleeding, especially if the patient has bleeding problems or is receiving anticoagulant therapy.
- Assess the extremity for signs of circulatory impairment: changes in the color, movement, temperature, sensation, and, if femoral site, pulses distal to the puncture site.
- Note on the laboratory slip whether the patient was breathing ambient (room) air or, if receiving supplemental oxygen, the oxygen flow.
- Report abnormal findings to the primary care provider.

• • • • • • • • • • • • • • • • •

Arteriography of the Lower Extremities
(Lower Extremity Angiography)

Angiography is a general term used to indicate visualization of any blood vessels, whether they be arteries or veins. The more precise term for visualization of the arteries is *arteriography*. Arteriograms are extremely valuable for observing the blood flow to a part of the body and to detect lesions that may be amenable to surgical treatment.

The primary purpose of arteriography of the lower extremities is to identify any occlusions within the femoral arteries and their branches. This is accomplished by introducing a radiopaque catheter into the femoral artery and injecting a contrast medium dye. This test is done for evaluation of peripheral vascular disease and in emergency situations in which blood flow to the extremity has suddenly stopped, as following some types of surgery.

Normal Values

Normal vascular anatomy

Possible Meanings of Abnormal Values

Aneurysm
Arterial disease (such as Buerger's disease)
Occlusion due to arteriosclerosis
Occlusion due to embolism
Occlusion due to neoplasm
Tumor neovascularity

Contributing Factors to Abnormal Values

- Any movement by the patient may alter quality of films taken.

CONTRAINDICATIONS

- Patients who are allergic to iodine, shellfish, or contrast medium dye
- Patients with bleeding disorders
- Pregnant women
  Caution: A woman in her childbearing years should undergo radiography only during her menses or 12 to 14 days after its onset to avoid any exposure to a fetus.

- Patients who are unable to cooperate owing to age, mental status, pain, or other factors
- Patients with renal failure or those susceptible to dye-induced renal failure (dehydrated patients)

Pre-Test Nursing Care

- Explain to the patient the purpose of the test. Provide any written teaching materials available on the subject. Note that discomfort involved with this test is primarily due to lying on a hard table for an extended period of time. Explain that an intense hot flushing may be experienced for 15 to 30 seconds when the dye is injected.
- Check for allergies to iodine, shellfish, or contrast medium dye. Inform the radiologist of such possible allergy and obtain order for an antihistamine and corticosteroid to be administered before the test.
- Baseline laboratory data (CBC, PT, PTT) are obtained.
- Note any medications, such as anticoagulants or aspirin, that may prolong bleeding.
- Patients receiving metformin (Glucophage) for non–insulin-dependent diabetes mellitus should discontine the drug 2 days before elective surgery or angiographic examinations. This is due to the possible occurrence of lactic acidosis, a potentially fatal complication of biguanide therapy.
- Fasting for at least 8 hours is required before the test.
- Obtain a signed informed consent.
- Administer any pre-test sedation after consent form is signed.
- Assess and document patient's peripheral pulses bilaterally before the test. Mark the location of the pulses with a marking pen.

Procedure

- The patient is assisted to a supine position on the examination table.
- A maintenance intravenous line is initiated.
- The area of the puncture site is cleansed and then anesthetized.
- The needle puncture of the artery is made and a guide wire is placed through the needle. The catheter is then inserted over the wire and into the artery.
- The radiopaque catheter is advanced into the desired artery. Positioning is monitored by fluoroscopy.
- Once the catheter is in the correct position, contrast dye is injected through the catheter.
- Radiographic films are taken.
- After films of satisfactory quality are obtained, the catheter is removed and pressure is held on the puncture site for at least 15 minutes.
- Gloves are worn throughout the procedure.

Post-Test Nursing Care

Possible complications:

    Allergic reaction to dye
    Arterial occlusion due to disruption of arteriosclerotic plaque or dissection of arterial lining
    Bleeding at puncture site
    Infection at the puncture site
    Renal failure

- Most allergic reactions to radiopaque dye occur within 30 minutes of administration of the contrast medium. Observe the patient closely for respiratory distress, hypotension, edema, hives, rash, tachycardia, and/or laryngeal stridor. Emergency resuscitation equipment must be readily accessible.
- A pressure dressing is applied to the puncture site. Check the dressing for bleeding and the area around the puncture site for swelling at frequent intervals.
- The patient is to remain on bed rest for 8 to 12 hours with the affected extremity immobilized.
- Maintain pressure on the puncture site with a sandbag.
- Monitor vital signs every 15 minutes for 1 hour, then every 30 minutes for 2 hours, then every hour for 4 hours, and then every 4 hours.
- Monitor urinary output.
- Assess the color, movement, temperature, and sensation (CMTS) and the pulse(s) of the affected extremity with each vital sign check. Compare with the other extremity.
- Encourage fluid intake to promote dye excretion.
- Renal function should be assessed before metformin is restarted.
- Report abnormal findings to the primary care provider.

• • • • • • • • • • • • • • • •

Arthrocentesis
(Synovial Fluid Analysis)

An arthrocentesis is the insertion of a sterile needle into a joint space to obtain a sample of synovial fluid for analysis. Although the procedure may be performed on any joint, the knee is the most common site. Arthrocentesis is used to assist in the differential diagnosis of arthritis, to investigate joint effusion, and to remove excess fluid from the joint that may be causing pain for the patient. If indicated, corticosteroids may be injected into the joint after fluid sample acquisition.

Normal Values

Synovial fluid is clear to straw colored with 0 to 200 white blood cells/µL, no crystals, and a good mucin clot. Values for protein, glucose, and uric acid are similar to serum values.

Possible Meanings of Abnormal Values

Gout
Osteoarthritis
Pseudogout
Rheumatic fever
Rheumatoid arthritis
Septic arthritis
Systemic lupus erythematosus
Traumatic arthritis
Tuberculous arthritis

CONTRAINDICATIONS

- Patients with joint infection or skin infection near proposed site of arthrocentesis

Pre-Test Nursing Care

- Explain to the patient the purpose of the test. Provide any written teaching materials available on the subject. Note that minimal discomfort during the test is due to the injection of the local anesthetic.
- Obtain a signed informed consent.
- No fasting is required before the test.

Procedure

- The patient is assisted to a supine position.
- The skin is cleansed with an antiseptic, and the skin overlying the puncture site is anesthetized.
- A needle is inserted into the joint space. A minimum of 10 mL of fluid is aspirated for analysis.
- If indicated, the needle is left in place and a syringe containing a steroid is attached.
- After the steroid is injected, the needle is withdrawn.
- Pressure is applied to the puncture site, followed by a sterile dressing.
- Gloves are worn throughout the procedure.

Post-Test Nursing Care

Possible complications:
Hemarthrosis
Joint infection

- The patient may experience discomfort after the procedure. The patient is instructed to rest the joint for 12 hours after the test. Elastic wraps, ice applications, and mild analgesics may be used. Strenuous activity should be avoided until approved by the physician.
- Assess the joint for redness, swelling, and tenderness.
- Report abnormal findings to the primary care provider.

• • • • • • • • • • • • • • • • • •

Arthrography
(Arthrogram)

A*rthrography* is the examination of the joint after injection of a radiopaque dye and/or air into a joint. Performed using local anesthesia, the arthrogram assists in the evaluation of joint damage, such as possible cartilage tears, by outlining the soft tissue structures and contour of the joint. Radiographs are taken as the joint is manipulated. This test is used primarily for persistent unexplained joint discomfort. If surgical intervention is anticipated, arthroscopy may be performed in place of arthrography.

Normal Values

Normal muscle, ligament, cartilage, synovial, and tendon structures of the joints

Possible Meanings of Abnormal Values

Arthritis
Cartilaginous abnormalities
Chondromalacia patellae
Disruption of the collateral ligaments
Disruption of the joint capsule
Meniscal tears/lacerations
Osteochondral fractures
Osteochondritis dissecans
Synovial abnormalities
Tears of the cruciate ligaments

CONTRAINDICATIONS

- Pregnant women
  Caution: A woman in her childbearing years should undergo radiography only during her menses or 12 to 14 days after its onset to avoid any exposure to a fetus.
- Patients who are allergic to iodine, shellfish, or contrast medium dye
- Patients with active arthritis
- Patients with joint infection

Pre-Test Nursing Care

- Explain to the patient the purpose of the test. Provide any written teaching materials available on the subject. Note that minimal discomfort during the test is due to the injection of the local anesthetic. Pressure or tingling may be felt during injection of the dye.
- Check for allergies to iodine, shellfish, or contrast medium dye. Inform the radiologist of such possible allergy and obtain order for an antihistamine and corticosteroid to be administered before the test.
- Obtain a signed informed consent.
- No fasting is required before the test.

Procedure

- The patient is assisted to a supine position.
- The skin is cleansed with an antiseptic, and the skin overlying the puncture site is anesthetized.
- A needle is inserted into the joint space. Fluid is usually aspirated for analysis.
- Leaving the needle in place, the radiopaque contrast dye is injected into the joint. Occasionally air is used in place of, or in addition to, the dye.
- The needle is removed and the joint is manipulated to spread the dye around the knee joints.
- Radiographs are taken with the joint in various positions.
- Gloves are worn throughout the procedure.

Post-Test Nursing Care

Possible complications:

Allergic reaction to dye
Infection
Persistent joint crepitus
Thrombophlebitis

- Most allergic reactions to radiopaque dye occur within 30 minutes of administration of the contrast medium. Observe the patient closely for respiratory distress, hypotension, edema, hives, rash, tachycardia, and/or laryngeal stridor. Emergency resuscitation equipment must be readily accessible.
- The patient may experience discomfort after the procedure. The patient is instructed to rest the joint for 12 hours after the test. Elastic wraps, ice applications, and mild analgesics may be used. Strenuous activity should be avoided until approved by the physician.
- Teach the patient to monitor the site and to notify the health care provider if signs or symptoms of infection occur, such as drainage, redness, warmth, edema, pain at the site, or fever.
- Report abnormal findings to the primary care provider.

• • • • • • • • • • • • • • • • •

Arthroscopy

Arthroscopy allows the physician to examine a joint directly with a fiberoptic endoscope. In addition to providing direct visualization of the joint structures, this endoscopic procedure also allows the performance of biopsy and simple repairs to the joint. Although this procedure might be performed on any joint, the knee is the most frequent site.

Normal Values

Normal muscle, ligament, cartilage, synovial, and tendon structures of the joints

Possible Meanings of Abnormal Values

Chondromalacia
Cysts
Degenerative joint changes
Fracture
Joint tumors
Meniscal disease
Osteoarthritis
Osteochondritis
Rheumatoid arthritis
Synovitis
Torn cartilage
Torn ligament
Trapped synovium

CONTRAINDICATIONS

- Patients with fibrous ankylosis of the joint, which prevents effective use of the arthroscope in the joint.
- Patients with joint infection or skin infection near proposed arthroscopic site.

Pre-Test Nursing Care

- Explain to the patient the purpose of the test. Provide any written teaching materials available on the subject. Note that discomfort during the test is due to the injection of the local anesthetic and penetration of the synovium with a blunt instrument. Pressure may be felt during the use of the arthroscope.
- Obtain a signed informed consent.
- The patient is kept NPO after midnight before the test.
- The area 5 to 6 inches above and below the joint is shaved.
- Administer a pre-procedure sedative as ordered.

Procedure

- The patient is assisted to a supine position.
- The extremity is scrubbed, elevated, and wrapped with an elastic bandage from the distal portion of the extremity to the proximal portion, to drain as much blood from the limb as possible.
- A pneumatic tourniquet placed around the proximal portion of the limb is inflated and the elastic bandage is removed.
- *Note:* If a tourniquet is not used, a normal saline solution containing 1% lidocaine and epinephrine is instilled into the joint to distend it and help reduce bleeding.
- The joint is bent to a 45-degree angle, and a local anesthetic is administered.
- A small incision is made in the skin in the lateral or medial aspect of the joint. An opening is made through the synovium using a blunt instrument.
- The arthroscope is then inserted into the joint spaces. The joint is manipulated as it is visualized. Additional puncture sites may be needed to provide a full view of the joint.
- Any biopsy or needed treatment can be performed at this time.
- The joint is irrigated, and the arthroscope is removed. Manual pressure is applied to the joint to remove remaining irrigating solution.
- The incision sites are sutured, and a pressure dressing is applied.
- Gloves are worn throughout the procedure.

Post-Test Nursing Care

Possible complications:

    Hemarthrosis
    Infection
    Infrapatellar anesthesia
    Joint injury
    Synovial rupture
    Thrombophlebitis

- Complications from this procedure are rare. Inform the patient to take an analgesic for knee discomfort after the procedure. Instruct the patient to observe the incision site for redness,

swelling, and tenderness. Strenuous activity involving the joint should be avoided until approved by the physician.
- Report abnormal findings to the primary care provider.

• • • • • • • • • • • • • • • • •

Asparate Aminotransferase
(AST, Formerly SGOT: Serum Glutamic Oxaloacetic Transaminase)

Asparate aminotransferase (AST) is the name now used for the substance that was formerly known as serum glutamic oxaloacetic transaminase, or SGOT. AST is an enzyme found primarily in the heart, liver, and muscle. It is released into the circulation after injury or death of cells. AST levels usually increase within 12 hours of the injury and remain elevated for 5 days. Thus, this test is one of several that is performed when there has been damage to the heart muscle, as in myocardial infarction, and in assessing liver damage. Other cardiac enzymes also assessed are the creatine kinase (CK) isoenzymes and lactic dehydrogenase (LDH, LD).

AST is assessed along with alanine aminotransferase (ALT) in monitoring liver damage. These two values normally exist in an approximately 1:1 ratio. The AST is greater than the ALT in alcohol-induced hepatitis, cirrhosis, and metastatic cancer of the liver. ALT is greater than AST in the case of viral or drug-induced hepatitis and hepatic obstruction due to causes other than malignancy.

The degree of increase of these enzymes may provide a clue as to the source of the problem. A twofold increase is suggestive of an obstructive problem, often requiring surgical intervention. A 10-fold increase of ALT and AST indicates a probable medical problem such as hepatitis.

Normal Values

Female:	9–25 U/L (0.15-0.42 µkat/L SI units)
Male:	10–40 U/L (0.17-0.67 µkat/L SI units)
Elderly:	Slightly higher norms
Newborn:	Norms two to three times higher

Possible Meanings of Abnormal Values

Increased	Decreased
Acute renal disease	Beriberi
Biliary obstruction	Diabetic ketoacidosis
Bone metastases	Hemodialysis
Brain trauma	Pregnancy
Cancer of the prostate	Uremia
Cirrhosis	
Eclampsia	
Gangrene	
Hemolytic disease	
Hepatitis	

Increased	Decreased
Infectious mononucleosis	
Liver cancer	
Malignant hyperthermia	
Muscle inflammation	
Myocardial infarction	
Pancreatitis	
Progressive muscular dystrophy	
Pulmonary infarction	
Reye's syndrome	
Shock	
Severe burns	
Trauma	

Contributing Factors to Abnormal Values

- Drugs that may *increase* AST levels: acetaminophen, allopurinol, antibiotics, ascorbic acid, chlorpropamide, cholestyramine, cholinergics, clofibrate, codeine, dicumarol, erythromycin, guanethidine analogs, hydralazine hydrochloride, isoniazid, meperidine hydrochloride, methyldopa, morphine, oral contraceptives, phenothiazines, procainamide hydrochloride, pyridoxine hydrochloride, salicylates, sulfonamides, verapamil hydrochloride, vitamin A.
- Drugs that may *decrease* AST levels: metronidazole, trifluoperazine hydrochloride.

Pre-Test Nursing Care

- Explain to the patient the purpose of the test and the need for a blood sample to be drawn.
- Inform the patient that this test is often performed on 3 consecutive days, and again in 1 week, necessitating multiple venipunctures.
- No fasting is required before the test.

Procedure

- A 5-mL blood sample is drawn in a collection tube containing a silicone gel.
- Gloves are worn throughout the procedure.

Post-Test Nursing Care

Possible complication: With liver dysfunction, patient may have prolonged clotting time.

- Apply pressure 3 to 5 minutes at venipuncture site. Apply dressing, periodically assessing for continued bleeding.
- Teach the patient to monitor the site. If the site begins to bleed, the patient should apply direct pressure and, if unable to control the bleeding, return to the laboratory or notify the nurse.
- Label the specimen and transport it to the laboratory.
- Report abnormal findings to the primary care provider.

• • • • • • • • • • • • • • • •

Barium Enema
(Large Bowel Study, Lower GI Series)

The barium enema is the fluoroscopic examination of the large intestine after instillation of barium sulfate into the rectum. If a "double contrast" or "air contrast" study is being used, air is also instilled. During this procedure, a fluoroscopic screen is positioned over the intestines. These structures are then projected onto the fluoroscopic screen. The image remains on the monitor for continuous observation; therefore, as the barium is instilled, the flow of barium can be monitored on the screen. The patient's position is changed throughout the examination to allow visualization of the structures and their function, including peristalsis. This test is especially useful in the evaluation of patients experiencing lower abdominal pain, changes in their bowel habits, or the passage of stools containing blood or mucus, and for visualizing polyps, diverticula, and tumors. Videotaping of the fluoroscopic procedure enables the movements to be studied at later times.

Normal Values

Normal size, shape, position, and functioning of the large intestine

Possible Meanings of Abnormal Values

Appendicitis
Carcinoma
Crohn's disease
Diverticulitis
Diverticulosis
Fistulas
Gastroenteritis
Granulomatous colitis
Hirschsprung's disease
Intussusception
Irritable bowel syndrome
Perforation of the colon
Polyps
Sigmoid torsion
Sigmoid volvulus
Telescoping of the bowel
Tumors
Ulcerative colitis

Contributing Factors to Abnormal Values

- Underexposure or overexposure of the film may alter film quality.
- When patients are unable to hold still, owing to pain or mental status, the quality of the film may be affected.
- Barium retained from other examinations and inadequate bowel preparation will interfere with the procedure.

B

CONTRAINDICATIONS

- Pregnant women
  Caution: A woman in her childbearing years should undergo radiography only during her menses or 12 to 14 days after its onset to avoid any exposure to a fetus.
- Patients with tachycardia
- Patients with severe active ulcerative colitis accompanied by systemic toxicity and megacolon
- Patients with suspected intestinal perforation
- Patients who are unable to cooperate in retaining the barium owing to age, mental status, pain, or other factors

Pre-Test Nursing Care

- *Note:* If a barium swallow or an upper gastrointestinal and small bowel series test is ordered, these should be completed *after* the barium enema is performed. Otherwise the barium sulfate ingested during the other examinations may obscure the films made during the barium enema.
- Explain to the patient the purpose of the test and the benefits and risks associated with the test. Provide any written teaching materials available on the subject. Explain to the patient that instillation of the barium and/or air may cause cramping and the urge to defecate.
- Explain to the patient the importance of all aspects of the preparation to ensure complete emptying of the intestinal tract. If fecal material has been retained, the test must be repeated at another time.
- Preparation of the patient includes:
  - A liquid diet with no dairy products for 24 hours before the examination
  - Intake of at least 1200 mL of fluids the day before the examination
  - Stool softeners, laxatives, and enemas as per institutional policy the evening before and the morning of the examination (*Note:* Enemas may occasionally be ordered "until clear". This means that enemas are given until the solution returned is clear and colorless.)
  - Being NPO (nothing by mouth) after midnight before the examination
- Carefully monitor the patient throughout the bowel preparation for fatigue and fluid and electrolyte imbalance.
- Instruct the patient to remove all objects containing metal, such as jewelry or undergarments, because these will show on the film.

Procedure

- The patient is first assisted to a supine position on the examination table, and a preliminary film is taken. This provides verification that no stool remains in the large intestine. If preparation is adequate, the test may continue.
- The patient is then turned to the side (Sims' position), and a lubricated rectal tube is inserted.
- The barium is allowed to flow slowly into the intestine until the entire intestine up to the ileocecal valve is filled. During this time, the flow of barium is observed on the fluoroscopic screen and periodic films are taken.
- Once the intestine is filled, the rectal tube is removed. The patient is assisted to the rest room, or provided a bed pan, and is instructed to expel as much barium as possible.
- After expulsion of the barium, an additional film is taken of the intestine.
- If a double-contrast barium enema has been ordered, air is then instilled in the intestine and additional films taken.
- The procedure takes 45 to 75 minutes.

Post-Test Nursing Care

Possible complications:
  Perforation of the colon
  Fluid and electrolyte imbalance
  Fecal impaction owing to retention of barium

- Resume the patient's diet and medications as taken before the test. Encourage fluid intake.
- Instruct the patient on the need to evacuate all of the barium. Administer a cathartic or enema as ordered. Check all stools for presence of barium, explaining to the patient that the stools will be white initially and return to normal color after passage of all of the barium.
- Instruct the patient to report any abdominal pain, fever, or weakness.
- Notify the physician if the barium is not expelled within 2 to 3 days.
- Report abnormal findings to the primary care provider.

• • • • • • • • • • • • • • • •

Barium Swallow
(Esophageal Radiography, Esophagography)

The barium swallow, which is usually included as a part of the upper gastrointestinal series, is the fluoroscopic examination of the pharynx and the esophagus after ingestion of barium sulfate mixtures. During this procedure, a fluoroscopic screen is positioned over the heart, lungs, and abdomen. These structures are then projected on the fluoroscopic screen. The image remains on the monitor for continuous observation; therefore, as the patient swallows barium, the flow of barium can be monitored on the screen. The patient's position is changed throughout the examination to allow visualization of the entire esophagus and to assess for such problems as gastric reflux. This test is especially useful in the evaluation of patients experiencing dysphagia and regurgitation. Videotaping of the fluoroscopic procedure enables the movements to be studied at later times.

Normal Values

Normal size, shape, position, and functioning of the esophagus

Possible Meanings of Abnormal Values

Achalasia
Cancer of the esophagus
Cancer of the stomach invading the esophagus
Chalasia
Congenital abnormalities
Diverticula
Esophageal motility disorders, such as spasms
Esophageal ulcers
Esophageal varices
Esophagitis
Hiatal hernia

B

Perforation of the esophagus
Polyps
Strictures

Contributing Factors to Abnormal Values

- Underexposure or overexposure of the film may alter film quality.
- When patients are unable to hold still, owing to pain or mental status, the quality of the film may be affected.

CONTRAINDICATIONS

- Pregnant women
  Caution: A woman in her childbearing years should undergo radiography only during her menses or 12 to 14 days after its onset to avoid any exposure to a fetus.
- Patients with intestinal obstruction
- Patients with a perforated esophagus (Gastrografin, a water-soluble contrast medium, would be used in place of barium).
- Patients who are unable to cooperate owing to age, mental status, pain, or other factors
- Patients with unstable vital signs

Pre-Test Nursing Care

- *Note:* If cholangiography and/or a barium enema test are ordered, these should be completed *before* the barium swallow is performed. Otherwise the barium sulfate ingested during the barium swallow may obscure the films made during the other examinations.
- Explain to the patient the purpose of the test and the benefits and risks associated with the test. Provide any written teaching materials available on the subject. Note that no discomfort is associated with this procedure. The barium, although in a milkshake-type solution, may taste chalky.
- Fasting for 8 hours is required before the test.
- Instruct the patient to remove all objects containing metal, such as jewelry or undergarments, because these will show on the film.

Procedure

- The patient is placed in an upright position for the first part of the procedure.
- The fluoroscopic screen is placed in front of the patient, and the heart, lungs, and abdomen are viewed.
- The patient is instructed to take one swallow of a thick barium mixture while the videotape is made of the pharyngeal action.
- As the patient then continues to drink the barium mixture, in addition to the fluoroscopic viewing, spot films are made of the esophageal area from a variety of angles.
- The patient is then placed in different positions and instructed to drink more of the barium. This allows for evaluation of the patient for such problems as gastric reflux.
- The test takes approximately 30 minutes.

Post-Test Nursing Care
Possible complication: Fecal impaction due to retention of barium.

- Resume the patient's diet and medications as taken before the test. Encourage fluid intake.
- Instruct the patient on the need to evacuate all of the barium. Administer a cathartic as ordered. Check all stools for the presence of barium, explaining to the patient that the stools will be white initially and will return to normal color after passage of all of the barium.
- Notify the physician if the barium is not expelled within 2 to 3 days.
- Report abnormal findings to the primary care provider.

• • • • • • • • • • • • • • • •

Barr Body Analysis
(Buccal Smear for Staining Sex Chromatin Mass, Sex Chromatin Body)

The *Barr body* is a tightly coiled, sex chromatin body. When stained, it appears in the shape of a half-moon. The number of Barr bodies in a person is one less than the number of X chromosomes present. Thus, it is absent in normal male cells, which are composed of one X and one Y chromosome. However, one or more Barr bodies are found in males with Klinefelter's syndrome.

This test is a screening test for sex chromosome abnormalities and to assist with the evaluation of a newborn with ambiguous genitalia. A more thorough analysis is provided through chromosomal analysis, called *chromosome karyotype testing*.

Normal Values
Normal female (XX): 1 Barr body
Normal male (XY): 0 Barr bodies

Abnormal Values
Female with Turner's syndrome (XO): 0 Barr bodies
Male with Klinefelter's syndrome (XXY, XXXY, XXXYY, XXXXY): 1–3 Barr bodies

Possible Meanings of Abnormal Values

Increased	Decreased
Klinefelter's syndrome	Turner's syndrome

Contributing Factors to Abnormal Values
- Obtaining saliva instead of buccal cells will lead to false test results.

Pre-Test Nursing Care

- Explain to the patient the purpose of the test and the need for a buccal mucosa scraping to be done.
- No fasting is required before the test.

Procedure

- The buccal mucosa is gently scraped with a metal or wooden spatula.
- The material is smeared on a glass slide, ensuring the cells are evenly distributed. An appropriate fixative or preservative is then applied.
- Gloves are worn throughout the procedure.

Post-Test Nursing Care

- Label the slide and transport it to the laboratory.
- Test results may not be available for up to 4 weeks.
- Report abnormal findings to the primary care provider.

• • • • • • • • • • • • • • • • •

Bilirubin, Blood
(Direct [Conjugated], Indirect [Unconjugated], Total)

Bilirubin, which is one of the components of bile, is formed in the liver, spleen, and bone marrow. It is also formed as a result of hemoglobin breakdown. There are three types of bilirubin: total, direct (conjugated), and indirect (unconjugated). *Total bilirubin* is composed of the direct bilirubin plus the indirect bilirubin. The total bilirubin level increases with any type of jaundice.

Normally, *direct, or conjugated, bilirubin* is excreted by the gastrointestinal (GI) tract, with only minimal amounts entering the bloodstream. It was originally named "direct" bilirubin, because this water-soluble type of bilirubin reacts directly with the reagents added to the blood sample. Its level rises in the blood when obstructive jaundice (as from gallstones) or hepatic jaundice occurs, because the bilirubin is unable to reach the intestines for excretion and, instead, enter the bloodstream for excretion by the kidneys. Direct bilirubin is the only type of bilirubin able to cross the glomerular filter; thus it is the only type of bilirubin that can be found in the urine.

Indirect bilirubin, also known as *free or unconjugated bilirubin,* is normally found in the bloodstream. Its name comes from the fact that this non–water-soluble bilirubin does not directly react with reagents added to a blood sample. Alcohol must be added for the reaction to occur. Indirect bilirubin rises in cases of hemolytic jaundice, in which the breakdown of hemoglobin results in a higher than normal level of indirect bilirubin being present in the bloodstream. This is the type of bilirubin elevated in cases of hepatocellular dysfunction, such as hepatitis. Both total bilirubin and direct bilirubin are directly measurable by laboratory testing. The indirect bilirubin is calculated thus:

Indirect bilirubin = Total bilirubin − direct bilirubin

Normal Values

Total bilirubin: 0.1–1.0 mg/dL (1–17 μmol/L SI units)
Unconjugated (indirect) bilirubin: 0.1–1.0 mg/dL (1–17 μmol/L SI units)
Conjugated (direct) bilirubin: 0.0-0.4 mg/dL (0–7 μmol/L SI units)

Possible Meanings of Abnormal Values

Increased Direct (Conjugated) Bilirubin

Biliary obstruction
Cancer of the head of the pancreas
Choledocholithiasis
Cirrhosis
Dubin-Johnson syndrome
Hepatitis
Obstructive jaundice
Pregnancy

Increased Indirect (Unconjugated) Bilirubin

Autoimmune hemolysis
Cirrhosis
Crigler-Najjar syndrome
Erythroblastosis fetalis
Gilbert's disease
Hemolytic transfusion reaction
Hepatitis
Malaria
Myocardial infarction
Pernicious anemia
Septicemia
Sickle cell disease
Tissue hemorrhage

Contributing Factors to Abnormal Values

- Hemolysis of the blood sample will alter test results.
- Testing with radioactive material within 24 hours will alter test results.
- Drugs that may *increase* total bilirubin: allopurinol, anabolic steroids, antimalarials, ascorbic acid, azathioprine, chlorpropamide, cholinergics, codeine, dextran, diuretics, epinephrine, isoproterenol, levodopa, MAO inhibitors, meperidine hydrochloride, methyldopa, methotrexate, morphine, novobiocin, oral contraceptives, phenelzine sulfate, phenazopyridine hydrochloride, phenothiazines, primaquine, quinidine, rifampin, streptomycin, theophylline, tyrosine, vitamin A.
- Drugs that may *decrease* total bilirubin: barbiturates, caffeine, chlorine, citrate, corticosteroids, ethanol, penicillin, protein, salicylates, sulfonamides, thioridazine hydrochloride, urea.

Pre-Test Nursing Care
- Explain to the patient the purpose of the test and the need for a blood sample to be drawn.
- Fasting for 4 to 8 hours is required before the test. Water is permitted.

Procedure
- A 5-mL blood sample is drawn in a collection tube containing a silicone gel.
- Gloves are worn throughout the procedure.

Post-Test Nursing Care
- Apply pressure at venipuncture site. Apply dressing, periodically assessing for continued bleeding.
- Protect the specimen from bright light by wrapping the sample tube in foil or placing in a refrigerator. Exposure to light causes breakdown of the bilirubin.
- Label the specimen and transport it to the laboratory.
- Report abnormal findings to the primary care provider.

• • • • • • • • • • • • • • • • •

Blastomycosis

Of the thousands of species of fungi known, very few are considered pathogenic to humans. Susceptibility to fungal infections is most frequently seen among those individuals with debilitating or chronic diseases, such as the acquired immunodeficiency syndrome (AIDS) or diabetes, and those undergoing certain types of drug therapy that may alter the immune system, such as steroids and antineoplastic agents. One fungus considered pathogenic is the organism *Blastomyces dermatitidis,* which is similar in structure to tuberculosis. It causes granulomatous skin lesions and may affect visceral organs.

Normal Values
Immunodiffusion: negative
Complement fixation titer: < 1:8

Abnormal Values
Titers of 1:8 to 1:16 indicate infection.
Titers > 1:32 indicate active disease.

Possible Meanings of Abnormal Values

Increased

Blastomycosis

B

Contributing Factors to Abnormal Values

- There may be a cross reaction with histoplasmosis, leading to a falsely high result.
- Skin tests can cause a serologic test to become positive. Thus, skin tests should be withheld until after the blood sample is drawn.
- Many mycoses cause immunosuppression, leading to low titers, or false-negative test results.
- Contamination of the blood sample will alter test results.
- Hemolysis of the sample due to excessive agitation may alter results.
- Antibodies may appear early in the disease and then disappear.

Pre-Test Nursing Care

- Obtain a travel and work history from the patient.
- Explain to the patient the purpose of the test, noting that it involves drawing a blood sample.
- The patient is to be NPO for 12 hours before the test.

Procedure

- The test should be conducted 2 to 4 weeks after exposure to the organism.
- A 7-mL blood sample is obtained in a collection tube containing a silicone gel.
- The venipuncture must not be performed on or near any fungal skin lesions.
- Gloves are worn during the procedure.

Post-Test Nursing Care

- Apply pressure at venipuncture site. Apply dressing, periodically assessing for continued bleeding.
- Label the specimen and transport it to to the laboratory immediately, taking care to avoid excessive agitation of the sample.
- Advise the patient that other procedures to test for this fungus may be done. Such testing might include smear and culture of material from lesions, biopsy, and skin testing.
- Report abnormal findings to the primary care provider.

• • • • • • • • • • • • • • • • •

Bleeding Time
(Aspirin Tolerance Test, Duke Bleeding Time, Ivy Bleeding Time, Modified Ivy, Template Bleeding Time)

Bleeding time measures the duration of bleeding after a standardized skin incision has been made. Commercially manufactured bleeding template devices predominate in the performance of bleeding times because of the standardization of testing that only they provide. In addition, they are cost effective, sterile, and disposable, and reduce scarring. With the template and modified template methods, one or two standardized incisions are made on the volar surface of the forearm and the time required for bleeding to stop is determined—this is the "bleeding time". Other methods for determining bleeding time include the Ivy method, which requires three small punctures, and the Duke method, which uses a puncture wound in the earlobe.

Bleeding time is a screening test for detecting disorders involving platelet function and for vascular (i.e., capillary) defects that interfere with the clotting process. The test is indicated when there is a personal or family history of bleeding tendencies, such as easy bleeding, and as a screening test for preoperative patients when a hemostatic defect is suspected.

Bleeding time is occasionally used before and after aspirin administration to determine the effects of the aspirin on bleeding time. Prolonged bleeding time in the absence of a low platelet count indicates that a qualitative platelet disorder exists. Further studies are then indicated.

Normal Values

Template method: < 9 minutes
Ivy method: 1–7 minutes
Duke method: 1–3 minutes

Possible Meanings of Abnormal Values

Increased (Prolonged)

Aplastic anemia
Bone marrow disorder
Collagen vascular disease
Cushing's disease
Disseminated intravascular coagulation (DIC)
Factor V, VII, XI deficiencies
Fibrinogen defects (e.g., dysfibrinogenemia, afibrinogenemia)
Folic acid deficiency anemia
Heat stroke
Hypocalcemia
Leukemia
Pernicious anemia
Platelet defects:
   Acquired (e.g., aspirin ingestion)
   Inherited (e.g., Von Willebrand's disease)
Renal failure
Severe liver disease
Thrombocytopenia
Uremia
Vascular abnormalities

Contributing Factors to Abnormal Values

- Drugs that may *prolong* bleeding time: alcohol, antibiotics, anticoagulants, antineoplastics, nitroglycerin, nonsteroidal anti-inflammatory medications, salicylates, thiazides, thrombolytics.

Contraindications

- Patients with platelet counts < 75,000/mm^3
- Patients with edematous arms, such as after mastectomy
- Patients who are unable to cooperate during the test

Pre-Test Nursing Care

- Obtain medication history. Aspirin, anticoagulants, and over-the-counter cold medications should be avoided a minimum of 7 days before the test.
- Explain the procedure to the patient.
- No fasting is required before the test.
- Advise the patient to abstain from drinking alcoholic beverages for 24 hours before the test.

Procedure

- The volar surface of the patient's forearm should be extended and inspected for superficial veins, scarring, bruises, and swelling. The muscular portion below the elbow fold is the site of choice. If visually satisfactory, the site is cleansed with an antiseptic and allowed to air dry completely.
- A blood pressure cuff is placed on the patient's arm and inflated to 40 mm Hg. This pressure should be maintained throughout the procedure.
- The commercially manufactured bleeding template device is placed in the prepared area on the forearm. Only enough pressure is applied to ensure that the entire device is touching the skin. Too much pressure will result in an incision that is too deep.
- Activate the device and start a stopwatch.
- As drops of blood form, they (not the wound) are blotted every 30 seconds with filter paper. Care must be taken not to touch the wound at any time during testing.
- When bleeding ceases, the watch is stopped and the blood pressure cuff is released.
- If two incisions are made, they must be in the same orientation, either parallel or perpendicular to the elbow, and the individual times obtained are averaged.
- If bleeding does not stop within 15 minutes, the test should be discontinued.
- Gloves are worn throughout the procedure.

Post-Test Nursing Care

Possible complications:
Bleeding
Scar formation
Skin infection at site

- Butterfly bandages are placed over each cut. These should remain in place for 48 hours to minimize scarring. Assess periodically for continued bleeding.
- If the patient has bleeding tendencies, apply a pressure dressing over the butterfly bandages. The pressure dressing can be removed after 12 hours, leaving the butterfly bandages in place.
- Notify the physician immediately if bleeding has not stopped within 15 minutes.
- Teach the patient to monitor the site. If the site begins to bleed, the patient should apply direct pressure and, if unable to control the bleeding, return to the laboratory or notify the nurse.
- Teach the patient to notify the health care provider if signs or symptoms of infection occur, such as drainage, redness, warmth, edema, pain at the site, or fever.
- Report abnormal findings to the primary care provider.

• • • • • • • • • • • • • • • •

B

Blood Alcohol
(Ethanol, Ethyl Alcohol, ETOH)

Ethanol is the type of alcohol found in alcoholic beverages. It is considered a central nervous system depressant. This depression can result in coma and death when blood levels reach 300 mg/dL or more. Testing for blood alcohol levels is usually done as part of a legal investigation regarding impaired driving. Each state establishes its own limit for what is considered intoxication. Because of its role as legal evidence, the blood sample must be handled very carefully. The specimen is transported in a sealed plastic bag and must be signed by each person handling the specimen.

Normal Values

0 mg/dL (0 mmol/L SI units)

Possible Meanings of Abnormal Values

Increased

Alcohol ingestion

Contributing Factors to Abnormal Values

- Blood alcohol levels may be *increased* when taken concomitantly with drugs such as antihistamines, barbiturates, chlordiazepoxide, diazepam, glutethimide, guanethidine sulfate, isoniazid, meprobamate, opiates, phenytoin, and tranquilizers.

Pre-Test Nursing Care

- Explain to the patient the purpose of the test and the need for a blood sample to be drawn.
- No fasting is required before the test.

Procedure

- If test is to be used as legal evidence, have specimen collection witnessed.
- Cleanse the venipuncture site with povidone-iodine solution instead of alcohol.
- A 5-mL blood sample is drawn in a collection tube containing no additives. *Do not* use alcohol to clean the top of the collection tube.
- Follow institutional policy regarding handling of legal evidence.
- Gloves are worn throughout the procedure.

Post-Test Nursing Care

- Apply pressure at venipuncture site. Apply dressing, periodically assessing for continued bleeding.
- Label the specimen and transport it in a sealed plastic bag to the laboratory. The bag must be signed by each person handling the specimen.
- Report abnormal findings to the primary care provider.

• • • • • • • • • • • • • • • •

Blood Culture and Sensitivity

Bacteria may enter the bloodstream in a variety of ways, including invasion by bacteria through the lymphatic system, through indwelling venous or arterial catheters, or owing to bacterial endocarditis associated with prosthetic heart valves. When bacteria enter the bloodstream, patients may experience chills and fever. It is usually at this point that a blood culture is performed to confirm the presence of bacteria in the blood, a condition called *bacteremia*. Ideally, the blood sample should be drawn before the beginning of antibiotic therapy. Once the blood sample is obtained, the blood is cultured, during which time the organisms are allowed to grow in special culture media. In 48 to 72 hours, the organism is usually identified. The sensitivity portion of the test involves the testing of the organism to identify drugs to which the organism is sensitive or resistant.

Once the specimen is obtained, the patient can be given a broad-spectrum antibiotic that is hoped to be effective against the suspected bacteria. After the blood culture and sensitivity results are available, the antibiotic in use should be verified as to its appropriateness according to the sensitivity report.

Normal Values

Negative

Possible Meanings of Abnormal Values

Positive

Bacteremia

Contributing Factors to Abnormal Values

- Improper technique while collecting the blood sample may alter test results.
- Drugs that may cause *false-negative* results: antibiotics.

Pre-Test Nursing Care

- Explain to the patient the purpose of the test and the need for a blood sample to be drawn. (*Note:* Some institutions require two samples to be drawn, each from a different site. This provides a verification of whether positive cultures are the result of contamination during sample collection or the actual presence of bacteria.)
- No fasting is required before the test.

Procedure

- The venipuncture site is cleansed, starting at the center and moving outward in a circular pattern, using first alcohol, and then iodine (provided the patient is not allergic to iodine).
- Allow the site to dry for 1 minute.
- Cleanse the tops of the culture bottles with alcohol or iodine and allow to dry.
- Apply the tourniquet and perform the venipuncture. A 10 to 20 mL blood sample is drawn.
- Remove the needle from the syringe and replace with a new sterile needle. Then transfer the blood from the syringe into the culture bottle.
- Mix the bottle gently.
- Gloves are worn throughout the procedure.

Post-Test Nursing Care

- Apply pressure at venipuncture site. Apply dressing, periodically assessing for continued bleeding.
- Begin antibiotic therapy, as ordered, after specimen collection is complete.
- Report results of the culture and sensitivity to the primary care provider so that modifications in drug therapy are made if the organism is found to be resistant to the prescribed antibiotic.

• • • • • • • • • • • • • • • • • •

Blood Smear
(Peripheral Blood Smear, RBC Smear, Red Blood Cell Smear)

There are many quantitative blood tests available to the health care worker that provide an enormous amount of information about the various blood components. However, the blood smear, a qualitative measure, is viewed as being equally, if not more, informative.

The test involves the preparation of a smear of peripheral blood on a slide. The smear is then microscopically examined to note the appearance of the red blood cells, white blood cells, and platelets. Red blood cells are examined in terms of size, shape, color, and structure. Examination of the white blood cells provides data regarding total quantity and differential count (see White Blood Cell Count and Differential). Platelets are also examined for number and the presence of abnormal appearance, or thrombocytopathy.

Normal Values

Normal quantity and appearance of red blood cells, white blood cells, and platelets

Possible Meanings of Abnormal Values

Red blood cells: See Table 4 on red blood cell abnormalities.
White blood cells: See White Blood Cell Count and Differential.
Platelets: See Platelet Count.

Contributing Factors to Abnormal Values

- The quality of the microscopic examination is highly dependent on the knowledge and experience of the individual performing the examination.
- Hemolysis of specimen may alter test results.

Pre-Test Nursing Care

- Explain to the patient the purpose of the test and the need for a blood sample to be drawn.
- No fasting is required before the test.

Procedure

- The blood smear may be prepared from blood obtained from a fingerstick or heelstick or from venipuncture.
- If a venipuncture is used, blood is drawn in a collection tube containing EDTA.
- Gloves are worn throughout the procedure.

TABLE 4
Red Blood Cell Abnormalities

Type of Abnormal Cell	Characteristic of Abnormal Cell	Conditions Exhibiting the Abnormality
Anisocytes	Vary in size	Any anemia
Basophilic stippling	Dark spots caused by abnormal hemoglobin synthesis	Thalassemia Lead or heavy-metal poisoning
Heinz-Ehrlich bodies	Particles of denatured hemoglobin attached to the cell membrane	Congenital glucose-6-phosphate dehydrogenase deficiency Other drug-induced hemolytic anemias Unstable hemoglobin disorders after splenectomy
Howell-Jolly bodies	Dark purple spherical bodies (remnants of nuclear material)	Occasionally in severe hemolytic anemias pernicious anemia Occasionally in leukemia, thalassemia, postsplenectomy state
Hyperchromic cells	Highly colored cells due to concentrated hemoglobin	Usually caused by dehydration
Hypochromic cells	Pale cells due to low hemoglobin content	Any anemias
Macrocytes	Abnormally large	Macrocytic anemias such as pernicious anemia, folic acid deficiency Increased erythropoiesis Postsplenectomy anemia
Microcytes	Anormally small	Microcytic anemias such as iron deficiency and thalassemia major
Ovalocytes (elliptocytes)	Oval, or elliptical shaped cells	Microcytic anemias (thalassemia, iron deficiency) Megaloblastic anemia Hemoglobinopathies
Poikilocytes	Irregular in shape	Any anemia
Rouleaux formation	Red blood cells stick to one another	Cryoglobulinemia Giant cell arteritis Macroglobulinemia Multiple myeloma
Schistocytes	Fragmented cells noted for their unusual shapes (helmet, spirals, triangles)	Hemolytic anemia Prosthetic heart valves or severe valvular heart disease Severe burns
Sickle cells	Cresecent-shaped (sickle-shaped) due to abnormal hemoglobin (Hb S)	Sickle cell anemia
Spherocytes	Small and round cells, instead of normal biconcave shape	Hereditary spherocytosis Immunohemolytic anemia
Stomatocytes	One or more slit-like areas of central pallor are present, producing a mouth-like appearance	Acute alcoholism Neoplastic, cardiovascular, hepatobiliary diseases Congenital stomatocytosis Drugs such as phenothiazines
Target cells	Thin cells, with less hemoglobin	Hemoglobin C disease or trait Thalassemia minor Iron-deficiency anemia Liver disease Postsplenectomy state

B

Post-Test Nursing Care

- Apply pressure at venipuncture site. Apply dressing, periodically assessing for continued bleeding.
- Report abnormal findings to the primary care provider.
- If blood smear is found to be abnormal, follow-up testing with bone marrow aspiration or biopsy may be done.

• • • • • • • • • • • • • • • • •

Blood Typing
(ABO Typing, ABO Red Cell Groups, Blood Groups, Rh Typing, Type and Crossmatch, T & C, Type and Screen)

The foundation of blood typing is the detection of ABO and Rh antigens on the red blood cells of an individual's blood. Each person has one blood type (A, B, AB, or O) that is genetically determined. These blood type designations specify the antigen present on the person's red blood cells. For example, a person with type B blood has the B antigen on the red blood cells and someone with type O blood has no antigens.

Another important aspect of blood typing is understanding the presence of antibodies in the blood and what they mean to blood transfusion therapy. For someone to receive blood from a donor with a minimum of risk for a transfusion reaction, the donor's blood must have no antibodies against the recipient's red blood cells and the recipient's blood must have no antibodies against the donor's red blood cells. For example, a person with type AB blood has no antibodies present and can therefore theoretically receive blood of any of the four blood types (A, B, AB, or O). Thus a person with type AB blood is often called the "universal recipient." A person with type O blood, on the other hand, has both anti-A and anti-B antibodies and can therefore receive type O blood, the only type with no antigen on its red blood cells. Individuals with type O blood are referred as "universal donors," because their blood, which has no antigens present on the red blood cells, will theoretically cause no reaction when administered to individuals with any of the four blood types.

The blood types with their associated antigens and antibodies, and a synopsis of donor and recipient blood types, are summarized in Table 5. Please note that although several blood types may be listed as being appropriate for use in a transfusion for a particular blood type, this applies to small volumes of blood being received. However, when large volumes of whole blood are transfused, ABO matching is essential.

Another component of blood typing is that of Rh typing. *Rh factor*, also known as D factor, was so named because the rhesus monkey was used in the initial investigations into this factor. An individual is either Rh positive or Rh negative. The Rh-positive individual has the Rh antigen present on the red blood cells and no antibodies against the Rh factor. The Rh-negative individual has no antigens present on the red blood cells and has anti-Rh antibodies *if* previously sensitized by Rh-positive blood. In Rh-negative males, this sensitization would have occurred through transfusion with Rh-positive blood. In Rh-negative females, the sensitization could have occurred either through transfusion with Rh-positive blood or through pregnancy in which the fetus was Rh positive.

Determination of the Rh factor is crucial for pregnant women. If the woman is Rh negative and her husband's blood is Rh positive, the fetus is Rh positive. If the woman is Rh negative, an indirect Coombs test, which screens for Rh antibodies, is ordered. If the test is positive, Rh antibodies are present and Rh antibody titers are then obtained. If the antibody test is negative both initially and again late in the pregnancy, there is no risk to the fetus. If, however, the test is positive, the Rh-negative mother is producing antibodies against the red blood cells of the Rh-positive fetus. These antibodies may cross the placenta and cause destruction of fetal red blood cells before or during birth. This results in a hemolytic disease known as hemolytic disease of the newborn or erythroblastosis fetalis. This disease can be prevented by administering an anti-Rh antibody preparation (RhoGAM) in the third trimester of pregnancy to women at risk.

RhoGAM acts to suppress the mother's production of antibodies in response to receiving the Rh-positive antigen. RhoGAM should be given to all Rh-negative women whenever there is a possibility of fetal-maternal transplacental hemorrhage, no matter how minor. Such hemorrhage may occur as a result of chorionic villus sampling, amniocentesis, spontaneous or therapeutic abortion, or delivery.

When a person receives an incompatible type of blood, that person's antibodies attack the antigens present on the red blood cells of the donor blood. For example, a person with type A blood has anti-B antibodies present in the blood. If this person is given type B blood, which has B antigens on the red blood cells, the recipient's anti-B antibodies will attack the donor's B antigens, resulting in a hemolytic, or transfusion reaction. Such a reaction can result in renal failure and death of the recipient. To avoid the occurrence of transfusion reactions, testing of both the recipient's blood and the donor's blood is done to ensure compatibility. Two tests that are conducted are the "type and crossmatch" and the "type and screen".

Type and crossmatch testing includes several components that take approximately 1 hour to complete. First, the ABO group and Rh type of the recipient are determined. Next, from the donated blood supply available, donor blood of the same ABO group and Rh type is chosen for compatibility testing. Indirect Coombs' testing, which is a general screening for antibodies, is performed on both the recipient and donor blood. More specific antibody testing may be required to identify unusual antibodies. Once these tests are completed, samples of the recipient's blood and the donor's blood are combined (crossmatched). If no antigen–antibody reaction occurs, the donor blood is considered to be compatible and thus acceptable for transfusion into the recipient.

Type and screen testing includes only testing to determine the ABO group and Rh type and the indirect Coombs test. Actual crossmatching with donor blood is not performed. Type and

TABLE 5
Blood Types

Blood Type	O	A	B	AB
Antigen(s) present on red blood cells	None	A	B	A and B
Antibodies present	Anti-A Anti-B	Anti-B	Anti-A	None
May receive what type blood	O	A, O	B, O	A, B, AB, O
May donate blood to people of what type	A, B, AB, O	A, AB	B, AB	AB

screen testing is conducted in situations in which there is only a slight change of the person requiring blood, or in emergency situations.

Normal Values

Compatible (no antigen–antibody reactions between donor and recipient blood samples)

Contributing Factors to Abnormal Values

- Hemolysis of the blood sample may alter test results.
- Administration of Dextran or intravenous contrast media before the test may alter test results.

Pre-Test Nursing Care

- Explain to the patient the purpose of the test and the need for a blood sample to be drawn.
- No fasting is required before the test.
- The blood sample should be drawn before administration of Dextran, a plasma volume expander.

Procedure

- A 10-mL blood sample is drawn in two collection tubes: one containing no additives and another containing EDTA.
- Gloves are worn throughout the procedure.

Post-Test Nursing Care

- Apply pressure at venipuncture site. Apply dressing, periodically assessing for continued bleeding.
- Report Rh status to the primary care provider.

• • • • • • • • • • • • • • • •

Bone Marrow Biopsy
(Bone Marrow Aspiration)

Bone marrow is the soft, sponge-like material contained in the medullary canals of the long bones and within the spaces between trabeculae of cancellous bone. The primary function of the bone marrow is the production of erythrocytes, leukocytes, and platelets. In this procedure, a sample of the bone marrow is removed through a needle inserted through the cortex of the bone and into the bone marrow. The preferred site for the bone marrow aspiration is the iliac crest, although the sternum is also occasionally used.

Normal Values

Red marrow contains connective tissue, fat cells, and hematopoietic cells. Yellow marrow contains connective tissue and fat cells.

Possible Meanings of Abnormal Values

Agranulocytosis
Amyloidosis
Cancer
Depressed hematopoiesis
Granuloma
Infection
Infectious mononucleosis
Iron-deficiency anemia
Leukemia
Lymphoma
Multiple myeloma
Myelofibrosis
Polycythemia vera
Sideroblastic anemia
Thalassemia

CONTRAINDICATIONS

- Patients with bleeding disorders
- Patients unable to cooperate with the examination

Pre-Test Nursing Care

- Explain to the patient the purpose of the test. Provide any written teaching materials available on the subject. Note that discomfort during the test is due to the injection of the local anesthetic and removal of the marrow sample. Pressure may be felt during insertion of the biopsy needle.
- Obtain baseline data regarding coagulation, such as prothrombin time, partial thromboplastin time, and platelet count.
- No fasting is required before the test.
- Obtain a signed informed consent.
- Administer a sedative before the procedure, if ordered.

Procedure

- The procedure is usually done at the bedside with the patient in the prone or lateral position.
- The skin overlying the proposed site of the aspiration is cleansed and draped. A local anesthetic is administered to the area.
- A large-bore needle is slowly advanced through the subcutaneous tissue and the cortex of the bone. Once inside the marrow, the stylet is removed from the needle and a syringe is attached.
- A sample of 0.2 to 0.5 mL of bone marrow is aspirated and slide preparation is completed.
- The needle is withdrawn, with pressure applied to the site for 10 to 15 minutes.
- A sterile dressing is applied.
- Gloves are worn throughout the procedure.

Post-Test Nursing Care

Possible complications:
> **Hemorrhage**
> **Infection**

- Observe the puncture site for bleeding.
- Assess for signs of infection: tenderness and erythema at the site, fever.
- Assess for signs of hemorrhage: increased pulse rate, decreased blood pressure, pain.
- Ideally, the patient should maintain bed rest for at least 1 hour. However, this procedure is now often done in clinic settings where this is not practical.
- Label the specimen and transport it to the laboratory immediately.
- Report abnormal findings to the primary care provider.

• • • • • • • • • • • • • • • •

Bone Scan

During a bone scan, the patient is given a radionuclide compound, usually a radiopharmaceutical such as technetium-99m, by means of intravenous injection. One to 3 hours later, a scintillation camera is used to take a radioactivity reading from the bone. These readings are fed into a computer, which translates these readings into a two-dimensional gray-scale picture. Normally, the bone has a fairly consistent uptake of the radionuclide, with the exception of areas of growing bone (epiphyseal plate). Such areas show as very dark spots on the scintigram and are called *hot spots* because more of the radionuclide was deposited in that spot. Abnormalities can also cause hot spots, including arthritis, fractures, osteomyelitis, and tumors. Spots without radionuclide uptake are known as *cold spots*.

The primary purpose for performing a bone scan is to detect metastatic cancer of the bone. It is also used to monitor the progression of degenerative bone disorders. Another use of a bone scan is to detect fractures in patients who continue to have pain, even though radiographs have proven negative. Further testing is warranted when abnormal findings are discovered in a bone scan, because the test is not specific. That is, all abnormalities are shown by increased radionuclide uptake, but the type of abnormality is not differentiated by the scan.

Normal Values

Normal patterns of bone uptake of the radionuclide

Possible Meanings of Abnormal Values

Bone necrosis
Degenerative arthritis
Fracture
Metastatic bone neoplasm
Osteomyelitis
Paget's disease
Primary bone malignancy
Renal osteodystrophy
Rheumatoid arthritis

B

Contributing Factors to Abnormal Values

- Any movement by the patient may alter the quality of films taken.

CONTRAINDICATIONS

- Pregnant women
  Caution: A woman in her childbearing years should undergo radiography only during her menses or 12 to 14 days after its onset to avoid any exposure to a fetus.
- Patients who are lactating
- Patients who are unable to cooperate owing to age, mental status, pain, or other factors

Pre-Test Nursing Care

- Explain to the patient the purpose of the test. Provide any written teaching materials available on the subject. Note that discomfort involved with this test is primarily due to lying on a hard table for an extended period of time and the needle puncture. Reassure the patient that only trace amounts of the radionuclide are involved in the test.
- The patient must remain still while the scan is being performed.
- No fasting is required before the test.
- Obtain a signed informed consent.

Procedure

- A radionuclide such as technetium-99m is administered by intravenous injection into a peripheral vein.
- The patient is to drink 4 to 6 glasses of water during the time between receiving the injection and undergoing the scan. This will help clear the body of excess radionuclide that the bone will not take up.
- The patient is to urinate just before the examination.
- The patient is assisted to a supine position on the examination table.
- A scintillation camera is positioned over the patient's body. This camera takes a radioactivity reading from the body. This information is transformed into a two-dimensional picture of the skeleton.
- Depending on the area of interest needing to be scanned, the patient may be placed in the prone and/or lateral positions for additional pictures to be taken.
- Gloves are worn during the radionuclide injection.

Post-Test Nursing Care

- Check the injection site for redness or swelling.
- If a woman who is lactating *must* have a nuclear scan, she should not breast feed the infant until the radionuclide has been eliminated, possibly for 3 days.
- Although the amount of diagnostic radionuclide excreted in the urine is low, the urine should not be used for any laboratory tests for the time period indicated by the nuclear medicine department. Clients should be told to flush the toilet three times after voiding.
- Gloves are worn when dealing with the urine.
- No other radionuclide tests should be scheduled for 24 to 48 hours.
- Encourage fluid intake by the patient to enhance excretion of the radionuclide.
- Report abnormal findings to the primary care provider.

• • • • • • • • • • • • • • • •

B

Brain Scan (Cerebral Blood Flow)

Normally, there is an impediment to blood coming in contact with the brain tissue. This hindrance is known as the *blood-brain barrier.* It is this barrier that normally prevents radionuclides from being taken up by the brain. However, in pathologic conditions, the blood-brain barrier is interrupted, allowing the radionuclide to become concentrated in the abnormal areas of the brain.

The primary use of the brain scan is to assess for brain abscesses, tumors, contusions, hematomas, and cerebrovascular accidents. An immediate scan after the injection of the radionuclide will show differences in the cerebral blood flow between the two sides of the brain. Allowing some time between the injection and the scanning will show pathogenic tissue. Such tissue will appear as a hot spot because more of the radionuclide will be deposited in that spot. Although a commonly used diagnostic test in the past, the brain scan is steadily being replaced with computed tomography and magnetic resonance imaging.

Normal Values

Negative

Possible Meanings of Abnormal Values

Alzheimer's disease
Aneurysm
Arteriovenous malformation
Brain abscess
Brain tumor
Cerebral hemorrhage
Cerebral thrombosis
Cerebrospinal fluid leak
Cerebrovascular accident
Contusion of the brain
Dementia
Hematoma
Huntington's disease
Metastatic cancer to the brain
Parkinson's disease
Seizure disorders

Contributing Factors to Abnormal Values

- Any movement by the patient may alter quality of films taken.

CONTRAINDICATIONS

- Pregnant women
  Caution: A woman in her childbearing years should undergo radiography only during her menses or 12 to 14 days after its onset to avoid any exposure to a fetus.
- Patients who are lactating
- Patients who are unable to cooperate owing to age, mental status, pain, or other factors

B

Pre-Test Nursing Care

- Explain to the patient the purpose of the test. Provide any written teaching materials available on the subject. Note that discomfort involved with this test is primarily due to lying on a hard table for an extended period of time and the needle puncture. Reassure the patient that only trace amounts of the radionuclide are involved in the test.
- The patient must remain still while the scan is being performed.
- No fasting is required before the test.
- Obtain a signed informed consent.
- Potassium chloride, a blocking agent, is administered by mouth 2 hours before the test to prevent an unusually high level of radionuclide uptake by the choroid plexus, which would mimic a pathologic condition in the brain.

Procedure

- The patient is assisted to a supine position on the examination table, with the scintillation camera positioned over the patient's head. This camera takes a radioactivity reading from the body. This information is transformed into a two-dimensional picture of the brain.
- A radionuclide such as technetium-99m is administered by intravenous injection into a peripheral vein.
- The scan is started immediately to provide a study of the cerebral blood flow.
- The scan is repeated 1 hour later to detect the presence of pathogenic tissue.
- Gloves are worn during the radionuclide injection.

Post-Test Nursing Care

- Check the injection site for redness or swelling.
- If a woman who is lactating *must* have a nuclear scan, she should not breast feed the infant until the radionuclide has been eliminated, possibly for 3 days.
- Although the amount of diagnostic radionuclide excreted in the urine is low, the urine should not be used for any laboratory tests for the time period indicated by the nuclear medicine department. Clients should be told to flush the toilet three times after voiding.
- Gloves are worn when dealing with the urine.
- No other radionuclide tests should be scheduled for 24 to 48 hours.
- Encourage fluid intake by the patient to enhance excretion of the radionuclide.
- Report abnormal findings to the primary care provider.

• • • • • • • • • • • • • • • • •

Breast Biopsy

Several diagnostic tests, including mammography and ultrasonography, are used in the diagnosis of breast masses. However, determination of whether a mass is malignant can be made only by obtaining a biopsy of the tissue. The tissue sample may be obtained by needle aspiration or by open incision. The needle aspiration, which can be either a needle biopsy or a fine-needle biopsy, is somewhat limited because of the small sample of tissue that is obtained. The open biopsy is the preferred method, because the entire lesion is able to be excised and thoroughly tested.

B

Breast biopsy is indicated when a breast lesion is found by palpation, mammography, or ultrasonography. It should also be used when there has been an observable change in the breast, such as skin ulceration or nipple drainage.

Normal Values

No abnormal cells or tissue present

Possible Meanings of Abnormal Values

Adenofibroma
Breast cancer
Fibrocystic disease
Intraductal papilloma
Mammary fat necrosis
Plasma cell mastitis

 CONTRAINDICATIONS

- Patients unable to cooperate with the examination

Pre-Test Nursing Care

- Explain to the patient the purpose of the test and the procedure to be done.
- The biopsy is usually obtained using a local anesthetic, although general anesthesia is an option.
- No fasting is required before the test.
- Obtain a signed informed consent.

Procedure

- The patient is assisted to a supine position.
- The skin is cleansed with an antiseptic and draped.
- A local anesthetic is administered.

Needle Biopsy

- A needle is inserted into the mass, and a sample of tissue or fluid is aspirated into the syringe.
- The tissue specimen is placed in a specimen container with normal saline solution or formaldehyde.
- The fluid sample is expelled into a collection tube containing heparin.
- If fine-needle aspiration is used, a slide is made for cytology and viewed immediately.
- A sterile dressing is applied.
- Gloves are worn throughout the procedure.

Open Biopsy

- An incision is made in the breast to expose the mass.
- The mass is then excised in entirety if it is smaller than 2 cm. If the mass is larger or appears malignant, a portion of the mass is excised.
- The tissue specimen is placed in a specimen container with normal saline solution or formaldehyde.
- If the mass appears malignant, the tissue sample is sent for frozen section and receptor assays. Do *not* place tissue for receptor assay testing in formaldehyde.
- The wound is sutured, and a sterile dressing is applied.

Post-Test Nursing Care

- For biopsy under local anesthesia, check vital signs after the procedure. If general anesthesia was used, check vital signs every 15 minutes for the first hour, every 30 minutes for the next hour after that, every hour for 4 additional hours, and then every 4 hours.
- Check the dressing for drainage.
- Teach the patient to monitor the site and to notify the health care provider if signs or symptoms of infection occur, such as drainage, redness, warmth, edema, pain at the site, or fever.
- Administer analgesics as needed.
- Provide emotional support as the patient awaits test results.
- Report abnormal findings to the primary care provider.

•   •   •   •   •   •   •   •   •   •   •   •   •   •   •   •   •   •

Breast Sonogram
(Ultrasonography of the Breast)

Ultrasonography is a noninvasive method of diagnostic testing in which ultrasound waves are sent into the body with a small transducer pressed against the skin. The transducer not only sends the sound waves into the body but also receives any returning sound waves, which are deflected back as they bounce off various structures. The transducer converts the returning sound waves into electric signals that are then transformed with a computer into a visual display on a monitor.

In this particular type of ultrasonography, the transducer is passed over all the skin of each breast. The purpose is to detect and measure breast cysts and tumors. It is especially useful as a screening method in low-risk persons, for screenings when mammography is not available, for use in pregnant women and in others who must avoid radiation, and in women who have breast implants. In women with fibrocystic breast disease, the water path method of ultrasonography may be used.

Normal Values

Normal breast tissue

Possible Meanings of Abnormal Values

Breast cyst
Breast tumor

Contributing Factors to Abnormal Values

- The transducer must be in good contact with the skin as it is being moved. A lubricant, such as mineral oil, glycerin, or a water-based jelly, is used to ensure good contact with the skin.

Pre-Test Nursing Care

- Explain to the patient the purpose of the test. Provide any written teaching materials available on the subject. Note that there is no discomfort involved with this test.
- No fasting is required before the test.

B

Procedure

- The patient is assisted to a supine position on the ultrasonography table and then rolled 35 degrees to the side of the breast to be examined.
- A coupling agent, such as a water-based gel, is applied to the area to be evaluated.
- A transducer is placed on the skin and moved as needed to provide good visualization of the breast tissue.
- The sound waves are transformed into a visual display on the monitor. Printed copies of this display are made.
- For the water path method, the patient is positioned prone on a special bed with the breast suspended into heated water. The scanning is performed through the water by a transducer located at the bottom of the water tank.

Post-Test Nursing Care

- Cleanse the patient's skin of remaining coupling agent, if used.
- Report abnormal findings to the primary care provider.

• • • • • • • • • • • • • • • • •

Bronchoscopy

Bronchoscopy is the direct visualization of the larynx, trachea, and bronchi through use of either a rigid bronchoscope or a flexible fiberoptic bronchoscope. This procedure is used diagnostically to visually examine abnormalities found on radiography and to obtain sputum specimens for bacteriologic and cytologic examination. Therapeutically, the procedure can be used to control tracheobronchial bleeding, to remove foreign bodies, to conduct endobronchial radiation therapy, and to obliterate neoplastic obstruction through use of a laser.

Normal Values

Normal larynx, trachea, bronchi, and alveoli

Possible Meanings of Abnormal Values

Abscesses
Carcinoma
Foreign body
Hemorrhage
Infection
Inflammation
Strictures
Tuberculosis

CONTRAINDICATIONS

- Patients with severe respiratory failure
- Patients who cannot tolerate interruption of high-flow oxygen

Pre-Test Nursing Care

- Explain to the patient the purpose of the test. Provide any written teaching materials available on the subject. Note that a local anesthetic will be used in the throat. Reassure the patient that breathing will not be obstructed during the procedure.
- Obtain a signed informed consent.
- Fasting for 8 to 12 hours is required before the test.
- Administer pre-procedure medications as ordered. An anticholinergic such as atropine may be used to decrease bronchial secretions. A medication such as meperidine, diazepam, or midazolam hydrochloride may be used for sedation and relief of anxiety.
- Dentures are removed.
- Resuscitation and suctioning equipment should be readily available.

Procedure

- The patient is assisted to either a sitting or supine position.
- A local anesthetic is sprayed into the patient's throat.
- The bronchoscope is then introduced through the patient's mouth or nose. When it is located just above the vocal cords, more local anesthetic is sprayed into the trachea to anesthetize deeper areas and to inhibit the cough reflex.
- The anatomy of the trachea and bronchi is inspected. Biopsy forceps may be used to remove a tissue specimen, or a bronchial brush may be used to obtain cells from the surface of a lesion.
- Removal of foreign bodies or mucus plugs is accomplished, if needed.
- Gloves are worn throughout the procedure.

Post-Test Nursing Care

Possible complications:

Aspiration	Hemorrhage from biopsy site
Bacteremia	Hypoxemia
Bronchial perforation	Laryngospasm
Bronchospasm	Pneumonia
Cardiac stress	Pneumothorax
Fever	

- Monitor vital signs until stable.
- Withhold fluids and food until the gag reflex returns (approximately 2 hours).
- Provide an emesis basis for the patient. Instruct the patient to spit out saliva rather than swallow it until the gag reflex returns. Observe the sputum for frank bleeding.
- Observe for and immediately report indications of respiratory dysfunction: laryngeal stridor, dyspnea, cyanosis, diminished breath sounds, wheezing. Assess for presence of subcutaneous crepitus around the face and neck, which would indicate tracheal or bronchial perforation.
- Inform that patient that normal temporary consequences of the procedure include hoarseness, loss of voice, and sore throat.
- Label the specimen and transport it to the laboratory immediately.
- Report abnormal findings to the primary care provider.

CA 15–3
(CA 15–3 Tumor Marker, Cancer Antigen 15–3)

C

A tumor marker is a substance produced by body cells in response to the presence of cancer. Cancer antigen 15–3 (CA 15–3) is a glycoprotein that has been found in benign and malignant disease of the breast, as well as breast carcinoma that has metastasized to the liver. However, CA 15–3 values are highest in metastatic breast disease. Testing for CA 15–3 is useful in the diagnosis of metastatic breast cancer and for the monitoring of patient response to breast cancer treatment. Because CA 15–3 values may not increase in early malignancy of the breast, it is not useful as a screening test. Elevated CA 15–3 levels have also been found in patients without cancer and in patients with other cancers such as liver, lung, and ovarian cancer.

Normal Values

< 22 U/mL (< 22 kU/L SI units)

Possible Meanings of Abnormal Values

Increased

Chronic hepatitis
Cirrhosis
Liver cancer
Lung cancer
Metastatic breast cancer
Ovarian cancer
Sarcoidosis
Systemic lupus erythematosus
Tuberculosis

Pre-Test Nursing Care

- Explain to the patient the purpose of the test and the need for a blood sample to be drawn.
- No fasting is required before the test.

Procedure

- A 5-mL blood sample is drawn in a collection tube containing a silicone gel.
- Gloves are worn throughout the procedure.

Post-Test Nursing Care

- Apply pressure at venipuncture site. Apply dressing, periodically assessing for continued bleeding.
- Label the specimen and transport it to the laboratory.
- Report abnormal findings to the primary care provider.

• • • • • • • • • • • • • • • •

CA 19–9
(CA 19–9 Tumor Marker, Cancer Antigen 19–9)

A tumor marker is a substance produced by body cells in response to the presence of cancer. Cancer antigen 19–9 (CA 19–9) is an antigen that has been found elevated in the blood of patients with tumors of the gastrointestinal tract. Monitoring the CA 19–9 levels can also be useful in assessing the effectiveness of treatment for such tumors. This test is especially useful in the diagnosis of pancreatic cancer. Caution must be used, however, in interpreting positive test results, because false-positive results have occurred when no gastrointestinal disease was present or when the problem was inflammatory, rather than neoplastic.

Normal Values

< 37 U/mL (< 37 kU/L SI units)

Possible Meanings of Abnormal Values

Increased

Cholecystitis
Cholelithiasis
Cirrhosis
Colorectal cancer
Cystic fibrosis
Gastric cancer
Hepatobiliary cancer
Intra-abdominal carcinoma
Liver disease
Lung cancer
Pancreatic carcinoma
Pancreatitis

Pre-Test Nursing Care

- Explain to the patient the purpose of the test and the need for a blood sample to be drawn.
- No fasting is required before the test.

Procedure

- A 5-mL blood sample is drawn in a collection tube containing a silicone gel.
- Gloves are worn throughout the procedure.

Post-Test Nursing Care

- Apply pressure at venipuncture site. Apply dressing, periodically assessing for continued bleeding.
- Label the specimen and transport it to the laboratory.
- Report abnormal findings to the primary care provider.

• • • • • • • • • • • • • • • •

CA–125
(CA–125 Tumor Marker, Cancer Antigen 125)

C

A tumor marker is a substance produced by body cells in response to the presence of cancer. Cancer antigen 125 (CA–125) is a glycoprotein normally present in endometrial tissue and in uterine fluid. It is *not* normally found in the bloodstream. It is only when there has been destruction of such tissue, as through endometrial or ovarian cancer, that CA–125 is detectible in the blood. There is a high incidence of false results with this test, making it inappropriate for use as a screening tool. However, sequential tests for this tumor marker can be useful in disclosing a change from normal to abnormal results or increasing values.

Normal Values
< 35 U/mL (< 35 kU/L SI units)

Possible Meanings of Abnormal Values

Increased

Acute pancreatitis
Breast cancer
Cirrhosis
Colon neoplasm
Endometrial malignancy
Endometriosis
Fallopian tube cancer
Liver cancer
Lung cancer
Menses
Ovarian cancer
Pancreatic cancer
Pancreatitis
Pelvic inflammatory disease
Peritonitis
Pregnancy
Uterine cancer

Pre-Test Nursing Care
- Explain to the patient the purpose of the test and the need for a blood sample to be drawn.
- No fasting is required before the test.

Procedure
- A 5-mL blood sample is drawn in a collection tube containing a silicone gel.
- Gloves are worn throughout the procedure.

Post-Test Nursing Care

- Apply pressure at venipuncture site. Apply dressing, periodically assessing for continued bleeding.
- Label the specimen and transport it to the laboratory.
- Report abnormal findings to the primary care provider.

• • • • • • • • • • • • • • • • • •

Calcitonin
(Thyrocalcitonin)

Calcitonin (thyrocalcitonin) is a polypeptide thyroid hormone that helps in the regulation of serum calcium and phosphorus levels. When an elevated level of calcium is present in the blood (hypercalcemia), calcitonin is secreted. This results in inhibition of calcium absorption from the gastrointestinal tract, inhibition of calcium resorption from the bone by osteoclasts and osteocytes, and increased excretion of calcium by the kidneys. These actions are antagonistic to parathyroid hormone and result in lowered serum calcium levels. The test is used to evaluate suspected medullary carcinoma of the thyroid, which is characterized by hypersecretion of calcitonin in the presence of normal serum calcium levels. In some patients who have medullary cancer of the thyroid, the fasting level of calcitonin is normal. If this occurs, a provocative test involving intravenous pentagastrin or calcium administration is used.

Normal Values

Basal:
    Female: < 14 pg/mL (14 ng/L SI units)
    Male: < 19 pg/mL (19 ng/L SI units)
Post–calcium infusion (administered at 2.4 mg/kg):
    Female: < 130 pg/mL (< 130 ng/L SI units)
    Male: < 190 pg/mL (< 190 ng/L SI units)
Post–pentagastrin injection (administered at 0.5 µg/kg):
    Female: < 35 pg/mL (< 35 ng/L SI units)
    Male: < 110 pg/mL (< 110 ng/L SI units)

Possible Meanings of Abnormal Values

Increased

Breast cancer
Chronic renal failure
Cushing's disease
Ectopic calcitonin production
Hypercalcemia
Islet cell tumors
Medullary cancer of the thyroid
Oat cell carcinoma of the lung

Increased

Parathyroid adenoma
Parathyroid hyperplasia
Pernicious anemia
Pheochromocytoma
Thyroiditis
Uremia
Zollinger-Ellison syndrome

Contributing Factors to Abnormal Values

- Hemolysis of the blood sample may alter test results.
- Drugs that may *increase* calcitonin levels: calcium, epinephrine, glucagon, oral contraceptives, pentagastrin.

Pre-Test Nursing Care

- Explain to the patient the purpose of the test and the need for a blood sample to be drawn.
- Fasting for 8 hours is required before the test. Water is permitted.

Procedure

- A 7-mL blood sample is drawn in a collection tube containing heparin.
- If calcium infusion is ordered, blood samples are drawn before and 3 to 4 hours after the infusion.
- If pentagastrin injection is ordered, blood samples are drawn before and 90 seconds and 5 minutes after the drug is administered.
- Gloves are worn throughout the procedure.

Post-Test Nursing Care

- Apply pressure at venipuncture site. Apply dressing, periodically assessing for continued bleeding.
- Label the specimen and transport it to the laboratory immediately.
- Report abnormal findings to the primary care provider.

• • • • • • • • • • • • • • • • •

Calcium, Blood

Calcium (Ca^{2+}) is present in the blood in two forms. Approximately 50% is present in a free state, and the other 50% is bound to plasma protein, primarily to albumin. The calcium that is circulating in the free state is biologically active. Its functions include important roles in muscle contraction, heart function, transmission of nerve impulses, and clotting of the blood.

The amount of calcium in the blood is minute compared with the 98% to 99% present in the teeth and bones. The storage of calcium in the bones provides an excellent reservoir that is readily available for release into the bloodstream to assist in maintaining a normal level of calcium in the blood.

Two hormones work together to control serum calcium levels. *Calcitonin,* which is secreted by the thyroid gland, causes calcium to be excreted by the kidneys, thus preventing a calcium excess in the blood. *Parathyroid hormone* (PTH) works directly on the bones to release calcium into the bloodstream when needed and also increases absorption of calcium by the intestines and kidneys. There is an inverse relationship between calcium and phosphorus; as serum calcium levels increase, serum phosphorus levels decrease.

This laboratory test measures the *total* calcium present in the blood. This provides information regarding parathyroid gland function and the metabolism of calcium. It is also used to evaluate malignancies, because cancer cells release calcium, often resulting in high calcium levels in the blood (*hypercalcemia*).

Because much of the circulating calcium is bound to albumin, calcium levels in the blood must be interpreted in relation to serum albumin levels. As serum albumin decreases 1 g, the total serum calcium decreases approximately 0.8 mg owing to the decrease in the bound calcium; the amount of free calcium would not change.

Patients with hypercalcemia may have deep bone pain, renal calculi, and muscle hypotonicity. Patients with *hypocalcemia,* or decreased serum calcium levels, may experience numbness and tingling in the hands, feet, and around the mouth; muscle twitching; cardiac arrhythmias; and possibly convulsions. These patients will also demonstrate Chvostek's sign and Trousseau's sign.

Normal Values

8.5–10.5 mg/dL (2.1–2.6 mmol/L SI units)
Elderly: decreased

Possible Meanings of Abnormal Values

Increased	Decreased
Acromegaly	Acute pancreatitis
Addison's disease	Chronic renal disease
Antacid abuse	Diarrhea
Dehydration	Early neonatal hypocalcemia
Hodgkin's disease	Hyperphosphatemia
Hyperparathyroidism	Hypoparathyroidism
Hyperthyroidism	Low albumin level
Prolonged immobilization	Malabsorption
Leukemia	Massive blood transfusions
Lung cancer	Metabolic alkalosis
Metastatic bone cancer	Osteomalacia
Multiple myeloma	Renal failure
Paget's disease	Rickets
Parathyroid tumor	Severe malnutrition
Renal cancer	Vitamin D deficiency
Respiratory acidosis	
Sarcoidosis	
Vitamin D intoxication	

C

Contributing Factors to Abnormal Values

- Use of a tourniquet during the acquisition of the blood sample causes venous stasis. This may alter test results.
- Drugs that may *increase* blood calcium levels: anabolic steroids, androgens, antacids, calcium carbonate, calcium gluconate, calcium salts, chlorothiazide sodium, chlorthalidone, ergocalciferol, estrogens, hydralazine hydrochloride, indomethacin, lithium carbonate, parathyroid hormone, progesterone, secretin, tamoxifen citrate, theophylline, thiazide diuretics, thyroid hormones, vitamin A, vitamin D.
- Drugs that may *decrease* blood calcium levels: acetazolamide, antacids, anticonvulsants, asparaginase, aspirin, barbiturates, calcitonin, cisplatin, corticosteroids, cholestyramine resin, furosemide, gastrin, gentamicin, glucagon, glucose, heparin, hydrocortisone, insulin, iron, laxatives, loop diuretics, magnesium salts, mercurial diuretics, mithramycin, methicillin sodium, phenobarbital, phenytoin, sulfonamides.

Pre-Test Nursing Care

- Explain to the patient the purpose of the test and the need for a blood sample to be drawn.
- No fasting is usually required before the test, although some laboratories do require a fast with water permitted.

Procedure

- A 7-mL blood sample is drawn in a collection tube containing a silicone gel. Use of a tourniquet is avoided, if possible.
- Gloves are worn throughout the procedure.

Post-Test Nursing Care

- Apply pressure at venipuncture site. Apply dressing, periodically assessing for continued bleeding.
- Label the specimen and transport it to the laboratory.
- Report abnormal findings to the primary care provider.
- Patients with low calcium levels should be informed of dietary sources of calcium: milk, cheese, turnip greens, collard greens, white beans, and lentils.

• • • • • • • • • • • • • • • •

Calcium, Urine

Calcium (Ca^{2+}) plays important roles in muscle contraction, heart function, transmission of nerve impulses, and clotting of the blood. Only 1% to 2% of the calcium is in the blood; the remaining 98% to 99% is stored in the teeth and bones, which can be released as needed to maintain normal serum calcium levels. Most of the calcium excreted from the body is lost in stool; 99% of the calcium filtered by the kidneys is reabsorbed. When increased levels of urinary calcium do exist, it is usually owing to elevated serum calcium levels.

Normal Values

0–300 mg/d (0–7.5 mmol/d SI units)

Possible Meanings of Abnormal Values

Increased	Decreased
Breast cancer	Hypoparathyroidism
Cushing's syndrome	Malabsorption
Fanconi's syndrome	Renal osteodystrophy
Hyperparathyroidism	Vitamin D deficiency
Lung cancer	
Metastatic cancer	
Milk-alkali syndrome	
Multiple myeloma	
Osteoporosis	
Renal tubular acidosis	
Sarcoidosis	
Vitamin D intoxication	
Wilson's disease	

Contributing Factors to Abnormal Values

- Urinary calcium levels are higher immediately after meals.
- False-negative results may occur with alkaline urine.
- Drugs that may *increase* urinary calcium levels: ammonium chloride, androgens, anabolic steroids, antacids, anticonvulsants, cholestyramine, furosemide, mercurial diuretics, parathyroid hormone, phosphates, vitamin D.
- Drugs that may *decrease* urinary calcium levels: corticosteroids, aspirin, indomethacin, oral contraceptives, thiazide diuretics.

Pre-Test Nursing Care

- Explain 24-hour urine collection procedure to the patient.
- Stress the importance of saving *all* urine in the 24-hour period. Instruct the patient to avoid contaminating the urine with toilet paper or feces.
- Inform the patient of the presence of a preservative in the collection bottle.

Procedure

- Obtain the proper container containing the appropriate preservative from the laboratory.
- Begin the testing period in the morning after the patient's first voiding, which is discarded.
- Timing of the 24-hour period begins at the time the first voiding is discarded.
- *All* urine for the next 24 hours is collected in the container, which is to be kept refrigerated or on ice.
- If any urine is accidentally discarded during the 24-hour period, the test must be discontinued and a new test begun.
- The ending time of the 24-hour collection period should be posted in the patient's room.
- Gloves are to be worn when dealing with the specimen collection.

C

Post-Test Nursing Care

- Label the container and transport it on ice to the laboratory as soon as possible after the end of the 24-hour collection period.
- Report abnormal findings to the primary care provider.

• • • • • • • • • • • • • • • •

Candida Antibody Test

Candidiasis, also known as moniliasis and thrush, is caused by the organism *Candida albicans*. It affects the mucous membranes, skin, and nails. The organism is a yeast-like fungus that is normally present in vaginal secretions. Under certain circumstances, rapid growth of the organism occurs. Such circumstances include long-term antibiotic therapy, corticosteroid therapy, pregnancy, use of oral contraceptives, diabetes, wearing nonventilated undergarments, and a compromised immune system. Oral candidiasis is often noted as the first sign of the acquired immunodeficiency syndrome (AIDS). The serologic test for the *Candida* antibody is used in conjunction with histologic study and culture to confirm the diagnosis.

Normal Values

Negative

Abnormal Values

Titer of > 1:8 indicates systemic infection
A fourfold increase in titers drawn 10 to 14 days apart indicate an acute infection.

Possible Meanings of Abnormal Values

Increased

Candida infection

Contributing Factors to Abnormal Values

- False-positive results occur in about 25% of the population.
- False-negative results may occur in immunocompromised patients owing to their inability to produce antibodies.
- Hemolysis due to excessive agitation of the blood sample or contamination of the sample may alter test results.

Pre-Test Nursing Care

- Explain to the patient the purpose of the test and the need for the drawing of a blood sample.
- The patient is to be NPO for 12 hours before the test.

Procedure

- A 5-mL blood sample is drawn into a collection tube containing no additives.
- Gloves are worn throughout the procedure.

Post-Test Nursing Care
- Apply pressure at venipuncture site. Apply dressing, periodically assessing for continued bleeding.
- Label the specimen and transport it to the laboratory as soon as possible.
- Inform the patient of the possible need for a second blood sample, should a comparison of titers be desired.
- Report abnormal findings to the primary care provider.

• • • • • • • • • • • • • • • •

Capillary Fragility Test
(Rumpel-Leede Positive-Pressure Test, Tourniquet Test)

Normally the walls of the capillaries are sufficiently strong to resist any increase in capillary pressure and thus remain intact. With certain conditions, such as defects in the capillary wall or thrombocytopenia, there is a decrease in the capillary resistance. When capillary pressure increases, the capillaries rupture; the bleeding results in the formation of *petechiae*, which are very small red spots on the skin.

The capillary fragility test is performed to determine the weakness of the capillary wall when outside pressure from a blood pressure cuff is applied. The degree of capillary fragility is measured by counting the number of petechiae present in a 5-cm area of the skin.

Normal Values

Negative: No petechiae present

Abnormal Values

Positive:
1+	1–10 petechiae/5 cm
2+	11–20 petechiae/5 cm
3+	21–50 petechiae/5 cm
4+	> 50 petechiae/5 cm

Possible Meanings of Abnormal Values

Increased

Acute leukemia
Aplastic anemia
Disseminated intravascular coagulation
Factor VII deficiency
Fibrinogen deficiency
Idiopathic thrombocytopenic purpura
Influenza
Liver disease
Measles
Menstruation

C

Increased

Polycythemia vera
Postmenopause
Prothrombin deficiency
Scarlet fever
Scurvy
Senile purpura
Thrombasthenia
Thrombocytopenia
Vascular purpura
Vitamin K deficiency
Von Willebrand's disease

Contributing Factors to Abnormal Values

- Failure to keep the blood pressure cuff inflated for 5 minutes will alter the test results.
- Conducting the test on the same arm a second time in less than 1 week from the time of the first test will affect test results.

 ## CONTRAINDICATIONS

- Patients with disseminated intravascular coagulation and other bleeding disorders
- Patient with platelet counts of < 50,000/mm^3
- Patients with significant petechiae present before the test
- Patients with edematous or very cold arms
- Patients receiving anticoagulant therapy
- Patients taking medications containing aspirin
- Patients in whom a tourniquet applied for blood tests causes petechiae

Pre-Test Nursing Care

- Explain to the patient the purpose of the test and how the test will be conducted.
- Do not apply the blood pressure cuff to an arm that has a cast, dressing, or arteriovenous fistula in place.
- Do not use the same arm on which the test has been done within the last week.

Procedure

- Delineate the 5-cm area of the arm to be used for counting any petechiae that might form.
- Observe the designated area for any petechiae present before the test.
- Apply a blood pressure cuff to the patient's upper arm.
- Inflate the cuff to 70 to 90 mm Hg or to a level equivalent to the midpoint between the patient's systolic and diastolic pressures. Do not inflate the cuff above 100 mm Hg.
- Keep the cuff inflated for 5 minutes; then deflate and remove the cuff.
- Count any new petechiae in the designated area that formed as a result of the cuff inflation.

Post-Test Nursing Care

- Observe the arm for any unusual bleeding or swelling.
- Report abnormal findings to the primary care provider.

Carboxyhemoglobin
(Carbon Monoxide [CO])

Carbon monoxide (CO) is a substance found in tobacco smoke, automobile exhaust, improperly functioning furnaces, and defective gas-burning appliances such as stoves. When the hemoglobin of the blood is exposed to carbon monoxide through inhalation, carboxyhemoglobin is formed. The affinity of hemoglobin for carbon monoxide is over 200 times greater than for oxygen. Thus, hemoglobin is prevented from combining with, and transporting, oxygen. This results in a lack of oxygen being released in the tissues of the body, a condition known as *hypoxia*.

Symptoms of carbon monoxide poisoning vary with the carboxyhemoglobin level. Levels of 20% to 30% cause dizziness, headache, and impaired judgment. Levels of 30% to 40% result in confusion, hyperpnea, hypotension, and tachycardia. When levels reach 50% to 60%, there is a loss of consciousness and convulsions, and, with values over 60%, respiratory arrest and death may occur.

Normal Values

Nonsmoker:	0.05%–2.5% of total hemoglobin
Smoker:	5%–10% of total hemoglobin
Newborn:	10%–12% of total hemoglobin

Possible Meanings of Abnormal Values

Increased

Carbon monoxide poisoning

Contributing Factors to Abnormal Values

- Contamination of the blood sample with room air will alter test results.

Pre-Test Nursing Care

- Explain to the patient the purpose of the test and the need for a blood sample to be drawn.
- No fasting is required before the test.

Procedure

- A 5 to 10 mL blood sample is drawn in a collection tube containing heparin.
- Gloves are worn throughout the procedure.

Post-Test Nursing Care

- Apply pressure at venipuncture site. Apply dressing, periodically assessing for continued bleeding.
- Label the specimen and transport it to the laboratory. The sample should be tested immediately or refrigerated.
- Report abnormal findings to the primary care provider.

• • • • • • • • • • • • • • • •

Carcinoembryonic Antigen
(CEA)

Carcinoembryonic antigen (CEA) is a glycoprotein that is normally produced by the fetus and secreted by gastrointestinal cells. In adults, it is normally found in trace amounts. However, CEA tends to increase in the case of malignancies. It is primarily nonspecific and thus is not used alone in cancer diagnosis. This test has been found effective in the early detection of colorectal cancer, with CEA levels rising several months before clinical symptoms appear. It can also be helpful in monitoring the response of the patient to cancer treatment.

Normal Values

Nonsmoker:	< 3 ng/mL (< 3 µg/L SI units)
Smoker:	< 5 ng/mL (< 5 µg/L SI units)

Possible Meanings of Abnormal Values

Increased

Acute pancreatitis
Acute renal failure
Bacterial pneumonia
Breast cancer
Colon cancer
Cirrhosis
Hypothyroidism
Inflammatory bowel disease
Inflammatory processes
Leukemia
Lung cancer
Neuroblastoma
Ovarian cancer
Peptic ulcer disease
Pulmonary emphysema
Radiation therapy
Smoking
Ulcerative colitis

Contributing Factors to Abnormal Values

- Smoking may *increase* CEA levels.
- Drugs that may *increase* CEA levels: antineoplastics, hepatotoxic drugs.

Pre-Test Nursing Care

- Explain to the patient the purpose of the test and the need for a blood sample to be drawn.
- No fasting is required before the test.

Procedure

- A 7-mL blood sample is drawn in a collection tube containing EDTA.
- Gloves are worn throughout the procedure.

Post-Test Nursing Care

- Apply pressure at venipuncture site. Apply dressing, periodically assessing for continued bleeding.
- Label the specimen and transport it to the laboratory.
- Report abnormal findings to the primary care provider.

• • • • • • • • • • • • • • • • • •

Cardiac Catheterization
(Angiocardiography, Coronary Angiography, Coronary Arteriography, Heart Catheterization)

Angiography is a general term used to indicate visualization of any blood vessels, whether they be arteries or veins. The more precise term for visualization of the arteries is *arteriography*. Arteriograms are extremely valuable for observing the blood flow to a part of the body and to detect lesions that may be amenable to surgical treatment.

The purposes of cardiac catheterization are to investigate congenital disorders of the heart and great vessels, to evaluate cardiac muscle function, and to assess valvular insufficiency. This procedure allows for determination of pressure readings within the heart chambers, for collection of blood samples, and for recording pictures of the cardiac structure and movement. The test involves the introduction of a radiopaque catheter into the femoral artery and injecting a contrast medium dye. Left-sided heart catheterization, in which the catheter is advanced retrograde through the aorta into the left ventricle, is used to evaluate patency of the coronary arteries, mitral and aortic valve function, and left ventricular function. Right-sided heart catheterization, used to evaluate tricuspid and pulmonary valve function and to measure pulmonary artery pressures, involves advancing the catheter through the vena cava, right atrium, and ventricle and into the pulmonary artery.

Normal Values

Normal heart size, structure, movement, and wall thickness
Normal blood flow and valve motion
Normal coronary vasculature

Possible Meanings of Abnormal Values

Aneurysm
Cardiomyopathy
Congenital anomalies
Coronary artery disease
Intracardiac tumors
Pulmonary emboli

Pulmonary hypertension
Septal defects
Valvular heart disease

Contributing Factors to Abnormal Values

- Any movement by the patient may alter quality of films taken.

CONTRAINDICATIONS

- Patients who are allergic to iodine, shellfish, or contrast medium dye
- Patients with bleeding disorders
- Pregnant women
  Caution: A woman in her childbearing years should undergo radiography only during her menses or 12 to 14 days after its onset to avoid any exposure to a fetus.
- Patients who are unable to cooperate owing to age, mental status, pain, or other factors
- Patients with renal failure or those susceptible to dye-induced renal failure (dehydrated patients)
- Patients who would refuse surgery if a surgically correctable problem was found during the procedure

Pre-Test Nursing Care

- Explain to the patient the purpose of the test. Provide any written teaching materials available on the subject. Note that discomfort involved with this test is primarily due to lying on a hard table for an extended period of time and the needle puncture. Explain that an intense hot flushing may be experienced for 15 to 30 seconds when the dye is injected.
- Check for allergies to iodine, shellfish, or contrast medium dye. Inform the radiologist of such possible allergy and obtain an order for an antihistamine and corticosteroid to be administered before the test.
- Baseline laboratory data (CBC, PT, PTT) are obtained.
- Note any medications, such as anticoagulants or aspirin, that may prolong bleeding.
- Patients receiving metformin (Glucophage) for non–insulin-dependent diabetes mellitus should discontinue the drug 2 days before elective surgery or angiographic examinations. This is due to the possible occurrence of lactic acidosis, a potentially fatal complication of biguanide therapy.
- Fasting for at least 8 hours is required before the test.
- Obtain a signed informed consent.
- Administer any pretest sedation after consent form is signed.
- Assess and document patient's peripheral pulses bilaterally before the test. Mark the location of the pulses with a marking pen.
- Perform and document a baseline neurologic assessment.

Procedure

- The patient is assisted to a supine position on the examination table.
- A maintenance intravenous line is initiated.
- Cardiac monitoring is initiated.
- Resuscitation and suctioning equipment should be readily available.
- The area of the puncture site is cleansed and then anesthetized.

C

- The needle puncture of the artery is made and a guide wire is placed through the needle. The catheter is then inserted over the wire and into the artery.
- The radiopaque catheter is advanced into the desired artery. Positioning is monitored with fluoroscopy.
- Once the catheter is in the correct position, contrast dye is injected through the catheter.
- Radiographic films are taken.
- After films of satisfactory quality are obtained, the catheter is removed and pressure held on the puncture site for at least 15 minutes.
- Gloves are worn throughout the procedure.

Post-Test Nursing Care

Possible complications:
 Allergic reaction to dye
 Arterial occlusion resulting in embolic stroke or myocardial infarction
 Bleeding at puncture site
 Cardiac arrhythmias
 Infection at the puncture site
 Perforation of the myocardium
 Pneumothorax
 Renal failure

- Most allergic reactions to radiopaque dye occur within 30 minutes of administration of the contrast medium. Observe the patient closely for respiratory distress, hypotension, edema, hives, rash, tachycardia, and/or laryngeal stridor. Emergency resuscitation equipment must be readily accessible.
- A pressure dressing is applied to the puncture site. Check the dressing for bleeding and the area around the puncture site for swelling at frequent intervals.
- The patient is to remain on bed rest for 8 to 12 hours with the affected extremity immobilized.
- Maintain pressure on the puncture site with a sandbag.
- Monitor vital signs and neurologic status every 15 minutes for 1 hour, then every 30 minutes for 2 hours, then every hour for 4 hours, and then every 4 hours.
- Monitor urinary output.
- Assess the color, movement, temperature, and sensation (CMTS) and the pulse(s) of the affected extremity with each vital sign check. Compare with the other extremity.
- Encourage fluid intake to promote dye excretion.
- Renal function should be assessed before metformin is restarted.
- Report abnormal findings to the primary care provider.

• • • • • • • • • • • • • • • • • •

C

Cardiac Enzymes

See:

Asparate Aminotransferase (AST) (Formerly SGOT: Serum Glutamic-Oxaloacetic Transaminase)

Creatine Kinase (CK) (Formerly CPK: Creatine Phosphokinase)

Lactic Dehydrogenase (LDH, LD)

• • • • • • • • • • • • • • •

Carotid Duplex Scanning
(Carotid Phonoangiography [CPA])

Ultrasonography is a noninvasive method of diagnostic testing in which ultrasound waves are sent into the body with a small transducer pressed against the skin. The transducer not only sends the sound waves into the body but also receives any returning sound waves, which are deflected back as they bounce off various structures. The transducer converts the returning sound waves into electric signals that are then transformed by a computer into audible sounds (Doppler method) which can be graphed. A visual image of the carotid artery can be seen on the monitor, as well as in a printed copy of the image.

In this particular type of ultrasonography, the blood flow through the carotid arteries is studied. This provides a noninvasive method of assessing bruits during systole and diastole. Sounds emitted during the examination change when turbulent blood flow caused by plaque, stenosis, or partial occlusion of the artery is encountered.

Normal Values

Normal carotid artery blood flow

Possible Meanings of Abnormal Values

Carotid artery occlusive disease

Contributing Factors to Abnormal Values

- The transducer must be in good contact with the skin as it is being moved. A lubricant, such as mineral oil, glycerin, or a water-based jelly, is used to ensure good contact with the skin.

Pre-Test Nursing Care

- Explain to the patient the purpose of the test. Provide any written teaching materials available on the subject. Note that there is no discomfort involved with this test.
- No fasting is required before the test.

Procedure

- The patient is assisted to a supine position on the ultrasonography table.
- A coupling agent, such as a water-based gel, is applied to the area to be evaluated.

- A transducer is placed on the skin and moved as needed to provide clearly emitted sounds.
- The sound waves are transformed into a visual display on the monitor. Printed copies of this display are made.

Post-Test Nursing Care
- Cleanse the patient's skin of remaining coupling agent.
- Report abnormal findings to the primary care provider.

• • • • • • • • • • • • • • • •

Cerebral Angiography
(Cerebral Arteriography)

Angiography is a general term used to indicate visualization of any blood vessels, whether they are arteries or veins. The more precise term for visualization of the arteries is *arteriography*. Arteriograms are extremely valuable for observing the blood flow to a part of the body and to detect lesions that may be amenable to surgical treatment.

The purposes of cerebral angiography are to detect cerebrovascular abnormalities such as aneurysm or arteriovenous malformation, to study vascular displacement due to such problems as tumor or hydrocephalus, and to evaluate the postoperative status of blood vessels. The test involves the introduction of a radiopaque catheter into either the femoral, carotid, or brachial artery and injecting a contrast medium dye. The most commonly used site is the femoral artery.

Normal Values
Normal cerebral vasculature

Possible Meanings of Abnormal Values
Arterial spasm
Arteriosclerosis
Arteriovenous malformations
Brain tumor
Cerebral aneurysm
Cerebral fistula
Cerebral occlusion
Cerebral thrombosis
Increased intracranial pressure

Contributing Factors to Abnormal Values
- Any movement by the patient may alter quality of films taken.

CONTRAINDICATIONS
- Patients who are allergic to iodine, shellfish, or contrast medium dye
- Patients with bleeding disorders

- Pregnant women
  Caution: A woman in her childbearing years should undergo radiography only during her menses or 12 to 14 days after its onset to avoid any exposure to a fetus.
- Patients who are unable to cooperate owing to age, mental status, pain, or other factors
- Patients with renal failure or those susceptible to dye-induced renal failure (dehydrated patients)

Pre-Test Nursing Care

- Explain to the patient the purpose of the test. Provide any written teaching materials available on the subject. Note that discomfort involved with this test is primarily due to lying on a hard table for an extended period of time and the needle puncture. Explain that an intense hot flushing may be experienced for 15 to 30 seconds when the dye is injected.
- Check for allergies to iodine, shellfish, or contrast medium dye. Inform the radiologist of such possible allergy and obtain order for an antihistamine and corticosteroid to be administered before the test.
- Baseline laboratory data (CBC, PT, PTT) are obtained.
- Note any medications, such as anticoagulants or aspirin, that may prolong bleeding.
- Patients receiving metformin (Glucophage) for non–insulin-dependent diabetes mellitus should discontinue the drug 2 days before elective surgery or angiographic examinations. This is due to the possible occurrence of lactic acidosis, a potentially fatal complication of biguanide therapy.
- Fasting for at least 8 hours is required before the test.
- Obtain a signed informed consent.
- Administer any pretest sedation after consent form is signed.
- Assess and document patient's peripheral pulses bilaterally before the test.
- Perform and document a baseline neurologic assessment.

Procedure

- The patient is assisted to a supine position on the examination table.
- A maintenance intravenous line is initiated.
- The area of the puncture site is cleansed and then anesthetized.
- The needle puncture of the artery is made and a guide wire is placed through the needle. The catheter is then inserted over the wire and into the artery.
- The radiopaque catheter is advanced into the desired artery. Positioning is monitored via fluoroscopy.
- Once the catheter is in the correct position, contrast dye is injected through the catheter.
- Radiographic films are taken.
- After films of satisfactory quality are obtained, the catheter is removed and pressure held on the puncture site for at least 15 minutes.
- Gloves are worn throughout the procedure.

Post-Test Nursing Care

Possible complications:

Allergic reaction to dye
Arterial occlusion due to disruption of arteriosclerotic plaque or dissection of arterial lining
Bleeding at puncture site

Infection at the puncture site
Renal failure

- Most allergic reactions to radiopaque dye occur within 30 minutes of administration of the contrast medium. Observe the patient closely for respiratory distress, hypotension, edema, hives, rash, tachycardia, and/or laryngeal stridor. Emergency resuscitation equipment must be readily accessible.
- A pressure dressing is applied to the puncture site. Check the dressing for bleeding and the area around the puncture site for swelling at frequent intervals.
- The patient is to remain on bed rest for 8 to 12 hours with the affected extremity immobilized.
- Maintain pressure on the puncture site with a sandbag.
- Monitor vital signs and neurologic status every 15 minutes for 1 hour, then every 30 minutes for 2 hours, then every hour for 4 hours, and then every 4 hours.
- Monitor urinary output.
- Assess the color, movement, temperature, and sensation (CMTS) and the pulse(s) of the affected extremity with each vital sign check. Compare with the other extremity.
- Encourage fluid intake to promote dye excretion.
- Renal function should be assessed before metformin is restarted.
- Report abnormal findings to the primary care provider.

• • • • • • • • • • • • • • • • •

Cerebrospinal Fluid (CSF) Analysis
(Cisternal Puncture, Lumbar Puncture, LP, Spinal Tap, Ventricular Puncture)

Cerebrospinal fluid (CSF) is a clear protein substance that circulates in the subarachnoid space. Its functions include protection of the brain and spinal cord from injury and the transportation of substances through the central nervous system (CNS). Samples of CSF are most commonly obtained by means of a lumbar puncture; however, they may also be obtained during myelography, cisternal puncture, or ventricular puncture. In a *lumbar puncture*, the spinal needle is inserted between two of the lumbar vertebrae. The *cisternal puncture* involves the insertion of the needle between the first cervical vertebra and the rim of the foramen magnum. The cisternal puncture is rarely used due to the needle's proximity to the brain stem. The *ventricular puncture*, also rarely used, involves drilling a hole in the skull and inserting a needle into a lateral ventricle. This procedure is used when the other methods might cause such complications as brain stem herniation. The analysis of the CSF provides information to assist in the diagnosis of a wide variety of CNS diseases, including infectious diseases.

Normal Values

Cell count:	0–5 mononuclear cells/μL (0–5×10^6 cells/L SI units)
Chloride:	120–130 mmol/L (120–130 mmol/L SI units)
Color:	clear, colorless
Glucose:	50–75 mg/dL (2.8–4.2 mmol/L SI units)
IgG:	8.0–8.6 mg/dL (0.08–0.086 g/L SI units)

Pressure: 70–180 mm Hg
Protein: 15–45 mg/dL (0.15–0.45 g/L SI units)

Possible Meanings of Abnormal Values

Cell Count

Increased	Decreased
Abscess	Hemorrhage
Acute infection	Traumatic tap
Demyelinating disease	
Meningitis	
Onset of chronic illness	
Tumor	

Chloride

	Decreased
	Meningitis
	Tuberculosis

Color

Bloody

Subarachnoid, intracerebral, or intraventricular hemorrhage
Spinal cord obstruction
Traumatic tap

Cloudy

Infection
Orange, yellow, or brown: Erythrocyte breakdown, elevated protein

Glucose

Increased	Decreased
Systemic hyperglycemia	Bacterial infection
	Fungal infection
	Meningitis
	Mumps
	Postsubarachnoid hemorrhage
	Systemic hypoglycemia

IgG

Increased

Demyelinating disease (e.g.,
    multiple sclerosis)
Guillain-Barré syndrome
Neurosyphilis

Pressure

Increased	Decreased
Hemorrhage	Spinal subarachnoid
Trauma	obstruction
Tumor	

Protein

Increased	Decreased
Blood in CSF	Rapid CSF production
Diabetes mellitus	
Hemorrhage	
Polyneuritis	
Syphilis	
Trauma	
Tumors	

Contributing Factors to Abnormal Values

- Coughing, crying, or straining during the procedure may increase the CSF pressure.

CONTRAINDICATIONS

- Patients with increased intracranial pressure (CSF removal can lead to brain stem herniation)
- Patients with infection at the puncture site

Pre-Test Nursing Care

- Explain to the patient the purpose of the test. Provide any written teaching materials available on the subject. Note that discomfort during the test is due to the injection of the local anesthetic and penetration of the dura mater with the needle.
- Obtain a signed informed consent.
- No fasting is required before the test.

Procedure

- The patient is assisted into a side-lying position with the knees drawn up to the abdomen and the chin on the chest. This flexion of the spine provides easy access to the lumbar subarachnoid space.
- Assist the patient in maintaining the proper position by placing one arm around the patient's knees and the other arm around his or her neck.
- The skin is cleansed and draped. A local anesthetic is administered to the area.
- Ask the patient to report any pain or tingling sensations throughout the procedure that may indicate irritation or puncture of a nerve root.
- The spinal needle is inserted in the midline, usually between the third and fourth lumbar vertebrae.
- The stylet is removed from the needle and a stopcock and manometer are attached to the needle to measure initial CSF pressure.
- A sample of the CSF is collected in a sterile container.
- A final pressure reading is taken, and the needle is removed.

- A sterile dressing is applied to the puncture site.
- Gloves are worn throughout the procedure.

Post-Test Nursing Care

Possible complications:

Bleeding into the spinal canal
Cerebellar tonsillar herniation
CSF leakage, causing severe headache
Meningitis
Retroperitoneal hemorrhage owing to puncture of the aorta or vena cava
Transient back or leg pain or paresthesia

- Instruct the patient to maintain bed rest for 8 hours with no more than a 30° elevation of the head of the bed. This will help to minimize the occurrence of headache.
- Encourage the patient to take in fluids.
- Observe the puncture site for swelling and drainage and assess the movement and sensation to the lower extremities frequently for the first 4 hours after the procedure.
- Report abnormal findings to the primary care provider.

• • • • • • • • • • • • • • • • •

Ceruloplasmin

Ceruloplasmin is an alpha$_2$-globulin protein that transports copper. It also regulates iron uptake by transferrin. Testing for ceruloplasmin gives direct information regarding the amount of copper in the blood serum. Ceruloplasmin levels increase during times of stress, infection, and pregnancy.

This test is used to aid in the diagnosis of *Wilson's disease,* a hereditary syndrome in which decreased levels of ceruloplasmin are manufactured by the liver. Without ceruloplasmin to transport the copper, Wilson's disease leads to an accumulation of copper in the tissue of the brain, eye, kidney, and liver. One of the hallmarks of this disease is the presence of Kayser-Fleischer rings around the iris of the eye, which are caused by copper deposits. Because of the types of tissue affected by Wilson's disease, this test is recommended for anyone younger than 30 with cirrhosis, hepatitis, or unexplained neurologic symptoms. Wilson's disease can be treated with penicillamine, an anticopper drug, that promotes the renal excretion of excess copper.

Normal Values

22.9–43.1 mg/dL (229–431 mg/L SI units)

Possible Meanings of Abnormal Values

Increased	Decreased
Cancer	Hypocupremia due to
Cirrhosis	hyperalimentation
Infection	Kwashiorkor
Inflammation	Liver disease

Increased	Decreased
Pregnancy	Malabsorption
Primary sclerosing cholangitis	Menkes' kinky hair syndrome
Rheumatoid arthritis	Nephrosis
Thyrotoxicosis	Nephrotic syndrome
	Normal infants
	Sprue
	Wilson's disease

Contributing Factors to Abnormal Values

- Hemolysis of the blood sample will alter test results.
- Drugs that may *increase* ceruloplasmin levels: estrogen, methadone, oral contraceptives, phenytoin.

Pre-Test Nursing Care

- Explain to the patient the purpose of the test and the need for a blood sample to be drawn.
- No fasting is required before the test.

Procedure

- A 7-mL blood sample is drawn in a collection tube containing no additives.
- Gloves are worn throughout the procedure.

Post-Test Nursing Care

- Apply pressure at venipuncture site. Apply dressing, periodically assessing for continued bleeding.
- Label the specimen and transport it to the laboratory.
- Report abnormal findings to the primary care provider.

• • • • • • • • • • • • • • • •

Chemistry Profile

See:
Alanine Aminotransferase (ALT)
Alkaline Phosphatase (ALP)
Asparate Aminotransferase (AST)
Bilirubin, Total
Calcium, Blood
Chloride, Blood
Cholesterol
Creatine Kinase (CK)
Creatinine, Blood
Gamma-glutamyl Transferase (GGT)
Glucose, Blood
Lactic Dehydrogenase (LDH)

C

Phosphorus
Potassium, Blood
Protein (Includes Total Protein and Albumin)
Sodium, Blood
Total Carbon Dioxide Content
Triglycerides
Urea Nitrogen, Blood
Uric Acid, Blood

• • • • • • • • • • • • • • • • •

Chest X-ray
(CXR, Chest Radiography)

Radiography is the use of radiation (roentgen rays, or "x-rays") to cause some substances to fluoresce and affect photographic plates. X-rays penetrate air easily; therefore, areas filled with air, such as the lungs, appear very dark on the film. Conversely, bones appear almost white on the film because the x-rays cannot penetrate them to reach the x-ray film. Organs and tissues such as the heart appear as shades of gray because they have more mass than air but not as much as bone.

Chest radiographs are used to identify abnormalities of the lungs and other structures in the thorax, including the heart, ribs, and diaphragm. Common pulmonary disorders detected are pneumonia, atelectasis, and pneumothorax. The chest x-ray may be performed in the radiology department or through use of a portable x-ray machine. When taken in the radiology department, the chest x-ray is a posteroanterior (PA) view, because the patient is positioned with the anterior part of the body next to the film. Portable x-rays are done with the film behind the person, resulting in an anteroposterior (AP) view. Other views such as lateral, oblique, supine, and lateral decubitus positions may also be obtained. Ideally, the part of the body that needs to be studied should be next to the film.

Normal Values

Normal lungs and other thoracic structures

Possible Meanings of Abnormal Values

Asthma
Atelectasis
Atherosclerosis
Bronchitis
Congestive heart failure
Cor pulmonale
Diaphragmatic hernia
Emphysema
Enlarged lymph nodes
Fractures of sternum or ribs
Kyphosis

Lung tumor
Mediastinal tumor
Pericardial effusion
Pericarditis
Phrenic nerve paresis
Pleural effusion
Pleurisy
Pneumonia
Pneumothorax
Pulmonary abscess
Pulmonary fibrosis
Pulmonary infiltrates
Scoliosis
Tuberculosis

Contributing Factors to Abnormal Values

- Portable chest x-rays are less reliable than those taken in the radiology department.
- Underexposure or overexposure of the film may alter film quality.
- When patients are unable to hold a deep breath due to pain or mental status, the quality of the film may be affected.

CONTRAINDICATIONS

- Pregnant women
  Caution: A woman in her childbearing years should undergo radiography only during her menses or 12 to 14 days after its onset to avoid any exposure to a fetus.

Pre-Test Nursing Care

- Explain to the patient the purpose of the test and the benefits and risks associated with the test. Provide any written teaching materials available on the subject. Note that no discomfort is associated with this procedure.
- No fasting is required before the test.
- Instruct the patient to remove all objects containing metal, such as jewelry or undergarments, because these will show on the film.

Procedure

- The patient's reproductive organs should be covered with a lead apron to prevent unnecessary exposure to radiation.
- Position the patient as ordered. If able, the patient stands during the procedure. The patient is instructed to take a deep breath and to hold it while the films are taken.

Post-Test Nursing Care

- No special physical post-test nursing care is needed.
- Report abnormal findings to the primary care provider.

• • • • • • • • • • • • • • • • •

Chlamydia

*C*hlamydia trachomatis is the most common cause of sexually transmitted disease in the United States. It is also responsible for trachoma, a serious eye infection. Mode of transmission for this bacteria includes direct contact through sexual activity or direct contact of the infant with the mother's cervix during birth. Although prevalent, the disease is often unrecognized. Many women with *Chlamydia* infections are asymptomatic. Thus, testing for the organism is very important. This is accomplished through either a culture of the cervix or eye or through detection of the antigen by enzyme-linked immunosorbent assay (ELISA) technique.

Normal Values

Culture: negative
Titer: < 1:16

Possible Meanings of Abnormal Values

Positive

Chlamydia infection

Contributing Factors to Abnormal Values

- Drugs that may cause *false-negative* results: antibiotics, immunosuppressive drugs.

Pre-Test Nursing Care

- Explain to the patient the purpose of the test and the need for a blood sample and/or culture to be collected.
- No fasting is required before the test.

Procedure

- *For titer:* A 7-mL blood sample is drawn in a collection tube containing a silicone gel.
- *For eye culture:*
  - Cleanse any mucus from the eye with a dry cotton swab.
  - Use a sterile swab to swab the inner canthus or lower conjunctive.
  - Place the swab in the medium required by the reference laboratory.
- *For cervical culture:*
  - The female patient is assisted into the lithotomy position, draped, and encouraged to relax through deep breathing techniques.
  - A vaginal speculum lubricated with warm water is inserted. (*Note:* The organism is sensitive to routinely used lubricants.)
  - Cervical mucus is removed using cotton balls held in ring forceps.
  - A dry, sterile cotton swab is then inserted into the endocervical canal and rotated from side to side.
  - Place the swab in the medium required by the reference laboratory.
  - Gloves are worn throughout any of the previous procedures.

Post-Test Nursing Care

- Apply pressure at venipuncture site. Apply dressing, periodically assessing for continued bleeding.
- Label any specimen and transport it to the laboratory as soon as possible.
- Report abnormal findings to the primary care provider.
- The sexual partners of patients with positive test results should be examined.

• • • • • • • • • • • • • • • • • •

Chloride, Blood

Chloride (Cl^-) is the major anion of the extracellular fluid. Chloride levels have an inverse relationship with those of bicarbonate; thus, they reflect acid–base status. Chloride has several functions, including maintaining electrical neutrality by counterbalancing cations such as sodium (NaCl, HCl), acting as one component of the buffering system, aiding in digestion, and helping to maintain osmotic pressure and water balance. Because chloride is most often seen in combination with sodium, shifts in sodium levels result in corresponding shifts in chloride levels.

Patients with elevated serum chloride levels (*hyperchloremia*) may experience weakness, deep rapid breathing, lethargy, and stupor, which may progress to coma. Patients with *hypochloremia*, or decreased serum chloride levels may exhibit hypertonicity of the muscles, tetany, and shallow breathing.

Normal Values

100–108 mEq/L (100–108 mmol/L SI units)

Possible Meanings of Abnormal Values

Increased (Hyperchloremia)	Decreased (Hypochloremia)
Acute renal failure	Acute infections
Alcoholism	Addison's disease
Anemia	Adrenal cortical
Cardiac decompensation	insufficiency
Cushing's syndrome	Burns
Dehydration	Chronic renal failure
Diabetes insipidus	Congestive heart failure
Eclampsia	Diabetic acidosis
Excessive saline infusion	Diarrhea
Hyperparathyroidism	Diaphoresis
Hyperventilation	Heat exhaustion
Metabolic acidosis	Hypokalemia
Multiple myeloma	Hyponatremia
Renal tubular acidosis	Metabolic alkalosis
Respiratory alkalosis	Nasogastric suctioning
Salicylate intoxication	Primary aldosteronism

Increased (Hyperchloremia)	Decreased (Hypochloremia)
	Pulmonary emphysema
	Pyloric obstruction
	Ulcerative colitis
	Vomiting

Contributing Factors to Abnormal Values

- Hemolysis of the blood sample may alter test results.
- Use of a tourniquet during acquisition of the blood sample may alter test results.
- Drugs that may *increase* serum chloride levels: acetazolamide, ammonium chloride, androgens, boracic acid, boric acid, chlorothiazide, cholestyramine, cyclosporine, estrogens, glucocorticoids, guanethidine sulfate, hydrochlorothiazide, imipenem-cilastatin sodium, methyldopa, nonsteroidal anti-inflammatory drugs, phenylbutazone, sodium bromide, sodium chloride, spironolactone
- Drugs that may *decrease* serum chloride levels: aldosterone, amiloride hydrochloride, bumetanide, corticosteroids, corticotropin, dextrose infusions, ethacrynic acid, furosemide, loop diuretics, mercurial diuretics, prednisolone, sodium bicarbonate, spironolactone, triamterene, thiazide diuretics.

Pre-Test Nursing Care

- Explain to the patient the purpose of the test and the need for a blood sample to be drawn.
- No fasting is required before the test.

Procedure

- A 7-mL blood sample is drawn in a collection tube containing a silicone gel, avoiding use of a tourniquet, if possible.
- Gloves are worn throughout the procedure.

Post-Test Nursing Care

- Apply pressure at venipuncture site. Apply dressing, periodically assessing for continued bleeding.
- Label the specimen and transport it to the laboratory.
- Report abnormal findings to the primary care provider.

• • • • • • • • • • • • • • • • •

Chloride, Urine

Chloride (Cl⁻) is the major anion of the extracellular fluid. Chloride levels have an inverse relationship with those of bicarbonate; thus, they reflect acid–base status. Chloride has several functions, including maintaining electrical neutrality by counterbalancing cations such as sodium (NaCl, HCl), acting as one component of the buffering system, aiding in digestion, and helping to maintain osmotic pressure and water balance. The amount of chloride excreted by the kidneys in a 24-hour period is an indication of the patient's electrolyte balance.

Normal Values

110–250 mEq/L (110–250 mmol/L SI units)

Possible Meanings of Abnormal Values

Increased	Decreased
Cushing's syndrome	Addison's disease
Dehydration	Congestive heart failure
Excessive salt intake	Diarrhea
Salicylate intoxication	Diaphoresis
Syndrome of inappropriate	Emphysema
ADH secretion (SIADH)	Low-sodium diet
Starvation	Malabsorption
	Nasogastric suctioning
	Pyloric obstruction
	Renal damage

Contributing Factors to Abnormal Findings

- Drugs that may *increase* urinary chloride levels: bromides, chlorothiazide diuretics, mercurial diuretics.

Pre-Test Nursing Care

- Explain 24-hour urine collection procedure to the patient.
- Stress the importance of saving *all* urine in the 24-hour period. Instruct the patient to avoid contaminating the urine with toilet paper or feces.

Procedure

- Obtain the proper container containing no preservative from the laboratory.
- Begin the testing period in the morning after the patient's first voiding, which is discarded.
- Timing of the 24-hour period begins at the time the first voiding is discarded.
- *All* urine for the next 24 hours is collected in the container, which is to be kept refrigerated or on ice.
- If any urine is accidentally discarded during the 24-hour period, the test must be discontinued and a new test begun.
- The ending time of the 24-hour collection period should be posted in the patient's room.
- Gloves are to be worn when dealing with the specimen collection.

Post-Test Nursing Care

- Label the container and transport it on ice to the laboratory as soon as possible after the end of the 24-hour collection period.
- Report abnormal findings to the primary care provider.

Cholecystography
(Gallbladder Radiography, Gallbladder [GB] Series, Oral Cholecystogram)

C

The oral cholecystogram is used when a patient is experiencing symptoms of biliary tract disease, such as upper right quadrant pain, fat intolerance, and jaundice, and is suspected of having gallbladder disease. This test is used to study the gallbladder after ingestion of a contrast medium, in this case, a radiopaque, iodinated dye. The dye is processed by the liver, excreted in the bile, and then accumulates in the gallbladder. The peak concentration of the dye in the gallbladder occurs 12 to 14 hours after ingestion, at which time films are taken. This test is often performed in conjunction with an ultrasound examination of the gallbladder.

Normal Values

Normal functioning of the gallbladder
No stones in gallbladder or ducts

Possible Meanings of Abnormal Values

Benign tumor
Cancer of the gallbladder
Cholecystitis
Cholesterol polyps
Cystic duct obstruction
Duct defects
Gallstones

Contributing Factors to Abnormal Values

- Underexposure or overexposure of the film may alter film quality.
- When patients are unable to hold still, owing to pain or mental status, the quality of the film may be affected.
- Retained barium from other examinations, vomiting, and diarrhea will affect test results.

CONTRAINDICATIONS

- Pregnant women
  Caution: A woman in her childbearing years should undergo radiography only during her menses or 12 to 14 days after its onset to avoid any exposure to a fetus.
- Patients with renal or hepatic failure
- Patients with hypersensitivity to iodine, seafood, or contrast media
- Patients with bilirubin of > 2 mg/dL (gallbladder will not be visualized by the dye)
- Patients who are unable to cooperate owing to age, mental status, pain, or other factors

Pre-Test Nursing Care

- *Note:* If a barium swallow or an upper gastrointestinal and small bowel series test is ordered, these should be completed *after* the cholecystography is performed. Otherwise the barium sulfate ingested during the other examinations may obscure the films made of the gallbladder.

- Explain to the patient the purpose of the test and the benefits and risks associated with the test. Provide any written teaching materials available on the subject. Note that no discomfort is associated with this procedure.
- The patient is given a low-fat or fat-free diet the evening before the test.
- Two hours after the meal and after assessing for allergy to the dye, the patient is given six tablets (3 g) of iopanoic acid. These should be taken at 5-minute intervals with at least 2 ounces of water each time.
- Fasting is required from the time of dye ingestion until the time of the test.
- Instruct the patient to remove all objects containing metal, such as jewelry or undergarments, because these will show on the film.

Procedure

- Films are taken of the right upper quadrant area with the patient in prone, left lateral decubitus, and erect positions.
- Occasionally, the patient is given a high-fat meal or a synthetic fat-containing agent such as Bilevac to stimulate and test for gallbladder contractility. Films are taken 1 to 2 hours after this fat stimulus.

Post-Test Nursing Care

Possible complication: Allergic reaction to dye

- Most allergic reactions to radiopaque dye occur within 30 minutes of administration of the contrast medium. Observe the patient closely for respiratory distress, hypotension, edema, hives, rash, tachycardia, and/or laryngeal stridor. Emergency resuscitation equipment must be readily accessible.
- Resume the patient's diet and medications as taken before the test. Encourage fluid intake to enhance excretion of the dye.
- Inform the patient that the dye is excreted in the urine and may cause mild dysuria.
- If the gallbladder does not visualize, the test may be repeated after ingestion of a double dose of the dye tablets.
- Report abnormal findings to the primary care provider.

• • • • • • • • • • • • • • • • •

Cholesterol

Cholesterol is synthesized in the liver from dietary fats. Its functions include being used in the production of bile salts and several of the steroid hormones and as a part of cell membranes. Cholesterol is transported in the blood by the low-density lipoproteins (LDLs, or "bad" cholesterol) and high-density lipoproteins (HDLs, or "good" cholesterol). A great deal of research has focused on the role of cholesterol in heart disease. High levels of cholesterol in the blood (*hypercholesterolemia*), especially in combination with low levels of HDL, have been found to increase the person's risk of atherosclerosis and heart disease. This test allows evaluation of this risk potential.

Normal Values

Desirable: < 200 mg/dL (< 5.18 mmol/L SI units)
Elderly: Increased

Abnormal Values

Borderline high: 200–239 mg/dL (5.18–6.19 mmol/L SI units)
High: > 239 mg/dL (> 6.20 mmol/L SI units)

Possible Meanings of Abnormal Values

Increased	Decreased
Atherosclerosis	Acquired immunodeficiency syndrome (AIDS)
Cardiovascular disease	Chronic anemia
Hypercholesterolemia	Hemolytic anemia
Hyperlipidemia	Hyperthyroidism
Hypertriglyceridemia	Hypolipoproteinemia
Hypothyroidism	Malabsorption
Liver disease/biliary obstruction	Malnutrition
Nephrotic syndrome	Pernicious anemia
Obesity	Sepsis
Pancreatic dysfunction	Severe infections
Preeclampsia	Severe liver damage
Pregnancy	Stress
Uncontrolled diabetes mellitus	
Xanthomatosis	

Contributing Factors to Abnormal Values

- Drugs that may *increase* cholesterol levels: anabolic steroids, androgens, bromides, chlorpromazine, chlorpropamide, corticosteroids, epinephrine, ergocalciferol, iodides, levodopa, oral contraceptives, phenytoin, sulfonamides, thiazides, trifluoperazine hydrochloride, trimethadione, vitamin A, vitamin C, vitamin D, vitamin E.
- Drugs that may *decrease* cholesterol levels: allopurinol, aminosalicylic acid, androgens, asparaginase, azathioprine, cholestyramine, chlorpropamide, chlortetracycline, clofibrate, clomiphene citrate, colchicine, colestipol hydrochloride, dextrothyroxine, erythromycin, estrogens, glucagon, haloperidol, heparin, isoniazid, kanamycin, levothyroxine sodium, MAO inhibitors, neomycin sulfate, niacin, phenformin, tetracyclines.

Pre-Test Nursing Care

- Explain to the patient the purpose of the test and the need for a blood sample to be drawn.
- Fasting for 12 hours is required before the test. Water is permitted.
- No alcohol is allowed for 24 hours before the test.

Procedure

- A 5-mL blood sample is drawn in a collection containing a silicone gel.
- Gloves are worn throughout the procedure.

Post-Test Nursing Care

- Apply pressure at venipuncture site. Apply dressing, periodically assessing for continued bleeding.
- Label the specimen and transport it to the laboratory.
- Report abnormal findings to the primary care provider.
- If the test result is > 200 mg/dL, patient education regarding needed dietary modifications and exercise should be conducted.

• • • • • • • • • • • • • • • •

Cholinesterase
(Acetylcholinesterase, Cholinesterase RBC, Pseudocholinesterase)

There are two enzymes that hydrolyze acetylcholine (ACh): acetylcholinesterase, or true cholinesterase, and pseudocholinesterase, or serum cholinesterase. *Acetylcholinesterase,* which is present in nerve tissue, the spleen, and the gray matter of the brain, helps with the transmission of impulses across nerve endings to muscle fibers. *Pseudocholinesterase,* produced mainly in the liver, appears in small amounts in the pancreas, intestine, heart, and white matter of the brain.

Two groups of anticholinesterase chemicals, organophosphates and muscle relaxants, either affect or are affected by these enzymes. Organophosphates, which inactivate acetylcholinesterase, are found in many insecticides and nerve gas. Muscle relaxants, such as succinylcholine, are normally destroyed by pseudocholinesterase. If, however, there is a lack of pseudocholinesterase, the patient may experience a prolonged period of apnea if given muscle relaxants during surgery. Thus, patients who are to receive such drugs during surgery should be pretested for cholinesterase.

Normal Values

7–19 U/mL (7–19 kU/L SI units)

Possible Meanings of Abnormal Values

Decreased

Acute infections
Anemia
Chronic malnutrition
Cirrhosis with jaundice
Dermatomyositis
Hepatitis
Inability to hydrolyze muscle relaxants in surgery
Infectious mononucleosis
Metastasis
Myocardial infarction

C

Decreased

Poisoning from organic phosphate insecticides
Tuberculosis
Uremia

Contributing Factors to Abnormal Values

- Hemolysis of the blood sample will alter test results.
- Drugs that may *decrease* cholinesterase levels: atropine, caffeine, chloroquine hydrochloride, codeine, cyclophosphamide, estrogens, folic acid, MAO inhibitors, morphine sulfate, neostigmine, oral contraceptives, phenothiazines, physostigmine, phospholine iodine, pyridostigmine bromide, quinidine, quinine sulfate, succinylcholine, theophylline, vitamin K.

Pre-Test Nursing Care

- Explain to the patient the purpose of the test and the need for a blood sample to be drawn.
- No fasting is required before the test.

Procedure

- A 5-mL blood sample is drawn in a collection tube containing a silicone gel.
- Gloves are worn throughout the procedure.

Post-Test Nursing Care

- Apply pressure at venipuncture site. Apply dressing, periodically assessing for continued bleeding.
- Label the specimen and transport it to the laboratory.
- Report abnormal findings to the primary care provider.

• • • • • • • • • • • • • • • •

Chorionic Villus Sampling
(CVS, Chorionic Villus Biopsy)

The chorionic villi are finger-like projections that surround the embryonic membrane. These projections establish a connection with the endometrium, leading to the development of the placenta. Chorionic villi sampling (CVS) is a test used for the detection of genetic and biochemical disorders. It is performed during the first trimester of pregnancy, usually between the 10th and 12th weeks of gestation. The test may be performed through transabdominal or transvaginal approaches, but the transvaginal one is most commonly used. Test results are available in 7 to 10 days.

Normal Values

Absence of genetic or biochemical disorders

Possible Meanings of Abnormal Values

Biochemical disorder
Genetic disorder

Pre-Test Nursing Care

- Explain to the patient the purpose of the test. Note that some mild discomfort may be felt during insertion of the cannula through the cervix.
- No fasting is required before the test.
- Obtain a signed written consent.

Procedure

- The patient is placed in the lithotomy position with her legs supported in the stirrups. Privacy is maintained with proper draping.
- The external genitalia are cleansed, and a vaginal speculum is inserted.
- The cervix is swabbed with an antiseptic solution.
- Under ultrasound guidance, the catheter is inserted through the cervix into the uterine cavity and rotated to the site of the developing placenta.
- Suction is applied to the catheter by a syringe to obtain a tissue sample from the villi.
- The sample is prepared per institutional policy.
- Gloves are worn throughout the procedure.

Post-Test Nursing Care

Possible complication:
> **Bleeding**
> **Infection**
> **Spontaneous abortion**

- Monitor the vital signs after the procedure and assess for vaginal bleeding.
- Inform the patient that mild cramping and vaginal discomfort may occur after the procedure. Instruct the patient to report immediately any excessive pain, cramping, or bleeding.
- Label the specimen and transport it to the laboratory immediately.
- Report abnormal findings to the primary care provider.
- An ultrasound examination of the fetus is usually performed 2 to 4 days after the chorionic villi sampling to assess continued fetal viability.

• • • • • • • • • • • • • • • •

Chromosome Analysis
(Chromosome Karyotype)

Chromosome analysis involves the study of an individual's chromosomal makeup, or karyotype. Both chromosomal number and structure are studied. The test is used to determine chromosomal abnormalities and to identify the child's sex in the case of ambiguous genitalia or before delivery. This test is considered part of the workup done for amenorrhea, infertility, and frequent miscarriages. It is also used in genetic counseling for individuals with a family history of genetic disease. Chromosome analysis usually involves a culture of leukocytes from peripheral blood. However, karyotyping may also be completed on other tissues, including amniotic fluid, bone marrow, buccal smear, placental tissue, skin, and tumor cells.

Normal Values

Female: 44 autosomes, plus 2 X chromosomes; karyotype: 46, XX
Male: 44 autosomes, plus 1X, 1Y chromosome karyotype: 46, XY

Possible Meanings of Abnormal Values

Ambiguous genitalia
Down syndrome
Hyperploidy (> 46 chromosomes)
Hypogonadism
Hypoploidy (< 46 chromosomes)
Kleinfelter's syndrome
Mental retardation
Physical retardation
Turner's syndrome

Contributing Factors to Abnormal Values

- Hemolysis of the blood sample will alter test results.

Pre-Test Nursing Care

- Explain to the patient the purpose of the test and the need for a blood sample to be drawn.
- No fasting is required before the test.

Procedure

- A 7-mL blood sample is drawn in a collection tube containing heparin.
- Gloves are worn throughout the procedure.

Post-Test Nursing Care

- Apply pressure at venipuncture site. Apply dressing, periodically assessing for continued bleeding.
- Label the specimen and transport it to the laboratory.
- Provide emotional support throughout the test and during the period of time spent waiting for results (time varies depending on type of tissue to be analyzed).
- Report abnormal findings to the primary care provider.
- Make appropriate referrals for genetic counseling, as needed.

• • • • • • • • • • • • • • • •

Clostridium difficile Toxin Assay
(C. Difficile, Clostridial Toxin Assay)

Clostridium difficile is a gram-positive bacterium that is normally present in the intestine. When patients are taking broad-spectrum antibiotics, especially ampicillin, cephalosporins, or clindamycin, the normal flora of the intestine are diminished. However, *C. difficile* is resistant to these antibiotics, so its presence actually increases under these circumstances. This particular bacterium releases two necrotizing toxins, one of which causes necrosis of the lining of the colon. This results in the development of *pseudomembranous colitis,* a potentially fatal condition, 4 to 10 days after the antibiotic therapy is initiated. Symptoms include complaints of abdominal cramping, fever, and copious amounts of watery diarrhea. Leukocytosis is also present. Through testing for this bacterial infection, treatment can be started, including discontinuance of the broad-spectrum antibiotics, administration of metronidazole or vancomycin, and intravenous infusion of fluids.

Normal Values

Negative

Possible Meanings of Abnormal Values

Increased

Antibiotic-related pseudomembranous enterocolitis

Contributing Factors to Abnormal Values

- Exposure of the specimen to carbon dioxide may deactivate the toxin.

Pre-Test Nursing Care

- Explain to the patient the purpose of the test and the need for a stool sample to be collected.
- Instruct the patient to avoid contaminating the stool with toilet paper or urine.
- No fasting is required before the test.

Procedure

- Obtain a fresh stool specimen of 25 g of solid or 25–50 mL of liquid stool in a sterile container.
- Gloves are to be worn when dealing with the specimen collection.

Post-Test Nursing Care

- Label the specimen and transport it to the laboratory as soon as possible after collection of the specimen.
- Report abnormal findings to the primary care provider.

• • • • • • • • • • • • • • • •

Clot Retraction Test

Platelets are very important components of hemostasis and blood clot formation. They make the clot form by shrinking, a process called *clot retraction.* If there is a problem with either the number of platelets present or in the ability of the platelets to function, or if there are fibrinolytic agents present in the blood, clot retraction does not take place, causing the clot to remain soft and semi-fluid. Testing for clot retraction is performed when thrombocytopenia is being considered as a cause of a bleeding disorder. Test results are an indication of platelet and fibrinogen quantity and functional ability.

Normal Values

50%–100% clot retraction within 2 hours (0.50–1.00/2 h SI units)
Complete clot retraction within 6 to 24 hours

Possible Meanings of Abnormal Values

Increased	Decreased
Hypofibrinogenemia	Acute leukemia
Severe anemia	Disseminated intravascular coagulation
	Glanzmann's thrombasthenia
	Multiple myeloma
	Thrombocytopenia
	von Willebrand's disease
	Waldenström's macroglobulinemia

Contributing Factors to Abnormal Values

- Hemolysis of the blood sample will alter test results.
- Drugs that may alter test results: aspirin, nonsteroidal anti-inflammatory drugs.

CONTRAINDICATIONS

- Patients with decreased platelet count ($< 50,000/mm^3$)
- Patients with hypofibrinogenemia
- Patients taking aspirin

Pre-Test Nursing Care

- Explain to the patient the purpose of the test and the need for a blood sample to be drawn.
- No fasting is required before the test.

Procedure

- A 5-mL blood sample is drawn in a collection tube containing no additives.
- Gloves are worn throughout the procedure.

Post-Test Nursing Care

Possible complication: Hematoma at site owing to prolonged bleeding time.

- Apply pressure 3 to 5 minutes at venipuncture site. Apply dressing, periodically assessing for continued bleeding.
- Teach the patient to monitor the site. If the site begins to bleed, the patient should apply direct pressure and, if unable to control the bleeding, return to the laboratory or notify the nurse.
- Report abnormal findings to the primary care provider.

• • • • • • • • • • • • • •

Coagulation Factor Assay
(Factor Assay, Clotting Factors)

The coagulation factor assay is conducted to determine whether a congenital or acquired deficiency of any blood clotting factor is present. This test is useful in diagnosing hemophilia and/or coagulation disorders. In the test, the patient's blood is mixed with either normal serum or a prepared serum with a known specific deficiency.

The coagulation factor assay is performed after the review of other test results that may indicate the factor that is possibly deficient. If the prothrombin time (PT) and activated partial thromboplastin time (APTT) are both abnormally prolonged, the deficiency is likely to involve factors II, V, or X. If the PT is abnormal, but the APTT is normal, factor VII may be deficient. And if the PT is normal, but the APTT is abnormal, the deficient factor(s) may be from among those in the intrinsic pathway (VIII, IX, XI, XII) (Table 6). (See Coagulation Studies for a description of the process of hemostasis.)

Normal Values

50%–150%

Possible Meanings of Abnormal Values

Factor I

Decreased

Congenital deficiency
Disseminated intravascular coagulation
Fibrinolysis
Liver disease

Factor II

Decreased

Congenital deficiency
Liver disease
Vitamin K deficiency

TABLE 6
Coagulation Factor Deficiencies

Prothrombin Time	Partial Thromboplastin Time	Factors Possibly Deficient
Prolonged	Prolonged	II, V, X
Prolonged	Normal	VII
Normal	Prolonged	VIII, IX, XI, XII

Factor V

Decreased

Congenital deficiency
Disseminated intravascular coagulation
Fibrinolysis
Liver disease

Factor VII

Decreased

Congenital deficiency
Hemorrhagic disease of the newborn
Kwashiorkor
Liver disease
Vitamin K deficiency

Factor VIII

Increased	Decreased
Coronary artery disease	Autoimmune disease
Cushing's syndrome	Congenital deficiency
Hyperthyroidism	Disseminated intravascular coagulation
Hypoglycemia	Fibrinolysis
Late pregnancy	Hemophilia A
Macroglobulinemia	Von Willebrand's disease
Myeloma	
Postoperative period	
Rebound activity after sudden cessation of warfarin	
Thromboembolic conditions	

Factor IX

Decreased

Cirrhosis
Congenital deficiency
Hemophilia B (Christmas disease)
Liver disease
Nephrotic syndrome
Normal newborn
Vitamin K deficiency

Factor X

Increased	Decreased
Pregnancy	Congenital deficiency
	Disseminated intravascular coagulation
	Liver disease
	Vitamin K deficiency

Factor XI

Decreased

Congenital deficiency
Congenital heart disease
Hemophilia C
Intestinal malabsorption of vitamin K
Liver disease
Normal newborn
Stress
Vitamin K deficiency

Factor XII

Increased	Decreased
Exercise	Congenital deficiency
	Nephrotic syndrome
	Normal newborn
	Pregnancy

Factor XIII

Decreased

Agammaglobulinemia
Hyperfibrinogenemia
Lead poisoning
Liver disease
Myeloma
Pernicious anemia
Postoperative period

Contributing Factors to Abnormal Values

- Hemolysis of the blood sample may alter test results.
- Drugs that may alter values on the coagulation factor assay: anticoagulants.

Pre-Test Nursing Care

- Explain to the patient the purpose of the test and the need for a blood sample to be drawn.
- No fasting is required before the test.
- If possible, the patient should receive no warfarin sodium for 2 weeks or heparin for 2 days before the test. Check with the physician regarding the appropriateness of withholding these medications from the patient.

Procedure

- A 7-mL blood sample is drawn in a collection tube containing sodium citrate and citric acid.
- Gloves are worn throughout the procedure.

C

Post-Test Nursing Care

Possible complication: Hematoma at site due to prolonged bleeding time

- Apply pressure 3 to 5 minutes at venipuncture site. Apply dressing, periodically assessing for continued bleeding.
- Teach the patient to monitor the site. If the site begins to bleed, the patient should apply direct pressure and, if unable to control the bleeding, return to the laboratory or notify the nurse.
- Resume any medications as taken before the test, if appropriate.
- Report abnormal findings to the primary care provider.

• • • • • • • • • • • • • • • •

Coagulation Studies

Coagulation Process

When there is tissue injury or injury to blood vessels, platelets aggregate at the area of the injury. These platelets release factors that begin the clotting process (hemostasis). The process of hemostasis is shown in Figure 4. The original type of injury dictates the pathway by which the process is initiated.

The *intrinsic pathway* is involved when there is damage to the blood or the blood is exposed to collagen in the walls of traumatized blood vessels. The intrinsic pathway requires the sequential activation of several *coagulation factors:* factor XII (Hageman factor), factor XI (plasma thromboplastin antecedent), factor IX (Christmas factor), and factor VIII (antihemophilic globulin).

The *extrinsic pathway* is launched when there is injury to tissue or to the vascular wall. In this pathway, clotting is triggered by the release of tissue thromboplastin (factor III) from the damaged vascular or tissue cells. When this substance encounters factor VII (stable factor), the extrinsic pathway is stimulated.

Both pathways ultimately lead to the activation of coagulation factor X (Stuart-Prower factor). This leads to the next step, in which prothrombin (factor II) is converted to thrombin (factor IIa [activated]). Thrombin then stimulates the formation of fibrin (factor Ia) from fibrinogen (factor I). This fibrin, with the addition of fibrin stabilizing factor (XIII), forms a stable fibrin clot at the site of injury. Once the fibrin clot is no longer needed, it is dissolved by fibrinolytic agents such as plasmin, resulting in fibrin degradation products.

Any excess amounts of clotting factors that remain after hemostasis are inactivated by fibrin inhibitors, such as antiplasmin, antithrombin III, and protein C. This prevents clotting from occurring indiscriminately.

Several laboratory tests are available for studying coagulation disorders. Platelet activity tests and the *clot retraction test* are used in studying the platelet factors that begin the clotting process. The *partial thromboplastin time (PTT)* is useful when evaluating the intrinsic and extrinsic pathways of the coagulation process, where the majority of clotting defects occurs. The step of the process during which prothrombin is converted to thrombin is evaluated through the *prothrombin time (Pro Time, PT)*. The next step, the conversion of fibrinogen to fibrin, as assessed with tests of *thrombin clotting time* and *fibrinogen*. Clot lysis is evaluated through tests of anti-thrombin III, D-dimer, euglobulin lysis time, fibrin degradation products, plasminogen, protein C, and protein S.

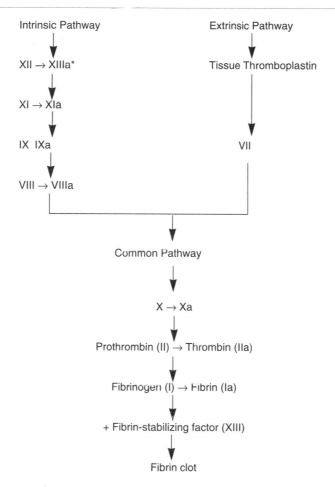

Figure 4 Process of Hemostasis.

For a discussion of each of these tests, please refer to the entry listed below:
Antithrombin III
Bleeding Time
Clot Retraction Test
Coagulation Factors
D-Dimer Test
Euglobulin Lysis Time
Fibrin Degradation Products
Fibrinogen
Partial Thromboplastin Time
Plasminogen
Protein C
Protein S
Prothrombin Time
Thrombin Clotting Time

• • • • • • • • • • • • • • •

Coccidioidomycosis

Coccidioidomycosis is a rare disease that carries a high mortality rate. It is caused by the organism *Coccidioides immitis*, which is endemic to Nevada, Utah, New Mexico, western Texas, Mexico, Central America, and South America. The person suffering from this disease usually presents with respiratory symptoms, fever, weight loss, and fatigue. Susceptibility to fungal infections is magnified by debilitating or chronic diseases, such as acquired immunodeficiency syndrome (AIDS) or diabetes, and by certain types of drug therapy that may alter the immune system, such as corticosteroids and antineoplastic agents.

Normal Values

Immunodiffusion: negative
Complement fixation titer: < 1:2

Abnormal Values

Titers of 1:2 to 1:4 indicate infection.
Titers > 1:16 indicate active disease.

Possible Meanings of Abnormal Values

Increased

Coccidioidomycosis

Contributing Factors to Abnormal Values

- Antibodies may be found normally in people who live where the fungus is considered endemic.
- Skin tests can cause a serologic test to become positive. Thus, skin tests should be withheld until after the blood sample is drawn.
- Many mycoses cause immunosuppression, leading to low titers, or false-negative test results.
- Contamination of the blood sample will alter test results.
- Hemolysis of the sample owing to excessive agitation may alter results.
- Antibodies may appear early in the disease and then disappear.

Pre-Test Nursing Care

- Obtain a travel and work history from the patient.
- Explain to the patient the purpose of the test, noting that it involves drawing a blood sample.
- The patient is to be NPO for 12 hours before the test.

Procedure

- The test should be conducted 2 to 4 weeks after exposure to the organism.
- A 7-mL blood sample is obtained in a collection tube containing no additives.
- Gloves are worn during the procedure.

Post-Test Nursing Care

- Apply pressure at venipuncture site. Apply dressing, periodically assessing for continued bleeding.
- Label the specimen and transport it immediately to the laboratory, taking care to avoid excessive agitation of the sample.
- Advise the patient that other procedures to test for this fungus may be done. Such testing might include sputum cultures, sputum smears, and skin testing.
- Report abnormal findings to the primary care provider.

• • • • • • • • • • • • • • • • • •

Cold Agglutinins

Cold agglutinins are antibodies that cause red blood cells to aggregate, or clump, at low temperatures. These antibodies, which are primarily of the IgM type, are most active at temperatures below 37°C, thus the term *cold* is used. This test is often used to diagnose primary atypical pneumonia caused by *Mycoplasma pneumoniae*. Cold agglutinins usually rise within 8 to 10 days after the onset of atypical pneumonia, peak in 12 to 25 days, and decrease 30 days after onset.

Normal Values

Negative or titers < 1:32

Possible Meanings of Abnormal Values

Increased

Hemolytic anemia
Hodgkin's disease
Infectious mononucleosis
Lymphoma
Malaria
Multiple myeloma
Mycoplasma pneumoniae infection
Primary atypical pneumonia
Scleroderma
Syphilitic cirrhosis
Viral pneumonia

Contributing Factors to Abnormal Values

- Hemolysis of the blood sample may alter test results.
- Antibiotics may interfere with the development of cold agglutinins.

C

Pre-Test Nursing Care

- Explain to the patient the purpose of the test and the need for a blood sample to be drawn. Inform the patient that additional blood samples may be needed in 12 to 25 days and again in 30 days.
- No fasting is required before the test.

Procedure

- A 7-mL blood sample is drawn in a collection tube containing no additives that has been prewarmed to 37°C.
- Gloves are worn throughout the procedure.

Post-Test Nursing Care

- Apply pressure at venipuncture site. Apply dressing, periodically assessing for continued bleeding.
- Label the specimen and transport to the laboratory immediately.
- Report abnormal findings to the primary care provider.

• • • • • • • • • • • • • • • •

Colonoscopy

Colonoscopy is the direct visualization of the large intestine through the use of a flexible fiberoptic endoscope. This endoscope is a multilumen instrument that allows viewing of the organ linings, insufflation of air, aspiration of fluid, removal of foreign objects, obtaining of tissue biopsy samples, and passage of a laser beam for obliteration of abnormal tissue or control of bleeding. This procedure is performed when the patient has experienced lower gastrointestinal bleeding or a change in bowel habits and when the patient is at high risk for colon cancer due to polyps, ulcerative colitis, or previous colon cancer.

Normal Values

Normal colon

Possible Meanings of Abnormal Values

Benign lesions
Colon cancer
Crohn's disease
Diverticulosis
Granulomatous colitis
Hemorrhoids
Polyps
Proctitis
Pseudomembranous colitis
Ulcerative colitis

Contributing Factors to Abnormal Values

- Retention of barium after previous tests, inadquate preparation of the colon resulting in retained feces, and active gastrointestinal bleeding hinders successful completion of this test.

CONTRAINDICATIONS

- Patients with acute diverticulitis, peritonitis, ischemic bowel disease, or fulminant ulcerative colitis
- Patients with suspected perforation of the colon
- Patients who are medically unstable
- Patients unable to cooperate with the examination

Pre-Test Nursing Care

- Explain to the patient the purpose of the test. Provide any written teaching materials available on the subject. Inform the patient that pressure in the colon may be experienced during movement of the endoscope and during insufflation with air or carbon dioxide.
- Obtain a signed informed consent.
- The colon is prepared for the examination as follows:
  - Clear liquid diet for 2 days before the test
  - Either a strong cathartic is given the evening before the test, followed by an enema the morning of the test,
    or the patient drinks a large volume of a solution such as Colyte the day before the test
- Monitor the patient for dehydration.
- Fasting for 8 to 12 hours is required before the test.
- Resuscitation and suctioning equipment should be readily available.
- Administer pre-procedure medications as ordered. An anticholinergic such as atropine and a medication such as meperidine, diazepam, or midazolam hydrochloride may be used for sedation and relief of anxiety.

Procedure

- The patient is assisted into the left lateral decubitus position on the endoscopy table.
- Baseline vital signs are obtained. Periodic vital sign assessment is performed during the procedure.
- A maintenance intravenous infusion is initiated.
- The endoscope is inserted through the anus and advanced through the rectum into the sigmoid colon and continuing to the cecum. The patient may need to be assisted to change positions to aid in advancement of the endoscope.
- During the procedure, insufflation of the bowel with air is used for better visualization.
- Encourage the patient to take slow, deep breaths to induce relaxation and to minimize the urge to defecate.
- Biopsy forceps may be used to remove a tissue specimen, or a cytology brush may be used to obtain cells from the surface of a lesion. Removal of foreign bodies or polyps is accomplished, if needed.
- Videotaping of the procedure is often done via a camera attached to the endoscope.
- Gloves are worn throughout the procedure.

Post-Test Nursing Care

Possible complications:
> **Bleeding**
> **Perforation of the bowel**
> **Oversedation**

- Monitor vital signs every 15 minutes until stable.
- Observe the patient for indications of bowel perforation: rectal bleeding, abdominal pain and distention, fever.
- Oversedation of the patient may require administration of a narcotic antagonist, such as naloxone.
- Once fully awake, fluids and food may be resumed.
- Inform the patient that passage of a large amount of flatus is normal after this procedure.
- Report abnormal findings to the primary care provider.

• • • • • • • • • • • • • • • •

Colposcopy
(Endometrial Biopsy)

Colposcopy is the direct visualization of the cervix and vagina with a colposcope, which is an instrument containing a magnifying lens and a light. When a patient has had abnormal cervical Papanicolaou smear results, this procedure is used to identify the area of cellular dysplasia. Any suspicious lesions that are found can then be accurately sampled.

Normal Values

Normal vagina and cervix

Possible Meanings of Abnormal Values

Atrophic changes
Cervical neoplasia
Condyloma
Erosion
Infection
Inflammation
Invasive carcinoma
Papilloma

Contributing Factors to Abnormal Values

- Scarring of the cervix and failure to thoroughly remove secretions from the cervix during the procedure may limit visualization of the cervix.

CONTRAINDICATIONS

- Patients with heavy menstrual flow
- Patients unable to cooperate with the examination

Pre-Test Nursing Care

- Explain to the patient the purpose of the test. Note that some discomfort will be felt during dilation of the cervix.
- No fasting is required before the test.
- Obtain a signed written consent.

Procedure

- The patient is placed in the lithotomy position with her legs supported in the stirrups. Privacy is maintained with proper draping.
- The external genitalia are cleansed and a vaginal speculum is inserted.
- If indicated, a Papanicolaou test is performed.
- The cervix is then swabbed with 3% acetic acid solution to remove secretions and medications.
- The colposcope is placed at the vaginal opening. It is not inserted into the vagina. The colposcope is focused on the cervix.
- The cervix is examined and a biopsy is taken of any suspicious lesions.
- The vagina is rinsed with sterile saline or water to remove the acetic acid, which can cause a burning sensation.
- Gloves are worn throughout the procedure.

Post-Test Nursing Care

Possible complication: Vaginal bleeding

- Cleanse the perineal area and assist the patient to a position of comfort. A tampon or a sanitary pad may be used in case of vaginal bleeding.
- Inform the patient that mild cramping, vaginal discomfort, and vaginal discharge may occur after the procedure. Note that the discharge may continue for several weeks.
- Instruct the patient to avoid strenuous exercise for 24 hours and that douching and intercourse should be avoided for 2 weeks.
- Instruct the patient to report immediately any abdominal pain, fever, or frank vaginal bleeding.
- Report abnormal findings to the primary care provider.

• • • • • • • • • • • • • • • •

Complement Assay
(C₃ and C₄ Complement)

The term *complement* refers to the 20 serum beta-globulin protein enzymes that are a part of the immune system response to antigen-antibody reactions. The complement system is necessary for phagocytosis, destruction of foreign bacteria, and mediation of the overall inflammatory response. Activation of the complement cascade may occur by way of the *classic pathway,* in which activation is stimulated by an antigen-antibody response, or by the *alternate pathway,* in which polysaccharides, endotoxins, or immunoglobulins are the stimulating forces. Regardless of the

C

stimulus, the final product of the complement cascade's work is a complex protein capable of destroying the cell membrane of the antigen.

To assess the functioning of the complement system, two of the components are typically measured. C_3 is involved in both the classic and alternate pathways and makes up about 70% of the total complement protein. C_4 is involved in only the classic pathway. Individuals found to be deficient in C_4 have a lowered resistance to infection.

Normal Values

C_3: 83–177 mg/dL (0.83–1.77 g/L SI units)
C_4: 15–45 mg/dL (0.15-0.45 g/L SI units)

Possible Meanings of Abnormal Values

C_3 Complement

Increased	Decreased
Infection	Anemia
Inflammatory	Acute glomerulonephritis
Malignancy with metastasis	Anorexia nervosa
Necrotizing disorders	Arthralgias
Rheumatic fever	Celiac disease
Rheumatoid arthritis	Chronic active hepatitis
	Chronic liver disease
	Cirrhosis
	Congenital C_3 deficiency
	Disseminated intravascular coagulation
	Immune complex disease
	Malnutrition
	Multiple myeloma
	Multiple sclerosis
	Renal transplant rejection
	Septicemia
	Serum sickness
	Subacute bacterial endocarditis
	Systemic lupus erythematosus
	Uremia

C_4 Complement

Increased	Decreased
Cancer	Chronic active hepatitis
Juvenile rheumatoid arthritis	Congenital C_4 deficiency
Rheumatoid spondylitis	Cryoglobulinemia
	Glomerulonephritis
	Hereditary angioedema
	Immune complex disease
	Lupus nephritis
	Renal transplant rejection

Increased	Decreased
	Serum sickness
	Subacute bacterial endocarditis
	Systemic lupus erythematosus

Contributing Factors to Abnormal Values
- Hemolysis of the sample may alter test results.

Pre-Test Nursing Care
- Explain to the patient the purpose of the test and the need for a blood sample to be drawn.
- No fasting is required before the test.

Procedure
- A 7-mL blood sample is drawn in a collection tube containing no additives.
- Gloves are worn throughout the procedure.

Post-Test Nursing Care
- Apply pressure at venipuncture site. Apply dressing, periodically assessing for continued bleeding.
- Label the specimen and transport it to the laboratory immediately.
- Report abnormal findings to the primary care provider.

• • • • • • • • • • • • • • • • •

Complete Blood Cell Count with Differential
(CBC with Diff)

The complete blood cell count with differential is one of the most commonly performed tests in health care. This is due to the vast amount of data obtained through the various components of this test.

If appropriate, the tests may be ordered individually. For example, a patient undergoing a total joint replacement has a complete blood cell count with differential drawn preoperatively. Postoperatively, the surgeon may choose to order a repeat testing of only the hematocrit to determine the extent of blood loss that may have occurred during surgery.

The test actually consists of several tests, which are discussed individually in this text.

See:
Blood Smear
Hematocrit
Hemoglobin
Platelet Count
Red Blood Cell Count
Red Blood Cell Indices (Includes Mean Corpuscular Volume [MCV], Mean Corpuscular Hemoglobin [MCH], and Mean Corpuscular Hemoglobin Concentration [MCHC])
White Blood Cell Count and Differential

• • • • • • • • • • • • • • • •

Computed Tomography of the Abdomen
(CT Scan of Abdomen, Computerized Axial Tomography [CAT] of the Abdomen)

Computed tomography (CT) is considered a radiographic procedure. X-rays are projected along the lines of the area of the body being assessed. An x-ray detector records the intensity of the x-rays as they are transmitted through the tissue. Different types of tissue cause differences in how the tissue decreases the x-ray beam as it passes through the tissue (tissue attenuation). This leads to an assignment of a density coefficient to the various tissues. The information is compiled and results in a visual display. The image may be enhanced by repeating the procedure after intravenous administration of iodine-based contrast dye.

CT of the abdomen is performed to diagnose pathologic conditions of the abdominal organs. Such conditions include inflammation, cysts, and tumors of the liver, gallbladder, pancreas, spleen, kidneys, and pelvic organs.

Normal Values

No abnormalities

Possible Meanings of Abnormal Values

Abdominal aortic aneurysm
Abscesses
Appendicitis
Bile duct dilation
Cysts
Diverticulitis
Gallstones
Hemorrhage
Infection
Laceration of spleen
Prostatic hypertrophy
Tumors

Contributing Factors to Abnormal Values

- Retained barium, gas, or stool in the intestines may result in poor quality films.
- Any movement by the patient may alter quality of films taken.

CONTRAINDICATIONS

- Patients who are allergic to iodine, shellfish, or contrast medium dye
- Pregnant women
  Caution: A woman in her childbearing years should undergo radiography only during her menses or 12 to 14 days after its onset to avoid any exposure to a fetus.
- Patients who are morbidly obese or claustrophobic
- Patients whose vital signs are unstable
- Patients who are unable to cooperate owing to age, mental status, pain, or other factors
- Patients with renal failure or those susceptible to dye-induced renal failure (dehydrated patients)

Pre-Test Nursing Care

- Explain to the patient the purpose of the test. Provide any written teaching materials available on the subject. Note that minimal discomfort during the test is owing to the venipuncture and that during injection of the dye transient sensations including warmth, flushing, a salty taste, and nausea may be experienced. Explain that no movement is allowed during the procedure.
- Check for allergies to iodine, shellfish, or contrast medium dye. Inform the radiologist of such possible allergy and obtain an order for an antihistamine and a corticosteroid to be administered before the test.
- Patients receiving metformin (Glucophage) for non–insulin-dependent diabetes mellitus should discontinue the drug 2 days before elective surgery or angiographic examinations. This is due to the possible occurrence of lactic acidosis, a potentially fatal complication of biguanide therapy.
- Fasting for at least 4 hours is required before the test if contrast dye is to be administered. The patient should be well hydrated before the beginning of the fasting period.
- Resuscitation and suctioning equipment should be readily available.
- Obtain a signed informed consent.

Procedure

- The patient is assisted to a supine position on the CT scan table.
- A maintenance intravenous line is initiated.
- The contrast dye is administered by intravenous injection.
- The patient is then placed in the body scanner.
- Films are made, during which the patient is asked to hold his or her breath.

Post-Test Nursing Care

Possible complications:
> **Allergic reaction to dye**
> **Acute renal failure from dye**

- Most allergic reactions to radiopaque dye occur within 30 minutes of administration of the contrast medium. Observe the patient closely for respiratory distress, hypotension, edema, hives, rash, tachycardia, and/or laryngeal stridor. Emergency resuscitation equipment must be readily accessible.
- Observe for allergic reaction to the dye for 24 hours.
- Discontinue the intravenous infusion. Apply pressure at venipuncture site. Apply dressing, periodically assessing for continued bleeding.
- Resume the patient's diet. Encourage fluid intake of at least three glasses of liquid to speed the excretion of the dye from the body.
- Monitor urinary output.
- Inform the patient that if oral contrast dye was ingested, diarrhea may occur.
- Renal function should be assessed before metformin is restarted.
- Report abnormal findings to the primary care provider.

• • • • • • • • • • • • • • • • • •

Computed Tomography of the Brain
(CT Scan of the Head, Computerized Axial Tomography [CAT] of the Head)

Computed tomography (CT) is considered a radiographic procedure. X-rays are projected along the lines of the area of the body being assessed. An x-ray detector records the intensity of the x-rays as they are transmitted through the tissue. Different types of tissue cause differences in how the tissue decreases the x-ray beam as it passes through the tissue (tissue attenuation). This leads to an assignment of a density coefficient to the various tissues. The information is compiled and results in a visual display. The image may be enhanced by repeating the procedure after intravenous administration of iodine-based contrast dye.

CT of the brain is performed to diagnose pathologic conditions such as neoplasms, cerebral infarctions, aneurysms, and intracranial hemorrhage.

Normal Values

No abnormalities

Possible Meanings of Abnormal Values

Abscess
Arteriovenous malformation
Cerebral aneurysms
Cerebral infarction
Hemorrhage/hematoma
Hydrocephalus
Meningiomas
Multiple sclerosis
Neoplasms
Ventricular displacement
Ventricular enlargement

Contributing Factors to Abnormal Values

- Any movement by the patient may alter quality of films taken.

CONTRAINDICATIONS

- Patients who are allergic to iodine, shellfish, or contrast medium dye
- Pregnant women
  Caution: A woman in her childbearing years should undergo radiography only during her menses or 12 to 14 days after its onset to avoid any exposure to a fetus.
- Patients who are morbidly obese or claustrophobic
- Patients whose vital signs are unstable
- Patients who are unable to cooperate owing to age, mental status, pain, or other factors
- Patients with renal failure or those susceptible to dye-induced renal failure (dehydrated patients)

Pre-Test Nursing Care

- Explain to the patient the purpose of the test. Provide any written teaching materials available on the subject. Note that minimal discomfort during the test is owing to the venipuncture and that during injection of the dye transient sensations including warmth, flushing, a salty taste, and nausea may be experienced. Explain that no movement is allowed during the procedure.
- Check for allergies to iodine, shellfish, or contrast medium dye. Inform the radiologist of such possible allergy and obtain an order for an antihistamine and a corticosteroid to be administered before the test.
- Patients receiving metformin (Glucophage) for non–insulin-dependent diabetes mellitus should discontinue the drug 2 days before elective surgery or angiographic examinations. This is due to the possible occurrence of lactic acidosis, a potentially fatal complication of biguanide therapy.
- Fasting for at least 4 hours is required before the test if contrast dye is to be administered. The patient should be well hydrated before the beginning of the fasting period.
- Resuscitation and suctioning equipment should be readily available.
- Obtain a signed informed consent.
- Instruct the patient to remove any metal items from the hair or mouth before the procedure.

Procedure

- The patient is assisted to a supine position on the CT scan table.
- The head is stabilized to prevent movement during the procedure.
- A maintenance intravenous line is initiated.
- The contrast dye is administered by intravenous injection.
- The patient is then placed in the body scanner.
- Films are made, during which the patient is asked to hold his or her breath.

Post-Test Nursing Care

Possible complications:
    Allergic reaction to dye
    Acute renal failure from dye

- Most allergic reactions to radiopaque dye occur within 30 minutes of administration of the contrast medium. Observe the patient closely for respiratory distress, hypotension, edema, hives, rash, tachycardia, and/or laryngeal stridor. Emergency resuscitation equipment must be readily accessible.
- Observe for allergic reaction to the dye for 24 hours.
- Discontinue the intravenous infusion. Apply pressure at venipuncture site. Apply dressing, periodically assessing for continued bleeding.
- Resume the patient's diet. Encourage fluid intake of at least three glasses of liquid to speed the excretion of the dye from the body.
- Monitor urinary output.
- Inform the patient that if oral contrast dye was ingested, diarrhea may occur.
- Renal function should be assessed before metformin is restarted.
- Report abnormal findings to the primary care provider.

• • • • • • • • • • • • • • • • •

Computed Tomography of the Chest
(CT Scan of the Chest, Computerized Axial Tomography [CAT] of the Chest)

Computed tomography (CT) is considered a radiographic procedure. X-rays are projected along the lines of the area of the body being assessed. An x-ray detector records the intensity of the x-rays as they are transmitted through the tissue. Different types of tissue cause differences in how the tissue decreases the x-ray beam as it passes through the tissue (tissue attenuation). This leads to an assignment of a density coefficient to the various tissues. The information is compiled and results in a visual display. The image may be enhanced by repeating the procedure after intravenous administration of iodine-based contrast dye.

CT of the chest is performed to diagnose pathologic conditions of the organs contained within the chest. Such conditions include inflammation, cysts, and tumors of the lungs, esophagus, and lymph nodes.

Normal Values
No abnormalities

Possible Meanings of Abnormal Values
Aortic aneurysm
Cyst
Enlarged lymph nodes
Esophageal tumors
Granuloma
Hiatal hernia
Inflammation
Mediastinal tumors
Metastatic tumors
Pleural effusion
Pneumonitis
Pulmonary tumor

Contributing Factors to Abnormal Values
- Any movement by the patient may alter quality of films taken.

CONTRAINDICATIONS

- Patients who are allergic to iodine, shellfish, or contrast medium dye
- Pregnant women
  Caution: A woman in her childbearing years should undergo radiography only during her menses or 12 to 14 days after its onset to avoid any exposure to a fetus.
- Patients who are morbidly obese or claustrophobic
- Patients whose vital signs are unstable
- Patients who are unable to cooperate owing to age, mental status, pain, or other factors
- Patients with renal failure or those susceptible to dye-induced renal failure (dehydrated patients)

Pre-Test Nursing Care

- Explain to the patient the purpose of the test. Provide any written teaching materials available on the subject. Note that minimal discomfort during the test is owing to the venipuncture and that during injection of the dye transient sensations including warmth, flushing, a salty taste, and nausea may be experienced. Explain that no movement is allowed during the procedure.
- Check for allergies to iodine, shellfish, or contrast medium dye. Inform the radiologist of such possible allergy and obtain an order for an antihistamine and a corticosteroid to be administered before the test.
- Patients receiving metformin (Glucophage) for non–insulin-dependent diabetes mellitus should discontinue the drug 2 days before elective surgery or angiographic examinations. This is due to the possible occurrence of lactic acidosis, a potentially fatal complication of biguanide therapy.
- Fasting for at least 4 hours is required before the test if contrast dye is to be administered. The patient should be well hydrated before the beginning of the fasting period.
- Resuscitation and suctioning equipment should be readily available.
- Obtain a signed informed consent.

Procedure

- The patient is assisted to a supine position on the CT scan table.
- A maintenance intravenous line is initiated.
- The contrast dye is administered by intravenous injection.
- The patient is then placed in the body scanner.
- Films are made, during which the patient is asked to hold his or her breath.

Post-Test Nursing Care

Possible complications:
   Allergic reaction to dye
   Acute renal failure from dye

- Most allergic reactions to radiopaque dye occur within 30 minutes of administration of the contrast medium. Observe the patient closely for respiratory distress, hypotension, edema, hives, rash, tachycardia, and/or laryngeal stridor. Emergency resuscitation equipment must be readily accessible.
- Observe for allergic reaction to the dye for 24 hours.
- Discontinue the intravenous infusion. Apply pressure at venipuncture site. Apply dressing, periodically assessing for continued bleeding.
- Resume the patient's diet. Encourage fluid intake of at least three glasses of liquid to speed the excretion of the dye from the body.
- Monitor urinary output.
- Inform the patient that if oral contrast dye was ingested, diarrhea may occur.
- Renal function should be assessed before metformin is restarted.
- Report abnormal findings to the primary care provider.

• • • • • • • • • • • • • • • • •

Contraction Stress Test
(CST, Contraction Challenge Test, Oxytocin Challenge Test, OCT)

C

The contraction stress test (CST) is used to evaluate the ability of the fetus to withstand the contractions of labor. It is usually administered to those patients whose nonstress test (NST) was nonreactive. The CST mimics labor, in that uterine contractions are stimulated either through nipple stimulation, which stimulates endogenous release of oxytocin , or through the administration of exogenous oxytocin. During normal labor, uterine contractions cause a decrease in the placental blood flow. It is important to know that the fetus will be able to withstand this decrease in placental blood flow, otherwise the fetus is at risk of intrauterine asphyxia.

A negative CST is considered the norm. In this case, the placental reserve is adequate, resulting in a normal fetal heart rate (FHR) during uterine contraction. When negative, the feto-placental units can be considered adequate for the next 7 days. The test can be repeated weekly until the onset of labor.

A CST is considered positive when the uterine contraction results in late deceleration of the FHR. This indicates intrauterine hypoxia due to inadequate placental reserve. There must be late deceleration with two or more uterine contractions for the test to be considered positive. Because of the possibility of false-positive results, a positive CST should be considered in conjunction with other test results, such as that of an amniocentesis, before the fetus is delivered before the anticipated due date.

The CST is used in high-risk pregnancies in which the fetus may be threatened. These include maternal diabetes mellitus or chronic hypertension, preeclampsia, intrauterine growth retardation, postmaturity syndrome, and Rh isoimmunization.

Normal Values

Negative (no late deceleration in the FHR after uterine contraction)

Possible Meanings of Abnormal Values

Inadequate placental reserve

Contributing Factors to Abnormal Values

- Maternal hypotension may cause a false-positive test result.

CONTRAINDICATIONS

- Patients with multiple pregnancy
- Patients with premature ruptured membranes
- Patients with placenta previa or abruptio placentae
- Patients with previous classic or low transverse cesarean sections
- Patients with pregnancies of less than 32 weeks' gestation
- Patients with a history of premature labor or incompetent cervix

Pre-Test Nursing Care

- Explain to the patient the purpose of the test and the procedure to be done. Note that discomfort associated with the test is due to mild labor contractions.

- Fasting for 4 to 8 hours is usually ordered in case premature labor occurs.
- Obtain a signed informed consent.

Procedure

- The patient is instructed to void.
- The patient is assisted into a semi-Fowler's, semi-side-lying position.
- An external fetal monitor is applied to the patient's abdomen, which will provide a graph of FHR and uterine contractions.
- Obtain baseline blood pressure. The blood pressure is monitored every 10 minutes during the procedure.
- Obtain a 20-minute baseline recording of the FHR. Assess for any uterine contractions.
  - If uterine contractions are present, withhold oxytocin and monitor fetal response to the spontaneous contractions.
  - If no uterine contractions are present, the nipples are stimulated for 15 minutes.
  - If no uterine contractions occur with nipple stimulation, oxytocin is administered intravenously by electronic infusion pump.
- The oxytocin is increased in rate until the patient is having 3 contractions per 10 minutes. The oxytocin is then discontinued while the FHR and uterine contractions continue to be monitored for 30 minutes. (*Note*: It usually takes 20 to 25 minutes for the body to metabolize the oxytocin.)

Post-Test Nursing Care

Possible complication: Premature labor

- Monitor the patient's blood pressure and the FHR until all uterine contractions have ceased.
- Discontinue the intravenous infusion and apply a dressing to the venipuncture site. Check the dressing periodically for continued bleeding.
- Report abnormal findings to the primary care provider.

• • • • • • • • • • • • • • • • •

Coombs' Test, Direct
(*Direct Antiglobulin Test, RBC Antibody Screen*)

In some types of diseases, such as infectious mononucleosis and systemic lupus erythematosus, and in sensitizations such as to the Rh factor, the red blood cells become coated with antibodies. The direct Coombs' test serves as a screening test to determine whether such antibodies are attached to the patient's red blood cells.

In this test a sample of the patient's blood is mixed with Coombs' anti–human globulin serum. This serum is actually a rabbit serum that contains antibodies against human globulins. When the patient's blood is mixed with the rabbit serum, clumping or agglutination occurs if antibodies are present on the patient's red blood cells. A common cause of a positive direct Coombs' test is autoimmune hemolytic anemia in which the person has antibodies against his or her own red blood cells.

The test has multiple purposes. It is used to screen blood during type and crossmatch procedures. It can also be used to detect red blood cell sensitization to drugs or blood transfusions, as in the testing for the occurrence of a hemolytic transfusion reaction. In cases of suspected erythroblastosis fetalis, the test can be used to determine the presence of antibodies to the newborn's red blood cells.

Normal Values

Negative

Possible Meanings of Abnormal Values

Positive	Negative
Elderly	Hemolytic anemia
Erythroblastosis fetalis	(nonautoimmune, non-
Hemolytic anemia (autoimmune,	drug-induced)
drug-induced)	Normal finding
Infectious mononucleosis	
Lymphomas	
Neoplasms	
Renal disorders	
Rheumatoid arthritis	
Systemic lupus erythematosus	
Transfusion reaction	

Contributing Factors to Abnormal Values

- Hemolysis of the blood sample may alter test results.
- Drugs that may cause a *positive* direct Coombs' test: ampicillin, captopril, cephalosporins, chlorpromazine, chlorpropamide, ethosuximide, hydralazine hydrochloride, indomethacin, insulin, isoniazid, levodopa, mefenamic acid, melphalan, methyldopa, para-aminosalicylic acid, penicillin, phenylbutazone, phenytoin, procainamide hydrochloride, quinidine, quinine sulfate, rifampin, streptomycin, sulfonamides, tetracyclines.

Pre-Test Nursing Care

- Explain to the patient the purpose of the test and the need for a blood sample to be drawn.
- No fasting is required before the test.

Procedure

- A 10-mL blood sample is drawn in a collection tube containing EDTA. For newborns, a 5-mL umbilical cord blood sample is sufficient.
- Gloves are worn throughout the procedure.

Post-Test Nursing Care

- Apply pressure at venipuncture site. Apply dressing, periodically assessing for continued bleeding.
- Label the specimen and transport it to the laboratory.
- Report abnormal findings to the primary care provider.

• • • • • • • • • • • • • • •

Coombs' Test, Indirect
(Antibody Screening Test)

The indirect Coombs test is used to detect unexpected circulating antibodies in the patient's serum that may react against transfused red blood cells. These antibodies are ones other than those of the ABO blood groups. This is different from the direct Coombs test, which detects antibodies already attached to the red blood cells.

In this test, the patient's serum is considered the antibody and the donor red blood cells as the antigen. The serum and antigenic red blood cells are brought together to allow any antibodies to attach to the red blood cells. Anti–human globulin is then added. If the patient's serum contains an antibody that reacted with and attached to the donor red blood cells, agglutination will occur and the test is considered positive. If no agglutination occurs, no antigen–antibody reaction has taken place. The serum may contain an antibody, but the donor red blood cells do not have the antigen against which the antibody would respond. Positive tests are followed with additional testing to identify the specific antibody present.

Normal Values

Negative

Possible Meanings of Abnormal Values

Positive

Erythroblastosis fetalis
Hemolytic anemia (drug induced)
Incompatible crossmatch
Maternal-fetal Rh incompatibility
Prior transfusion reaction

Contributing Factors to Abnormal Values

- Hemolysis of the blood sample may alter test results.
- Administration of dextran or intravenous contrast media before the test may alter test results.
- Drugs that may cause a *positive* indirect Coombs' test: cephalosporins, chlorpromazine, insulin, isoniazid, levodopa, mefenamic acid, methyldopa, penicillin, phenytoin, procainamide hydrochloride, quinidine, sulfonamides, tetracyclines.

Pre-Test Nursing Care

- Explain to the patient the purpose of the test and the need for a blood sample to be drawn.
- No fasting is required before the test.

Procedure

- A 10-mL sample is drawn in a collection tube containing either no additives or a silicone gel.
- Gloves are worn throughout the procedure.

C

Post-Test Nursing Care

- Apply pressure at venipuncture site. Apply dressing, periodically assessing for continued bleeding.
- Label the specimen and transport it to the laboratory.
- Report abnormal findings to the primary care provider.
- Positive indirect Coombs' tests indicate the need for antibody identification testing.

• • • • • • • • • • • • • • • • • •

Copper

Copper is an essential trace element needed in the synthesis of hemoglobin and oxidation reduction. Normally, urine contains a very small amount of free copper, because most copper in the plasma is bound to ceruloplasmin, an alpha$_2$-globulin protein. Testing for urine copper content is used to aid in the diagnosis of *Wilson's disease*, a hereditary syndrome transmitted as an autosomal recessive trait. In this condition, decreased levels of ceruloplasmin are manufactured by the liver, serum copper levels are low, and urine copper levels are high. Without ceruloplasmin to transport the copper, Wilson's disease leads to an accumulation of copper in the tissue of the brain, eye, kidney, and liver. One of the hallmarks of this disease is the presence of Kayser-Fleischer rings around the iris of the eye, which are caused by copper deposits. Wilson's disease can be treated with penicillamine, an anticopper drug, which promotes the renal excretion of excess copper.

Normal Values

0–60 µg/24 hr (0-0.96 µmol/d SI units)
Elderly: increased

Possible Meanings of Abnormal Values

Increased

Alzheimer's disease
Biliary cirrhosis
Chronic, active hepatitis
Hyperceruloplasminemia
Nephrotic syndrome
Pellagra
Proteinuria
Wilson's disease

Pre-Test Nursing Care

- Explain 24-hour urine collection procedure to the patient.
- Stress the importance of saving *all* urine in the 24-hour period. Instruct the patient to avoid contaminating the urine with toilet paper or feces.
- Inform the patient of the presence of a preservative in the collection bottle.

Procedure

- Obtain the proper container containing the appropriate preservative from the laboratory.
- Begin the testing period in the morning after the patient's first voiding, which is discarded.
- Timing of the 24-hour period begins at the time the first voiding is discarded.
- *All* urine for the next 24 hours is collected in the container, which is to be kept refrigerated or on ice.
- If any urine is accidentally discarded during the 24-hour period, the test must be discontinued and a new test begun.
- The ending time of the 24-hour collection period should be posted in the patient's room.
- Gloves are to be worn when dealing with the specimen collection.

Post-Test Nursing Care

- Label the container and transport it on ice to the laboratory as soon as possible after the end of the 24-hour collection period.
- Report abnormal values to the primary care provider.

• • • • • • • • • • • • • • • • • •

Cortisol, Blood

In response to a stimulus such as stress, the hypothalamus secretes corticotropin-releasing hormone. This hormone stimulates the secretion of *adrenocorticotropic hormone* (ACTH) by the anterior pituitary gland. ACTH, in turn, causes the adrenal cortex to release the glucocorticoid hormone, *cortisol.* Cortisol has several functions:

- Stimulation of glucose formation (gluconeogenesis)
- Stimulation of stored energy molecular breakdown (fats, proteins, carbohydrates)
- Promotion of sympathetic responses to stressors
- Reduction of inflammation and immune function
- Stimulation of gastric acid secretion

Cortisol levels in the blood provide valuable information regarding the functioning of the adrenal cortex. Cortisol is normally secreted in a diurnal pattern, with the peak or highest levels being between 5 and 10 AM and trough, or lowest, levels being between 4 and 8 PM.

Normal Values

8 AM–12 noon	5.0–25.0 µg/dL (138–690 nmol/L SI units)
12 noon–8 PM	5.0–15.0 µg/dL (138–410 nmol/L SI units)
8 PM–8 AM	0.0–10.0 µg/dL (0–276 nmol/L SI units)

Possible Meanings of Abnormal Values

Increased	Decreased
Adrenal adenoma	Addison's disease
Burns	Adrenal insufficiency

Increased	Decreased
Cushing's disease	Hypoglycemia
Cushing's syndrome	Hypopituitarism
Eclampsia	Hypothyroidism
Ectopic ACTH-producing tumors	Liver disease
Exercise	Postpartum pituitary necrosis
Hyperpituitarism	
Hypertension	
Hyperthyroidism	
Infectious disease	
Obesity	
Pancreatitis (acute)	
Pregnancy	
Shock	
Stress	
Surgery	

Contributing Factors to Abnormal Values

- Levels of ACTH may vary with exercise, sleep, and stress.
- Hemolysis of the sample may alter test results.
- Drugs that may *increase* cortisol levels: amphetamines, estrogens, ethyl alcohol, lithium carbonate, methadone, nicotine, oral contraceptives, spironolactone.
- Drugs that may *decrease* cortisol levels: androgens, barbiturates, dexamethasone, levodopa, phenytoin.

Pre-Test Nursing Care

- Explain to the patient the purpose of the test and the need for a blood sample to be drawn.
- Fasting and limited physical activity for 10 to 12 hours is required before the test.

Procedure

- A 5-mL blood sample is drawn in a collection tube containing no additives.
- Gloves are worn throughout the procedure.

Post-Test Nursing Care

- Apply pressure at venipuncture site. Apply dressing, periodically assessing for continued bleeding.
- Label the specimen and transport it to the laboratory as soon as possible.
- Report abnormal findings to the primary care provider.

• • • • • • • • • • • • • • • •

Cortisol, Urine
(Free Cortisol)

In response to a stimulus such as stress, the hypothalamus secretes corticotropin-releasing hormone. This hormone stimulates the secretion of *adrenocorticotropic hormone* (ACTH) by the anterior pituitary gland. ACTH, in turn, causes the adrenal cortex to release the glucocorticoid hormone, *cortisol.* Cortisol has several functions:

- Stimulation of glucose formation (gluconeogenesis)
- Stimulation of stored energy molecular breakdown (fats, proteins, carbohydrates)
- Promotion of sympathetic responses to stressors
- Reduction of inflammation and immune function
- Stimulation of gastric acid secretion

Most of the cortisol present in the body is bound to cortisol-binding globulin and albumin. Five to 10% is "free" or unconjugated and is thus filtered by the kidneys into the urine. It is the free urinary cortisol that is measured by this test, which is used to evaluate adrenal function, especially hyperfunction. Generally, the urinary cortisol level will increase when the plasma cortisol level increases and will decrease when the plasma cortisol level decreases. The creatinine level in the 24-hour urine specimen is usually measured along with the urinary cortisol level to confirm that the urine volume is adequate.

Normal Values

20–70 µg/d (55–193 nmol/d SI units)

Possible Meanings of Abnormal Values

Increased	Decreased
Amenorrhea	Addison's disease
Cushing's syndrome	Hypopituitarism
Hyperthyroidism	Hypothyroidism
Lung cancer	Renal glomerular dysfunction
Pituitary tumor	
Pregnancy	
Stress	

Contributing Factors to Abnormal Values

- Drugs that may *increase* urinary cortisol levels: amphetamines, corticotropin, estrogens, nicotine, oral contraceptives, quinacrine hydrochloride, spironolactone.
- The drug dexamethasone may *decrease* urinary cortisol levels.

Pre-Test Nursing Care

- Explain 24-hour urine collection procedure to the patient.
- Stress the importance of saving *all* urine in the 24-hour period. Instruct the patient to avoid contaminating the urine with toilet paper or feces.
- Inform the patient of the presence of a preservative in the collection bottle.

Procedure

- Obtain the proper container containing the appropriate preservative from the laboratory.
- Begin the testing period in the morning after the patient's first voiding, which is discarded.
- Timing of the 24-hour period begins at the time the first voiding is discarded.
- *All* urine for the next 24 hours is collected in the container, which is to be kept refrigerated or on ice.
- If any urine is accidentally discarded during the 24-hour period, the test must be discontinued and a new test begun.
- The ending time of the 24-hour collection period should be posted in the patient's room.
- Gloves are to be worn when dealing with the specimen collection.

Post-Test Nursing Care

- Label the container and transport it on ice to the laboratory as soon as possible after the end of the 24-hour collection period.
- Report abnormal values to the primary care provider.

• • • • • • • • • • • • • • • • • •

C-Peptide
(Connecting Peptide)

Proinsulin is converted to insulin in the beta cells of the pancreas. A by-product of this conversion is C-peptide, an inactive amino acid. C-peptide levels usually correlate with endogenous insulin levels and are not affected by exogenous insulin administration. Thus, this test is useful in determining endogenous insulin levels.

Normal Values

0.30–3.70 µg/L (0.10–1.22 nmol/L SI units)

Possible Meanings of Abnormal Values

Increased	Decreased
Insulinoma	Diabetes mellitus
Islet cell tumor	Hypoglycemia owing to
Pancreas transplants	insulin overdose/abuse
Renal failure	Pancreatectomy

Contributing Factors to Abnormal Values

- Hemolysis of the blood sample may alter test results.
- C-peptide levels may not correlate with endogenous insulin levels in the presence of obesity or islet cell tumors.
- Drugs that may *increase* C-peptide levels: oral hypoglycemic agents, sulfonylureas.

Pre-Test Nursing Care

- Explain to the patient the purpose of the test and the need for a blood sample to be drawn.
- Fasting for 8 to 10 hours is required before the test. Water is permitted.

Procedure

- A 7-mL blood sample is drawn in a collection tube containing a silicone gel.
- Gloves are worn throughout the procedure.

Post-Test Nursing Care

- Apply pressure at venipuncture site. Apply dressing, periodically assessing for continued bleeding.
- Label the specimen and transport it to the laboratory.
- Report abnormal findings to the primary care provider.

• • • • • • • • • • • • • • • • •

C-Reactive Protein Test
(CRP)

C-reactive protein (CRP) is a glycoprotein produced by the liver. It is normally absent from the blood. The presence of acute inflammation with tissue destruction within the body stimulates its production. Therefore, a positive CRP indicates the presence of an inflammatory process. When the acute inflammation is no longer present, the CRP rapidly dissipates from the body.

The CRP is considered a nonspecific test in that it does not identify specific disease processes as the cause of the inflammatory process. However, CRP is considered a more sensitive test than the erythrocyte sedimentation rate (ESR), which is considered very nonspecific. Uses of the CRP include the monitoring of postoperative wound healing for indications of infection and the evaluation of patients after a suspected myocardial infarction.

Normal Values

Qualitative: negative
Quantitative: 0–8 mg/dL (0–8 µg/mL SI units)

Possible Meanings of Abnormal Values

Positive

Acute bacterial infection
Acute rheumatic fever
Acute viral infection
Crohn's disease
Gout
Hodgkin's disease
Inflammation
Malignancies
Meningitis

Positive

Myocardial infarction
Nephritis
Peritonitis
Pharyngitis
Pneumonia
Postoperative period (1–3 days)
Postoperative wound infection
Rheumatoid arthritis
Systemic lupus erythematosus
Tissue trauma/necrosis
Tuberculosis

Contributing Factors to Abnormal Values

- The presence of an intrauterine device may cause a false-positive CRP result owing to inflammation.
- Drugs that may cause a *false-positive* CRP: oral contraceptives.
- Drugs that may cause a *false-negative* CRP: nonsteroidal anti-inflammatory drugs, salicylates, steroids.

Pre-Test Nursing Care

- Explain to the patient the purpose of the test and the need for a blood sample to be drawn.
- Fasting for 4 to 12 hours is usually required before the test.

Procedure

- A 5-mL blood sample is drawn in a collection tube containing no additives.
- Gloves are worn throughout the procedure.

Post-Test Nursing Care

- Apply pressure at venipuncture site. Apply dressing, periodically assessing for continued bleeding.
- Label the specimen and transport it to the laboratory immediately.
- Report abnormal findings to the primary care provider.

• • • • • • • • • • • • • • • •

Creatine Kinase and Isoenzymes
(CK, Formerly: Creatine Phosphokinase [CPK])

Creatine kinase and isoenzymes (CK) is the name now used for the test that was formerly known as creatine phosphokinase (CPK). CK is an enzyme found primarily in the heart and skeletal muscles and in smaller amounts in the brain. It is involved in the reaction that changes creatine to creatinine.

CK can be measured as the total enzyme in the serum, or each of its three isoenzymes may be measured. The isoenzymes include

CK$_1$ (CPK-BB):   produced primarily by brain tissue and smooth muscle of the lungs
CK$_2$ (CPK-MB):   produced primarily by heart tissue
CK$_3$ (CPK-MM):   produced primarily by skeletal muscle

CK, along with asparate aminotransferase (AST) and lactic dehydrogenase (LDH, LD), is assessed in the case of suspected myocardial infarction. It typically appears in the bloodstream within 3 to 6 hours of the tissue injury, with peak values occurring 18 to 24 hours post injury. CK levels are usually elevated for approximately 3 days. Thus, CK is the first of the cardiac enzymes to become elevated after a myocardial infarction.

Normal Values

Total CK

Female: 40–150 U/L (0.67–2.50 μkat/L SI units)
Male: 60–400 U/L (1.00–6.67 μkat/L SI units)

Isoenzymes

CK$_1$ (CPK-BB):   0–1%
CK$_2$ (CPK-MB):   < 3%
CK$_3$ (CPK-MM):   95%–100%

Possible Meanings of Abnormal Values

Increased Total CK

Acute cerebrovascular disease
Acute psychosis
Alcoholism
Brain trauma
Cardiac defibrillation
Cardiac surgery
Convulsions
Dermatomyositis
Electrical shock
Hypokalemia
Hypothyroidism
Intramuscular injections
Muscle inflammation
Myocardial infarction
Myxedema
Polymyositis
Progressive muscular dystrophy
Pulmonary infarction

Decreased Total CK

Addison's disease
Anterior pituitary
   hyposecretion
Connective tissue disease
Early pregnancy
Hepatic disease
Low muscle mass
Metastatic neoplasia

Increased CK$_1$ (CPK-BB) Isoenzyme

Biliary atresia
Brain tissue injury
Brain tumors

C

Increased CK₁ (CPK-BB) Isoenzyme

Cancer of breast, lung, prostate
Cerebrovascular accident
Pulmonary infarction
Shock

Increased CK₂ (CPK-MB) Isoenzyme

Acute myocardial infarction
Duchenne's muscular dystrophy
Malignant hyperthermia
Polymyositis
Reye's syndrome

Increased CK₃ (CPK-MM) Isoenzyme

Hypokalemia
Hypothyroidism
Intramuscular injections
Myocardial infarction
Muscle inflammation
Muscle necrosis
Muscular dystrophy
Postoperative period
Shock

Contributing Factors to Abnormal Values

- Hemolysis of the blood sample or strenuous exercise before the test will alter test results.
- Drugs that may *increase* total CK: aminocaproic acid, amphotericin B, ampicillin, anticoagulants, aspirin, clofibrate, codeine, dexamethasone, digoxin, ethanol, furosemide, glutethimide, guanethidine sulfate, halothane, heroin, imipramine hydrochloride, lithium, meperidine hydrochloride, morphine, phenobarbital, succinylcholine chloride.
- Drugs that may *decrease* total CK: steroids.

Pre-Test Nursing Care

- Explain to the patient the purpose of the test and the need for a blood sample to be drawn.
- Inform the patient that this test is often performed on 3 consecutive days, and again in 1 week, necessitating multiple venipunctures.
- No fasting is required before the test.
- Do not administer any intramuscular injections for 1 hour before the test.

Procedure

- A 5-mL blood sample is drawn in a collection tube containing a silicone gel or in a plasma separation tube.
- Gloves are worn throughout the procedure.

Post-Test Nursing Care

- Apply pressure at venipuncture site. Apply dressing, periodically assessing for continued bleeding.
- Label the specimen and transport it to the laboratory immediately.
- Report abnormal findings to the primary care provider.

• • • • • • • • • • • • • • • •

Creatinine, Blood
(Serum Creatinine)

Creatinine is the waste product of creatine phosphate, a compound found in the skeletal muscle tissue. It is excreted entirely by the kidneys. The creatinine level is affected primarily by renal dysfunction and is thus very useful in evaluating renal function. Increased levels of creatinine indicate a slowing of the glomerular filtration rate. Because creatinine levels normally remain constant, even with aging, this test is particularly useful in evaluating renal dysfunction in which a large number of nephrons have been destroyed. The creatinine level is usually determined in conjunction with the blood urea nitrogen (BUN) in assessing renal function. The normal ratio of BUN to creatinine ranges from 6:1 to 20:1. Testing of the creatinine level in the blood is also used to monitor patients on drugs known to be nephrotoxic, such as the aminoglycosides. Both BUN and creatinine should be assessed before administration of any aminoglycoside to the patient.

Normal Values

Female: 0.6–1.1 mg/dL (53–97 μmol/L SI units)
Male: 0.6–1.5 mg/dL (53–133 μmol/L SI units)
Children: 0.2–1.0 mg/dL (18–88 μmol/L SI units)

Possible Meanings of Abnormal Values

Increased	Decreased
Congestive heart failure	Atrophy of muscle tissue
Dehydration	Pregnancy
Diabetes mellitus	
Glomerulonephritis	
Gout	
Hyperthyroidism	
Multiple myeloma	
Nephritis	
Pyelonephritis	
Renal failure	
Rheumatoid arthritis	
Shock	
Subacute bacterial endocarditis	
Systemic lupus erythematosus	
Uremia	
Urinary obstruction	

C

Contributing Factors to Abnormal Values

- Creatinine levels are 20% to 40% higher in the late afternoon than in the morning.
- Test results may be altered by hemolysis of the blood sample and by ingestion of a high-meat diet.
- Drugs that may *increase* creatinine levels: acetohexamide, amphotericin B, androgens, arginine hydrochloride, ascorbic acid, barbiturates, captopril, cephalosporins, chlorthalidone, cimetidine, clofibrate, clonidine hydrochloride, corticosteroids, dextran, diacetic acid, disopyramide phosphate, doxycycline hyclate, fructose, gentamicin, glucose, hydralazine hydrochloride, hydroxyurea, kanamycin, levodopa, lithium carbonate, mannitol, meclofenamate sodium, methicillin sodium, methyldopa, metoprolol tartrate, minoxidil, mithramycin, nitrofurantoin, phenolsulfonphthalein, propranolol hydrochloride, protein, pyruvate, sulfonamides, streptokinase, testosterone, triamterene, trimethoprim.
- Drugs that may *decrease* creatinine levels: cefoxitin sodium, cimetidine, chlorpromazine, chlorprothixene, marijuana, thiazide diuretics, vancomycin.

Pre-Test Nursing Care

- Explain to the patient the purpose of the test and the need for a blood sample to be drawn.
- Fasting is required for 8 hours before the test.
- Instruct the patient to avoid excessive exercise for 8 hours before the test.
- Instruct the patient to avoid red meat intake for 24 hours before the test.

Procedure

- A 7-mL blood sample is drawn in a collection tube containing a silicone gel.
- Gloves are worn throughout the procedure.

Post-Test Nursing Care

- Apply pressure at venipuncture site. Apply dressing, periodically assessing for continued bleeding.
- Label the specimen and transport it to the laboratory immediately.
- Report abnormal findings to the primary care provider.
- If the creatinine level is elevated, check with the primary care provider before administering any aminoglycoside.

• • • • • • • • • • • • • • • •

Creatinine Clearance

Creatinine is the waste product of creatine phosphate, a compound found in the skeletal muscle tissue. It is excreted entirely by the kidneys. Increased levels of creatinine indicate a slowing of the glomerular filtration rate. The creatinine clearance test consists of two components: a 24-hour urine collection and a blood sample. Conducting both urine and blood testing allows for the comparison of the serum creatinine level with the amount of creatinine excreted in the urine. This is a more sensitive indicator of kidney function than serum creatinine alone. The creatinine clearance normally decreases with aging owing to a decline in the glomerular filtration rate.

Because "clearance" means the amount of blood cleared of creatinine in 1 minute, a monitoring of the creatinine clearance rate provides valuable information regarding the progression of renal disease. A minimum creatinine clearance of 10 mL/min is necessary to maintain life without the use of hemodialysis or peritoneal dialysis. The creatinine clearance rate is calculated by the following formula:

$$\frac{\text{Urine creatinine} \times \text{urine volume}}{\text{Creatinine in serum}} = \begin{array}{l}\text{Creatinine clearance rate} \\ \text{(expressed in mL/min/1.73 m}^2 \\ \text{of body surface)}\end{array}$$

Normal Values

Female:	85–125 mL/min (0.8–1.2 mL/s SI units)
Male:	95–135 mL/min (0.9–1.3 mL/s SI units)
Pregnancy:	increased
Elderly:	decreased
Children:	decreased

Possible Meanings of Abnormal Values

Increased	Decreased
Exercise	Acute tubular necrosis
Pregnancy	Congestive heart failure
	Dehydration
	Glomerulonephritis
	Obstruction of renal artery
	Polycystic kidney disease
	Preeclampsia
	Pyelonephritis
	Renal malignancy
	Renal tuberculosis
	Shock

Contributing Factors to Abnormal Values

- Test results may be altered if urine collection is not kept on ice.
- Drugs that may *increase* creatinine clearance rate: acetohexamide, amphotericin B, androgens, arginine hydrochloride, ascorbic acid, barbiturates, captopril, cephalosporins, chlorthalidone, cimetidine, clofibrate, clonidine hydrochloride, corticosteroids, dextran, diacetic acid, disopyramide phosphate, doxycycline hyclate, fructose, gentamicin, glucose, hydralazine hydrochloride, hydroxyurea, kanamycin, levodopa, lithium carbonate, mannitol, meclofenamate sodium, methicillin sodium, methyldopa, metoprolol tartrate, minoxidil, mithramycin, nitrofurantoin, phenolsulfonphthalein, propranolol hydrochloride, protein, pyruvate, sulfonamides, streptokinase, testosterone, triamterene, trimethoprim.
- Drugs that may *decrease* creatinine clearance rate: anabolic steroids, androgens, cefoxitin sodium, cimetidine, chlorpromazine, chlorprothixene, marijuana, thiazide diuretics, vancomycin.

C

Pre-Test Nursing Care

- Explain 24-hour urine collection procedure to the patient.
- Stress the importance of saving *all* urine in the 24-hour period. Instruct the patient to avoid contaminating the urine with toilet paper or feces.
- Explain that a blood sample will also need to be drawn during the period of the urine collection.
- Instruct the patient to avoid excessive exercise for 8 hours before the test.

Procedure

- Although a 2-hour, 6-hour, or 12-hour urine collection can be used, a 24-hour urine collection is preferred.
- Obtain the proper container from the laboratory.
- Begin the testing period in the morning after the patient's first voiding, which is discarded.
- Timing of the 24-hour period begins at the time the first voiding is discarded.
- *All* urine for the next 24 hours is collected in the container and kept on ice.
- If any urine is accidentally discarded during the 24-hour period, the test must be discontinued and a new test begun.
- The ending time of the 24-hour collection period should be posted in the patient's room.
- A 7-mL blood sample is drawn in a collection tube containing a silicone gel anytime during the test period.
- Gloves are worn throughout the procedure.

Post-Test Nursing Care

- Label the urine container and transport it on ice to the laboratory as soon as possible after the end of the 24-hour collection period.
- Apply pressure at venipuncture site. Apply dressing, periodically assessing for continued bleeding.
- Label the blood sample and transport it to the laboratory.
- Report abnormal findings to the primary care provider.

• • • • • • • • • • • • • • • • •

Creatinine, Urine
(Urine Creatinine)

Creatinine is the waste product of creatine phosphate, a compound found in the skeletal muscle tissue. It is excreted entirely by the kidneys. The creatinine level is affected primarily by renal dysfunction and is thus very useful in evaluating renal function.

Normal Values

Female: 600–1800 mg/24 h (5.3–16 mmol/24 h SI units)
Male: 800–2000 mg/24 h (7–17.6 mmol/24 h SI units)

Possible Meanings of Abnormal Values

Increased	Decreased
Salmonella infection	Anemia
Tetanus	Glomerulonephritis
Typhoid fever	Hyperthyroidism
	Hypovolemic shock
	Leukemia
	Muscular atrophy
	Polycystic kidney disease
	Pyelonephritis
	Urinary tract obstruction

Contributing Factors to Abnormal Findings

- Creatinine levels are 20% to 40% higher in the late afternoon than in the morning.
- Test results may be altered if urine collection is not kept on ice.
- Drugs that may *increase* urine creatinine levels: acetohexamide, amphotericin B, androgens, arginine hydrochloride, ascorbic acid, barbiturates, captopril, cephalosporins, chlorthalidone, cimetidine, clofibrate, clonidine hydrochloride, corticosteroids, dextran, diacetic acid, disopyramide phosphate, doxycycline hyclate, fructose, gentamicin, glucose, hydralazine hydrochloride, hydroxyurea, kanamycin, levodopa, lithium carbonate, mannitol, meclofenamate sodium, methicillin sodium, methyldopa, metoprolol tartrate, minoxidil, mithramycin, nitrofurantoin, phenolsulfonphthalein, propranolol hydrochloride, protein, pyruvate, sulfonamides, streptokinase, testosterone, triamterene, trimethoprim.
- Drugs that may *decrease* urine creatinine levels: anabolic steroids, androgens, cefoxitin sodium, cimetidine, chlorpromazine, chlorprothixene, marijuana, thiazide diuretics, vancomycin.

Pre-Test Nursing Care

- Explain 24-hour urine collection procedure to the patient.
- Stress the importance of saving *all* urine in the 24-hour period. Instruct the patient to avoid contaminating the urine with toilet paper or feces.

Procedure

- Obtain the proper container from the laboratory.
- Begin the testing period in the morning after the patient's first voiding, which is discarded.
- Timing of the 24-hour period begins at the time the first voiding is discarded.
- *All* urine for the next 24 hours is collected in the container and kept on ice.
- If any urine is accidentally discarded during the 24 hour period, the test must be discontinued and a new test begun.
- The ending time of the 24-hour collection period should be posted in the patient's room.
- During the 24-hour collection period, all food intake must be accurately recorded by the nurse and the protein intake determined by the dietitian.
- Gloves are worn throughout the procedure.

Post-Test Nursing Care

- Label the container and transport it on ice to the laboratory as soon as possible after the end of the 24-hour collection period.
- Report abnormal findings to the primary care provider.

• • • • • • • • • • • • • • • • •

Cryoglobulin

Cryoglobulins are abnormal serum proteins that precipitate at low laboratory temperatures and re-dissolve after being warmed. When patients with cryoglobulins present in their blood are subjected to cold, they may experience vascular problems of their extremities, with Raynaud's syndrome–like symptoms such as pain, cyanosis, and coldness of the fingers and toes. The presence of cryoglobulins in the blood (cryoglobulinemia) is usually associated with immunologic disease. There are three types of cryoglobulins; delineating these types assists in differntiating the disease involved.

The test is conducted by refrigerating a serum sample at 4°C for at least 72 hours and observing for the formation of a precipitate. The reversibility of the reaction is verified by rewarming the serum sample. If the presence of cryoglobulins is thus shown, further study is done to identify the cryoglobulin components.

Normal Values

Negative

Possible Meanings of Abnormal Values

Type I Cryoglobulins

Positive

Chronic lymphocytic leukemia
Lymphoma
Multiple myeloma
Waldenström's macroglobulinemia

Type II Cryoglobulins

Positive Lymphoma

Mixed essential cryoglobulinemia
Multiple myeloma
Rheumatoid arthritis
Sjögren's syndrome

Type III Cryoglobulins

Positive

Chronic infection
Cytomegalovirus infection

Positive

Hepatitis
Infectious mononucleosis
Infective endocarditis
Kala-azar
Leprosy
Polymyalgia rheumatica
Poststreptococcal glomerulonephritis
Primary biliary cirrhosis
Rheumatoid arthritis
Scleroderma
Sjögren's syndrome
Systemic lupus erythematosus
Tropical splenomegaly syndrome

Type I, II, or III Cryoglobulins

Positive

Hodgkin's disease
Raynaud's disease
Viral infection

Pre-Test Nursing Care

- Explain to the patient the purpose of the test and the need for a blood sample to be drawn.
- Fasting for 8 hours is required before the test.

Procedure

- A 10-mL blood sample is drawn in a collection tube containing a silicone gel prewarmed to 37°C.
- Gloves are worn throughout the procedure.

Post-Test Nursing Care

- Apply pressure at venipuncture site. Apply dressing, periodically assessing for continued bleeding.
- Label the specimen and transport it to the laboratory immediately.
- Report abnormal findings to the primary care provider.

• • • • • • • • • • • • • • • • • •

Cryptococcosis

Cryptococcosis is caused by the organism *Cryptococcus neoformans*. It is one of the most frequent fungal infections (mycoses) of the central nervous system (CNS). Susceptibility to this infection is higher in those with chronic or debilitating diseases, such as acquired immunodeficiency sydrome (AIDS), and by certain types of drug therapy that may alter the immune system, such as corticosteroids and antineoplastic agents. The disease usually begins as a respiratory infection,

C

which then disseminates to the CNS. The organism is carried by pigeons, with the probable mode of transmission being inhalation. Symptoms range from headache and subtle changes in mental status to fever, seizures, and coma. If untreated, the disease can be fatal within a few weeks.

Normal Values

Immunodiffusion: negative
Complement fixation titer: < 1:4

Abnormal Values

Titers of 1:4 are suggestive of cryptococcal infection. Titers > 1:8 indicate active cryptococcal infection.

Possible Meanings of Abnormal Values

Increased

Cryptococcosis

Contributing Factors to Abnormal Values

- False-positive test results have occurred in patients with elevated rheumatoid factor levels.
- Skin tests can cause a serologic test to become positive. Thus, skin tests should be withheld until after the blood sample is drawn.
- Many mycoses cause immunosuppression, leading to low titers, or false-negative test results.
- Contamination of the blood sample will alter test results.
- Hemolysis of the sample owing to excessive agitation may alter results.
- Antibodies may appear early in the disease and then disappear.

Pre-Test Nursing Care

- Assess neurologic status. Report headache, changes in mental status or motor function.
- Explain to the patient the purpose of the test, noting that it involves drawing a blood sample.
- The patient is to be NPO for 12 hours before the test.

Procedure

- The test should be conducted 2 to 4 weeks after exposure to the organism.
- A 7-mL blood sample is obtained in a collection tube containing no additives.
- Gloves are worn throughout the procedure.

Post-Test Nursing Care

- Apply pressure at venipuncture site. Apply dressing, periodically assessing for continued bleeding.
- Label the specimen and transport it immediately to the laboratory, taking care to avoid excessive agitation of the sample.
- Advise the patient that other procedures to test for this fungus may be done. Such testing might include the need for a lumbar puncture to obtain a sample of cerebrospinal fluid for culturing.
- Report abnormal findings to the primary care provider.

• • • • • • • • • • • • • • • •

Cutaneous Immunofluorescence Biopsy
(Skin Biopsy)

Immunofluorescence is a histologic technique in which fluorescent dyes are attached to antibody molecules. When viewed under an ultraviolet microscope, these antibody molecules appear as a colored fluorescence when they have become complexed with an antigen. This technique is used when performing a biopsy of the skin. This test is indicated in the evaluation of skin disorders such as lupus erythematosus and blistering diseases such as pemphigus and pemphigoid.

Normal Values

Normal skin histology
Absence of antibody–antigen complexes

Possible Meanings of Abnormal Values

Bullous pemphigoid
Dermatitis herpetiformis
Discoid lupus erythematosus
Pemphigus
Systemic lupus erythematosus

Pre-Test Nursing Care

- Explain to the patient the purpose of the test and the need for a skin sample to be obtained.
- No fasting is required before the test.
- Obtain a signed informed consent.

Procedure

- A 4-mm punch biopsy or tissue excision specimen of skin is obtained.
- Gloves are worn throughout the procedure.

Post-Test Nursing Care

- Label the specimen and transport it on ice to the laboratory immediately to be quick frozen in liquid nitrogen.
- Apply a sterile dressing to the biopsy site.
- Teach the patient to monitor the site and to notify the health care provider if signs or symptoms of infection occur, such as drainage, redness, warmth, edema, pain at the site, or fever.
- Test results will not be available for 3 days.
- Report abnormal findings to the primary care provider.

• • • • • • • • • • • • • • • • •

Cystometry
(Cystometrography, CMG)

Cystometry is used to evaluate detrusor muscle function and tone and to determine the cause of bladder dysfunction. The test involves the instillation of fluid and/or air into the patient's bladder. Assessments are made of the patient's neurologic sensations and muscular responses to this filling of the bladder and also assesses the patient's voiding for abnormalities. The results of this test are considered in conjunction with those of other urinary diagnostic tests, such as excretory urography and cystourethrography.

Normal Values

Normal filling pattern of the bladder and ability to distinguish temperature of solution instilled

Residual urine:	0 mL
First urge to void:	150–200 mL
Bladder capacity:	400–500 mL

Possible Meanings of Abnormal Values

Bladder hypertonicity
Bladder infection
Bladder obstruction
Diminished bladder capacity
Neurogenic bladder

CONTRAINDICATIONS

- Patients with acute urinary tract infection
- Patients with urinary tract obstruction

Pre-Test Nursing Care

- Explain to the patient the purpose of the test and the procedure to be done. Explain that even though a catheter will be in place during the procedure, the patient will feel the urge to void as fluid or gas fills the bladder.
- Obtain a signed informed consent.
- No fasting is required before the test.

Procedure

- The patient is asked to void to empty the bladder.
- The patient is assisted into the supine position.
- A Foley catheter is inserted into the bladder, and the residual urine volume is measured.
- Thermal sensation is assessed by instilling 30 mL of room temperature sterile saline or water into the bladder, followed by 30 mL of warm fluid. Any sensations reported by the patient are recorded.
- The fluid is drained from the bladder, and a cystometer is connected to the catheter. This instrument graphically displays pressures and volumes within the bladder.
- Sterile saline or water or a gas, such as carbon dioxide, is slowly introduced into the bladder.

- Notations are made on the cystometrogram printout as to the point when the patient first feels an urge to void and again when the patient feels that the bladder is completely full and that he or she must void.
- The patient is then requested to urinate, which permits recording of the maximal intravesical voiding pressure.
- The bladder is then drained and the catheter is removed.
- Other testing may involve repeating the above procedure with the patient in a standing or sitting position or after administration of a bladder tone stimulant such as bethanechol chloride.

Post-Test Nursing Care

Possible complication: Urinary tract infection

- Assess the patient for complaints of burning on urination, frequency of urination, and bladder spasms. Interventions should include:
  - Assessing vital signs (elevated temperature may indicate infection)
  - Encouraging the patient to increase fluid intake
  - Administering analgesics as ordered
  - Administering antibiotics as ordered
  - Suggesting warm tub baths
- Monitor intake and output for 24 hours. Observe urine for frank bleeding.
- Report abnormal findings to the primary care provider.

Cystourethrography
(Cystography, Voiding Cystourethrography)

Cystourethrography involves the instillation of a contrast medium into the bladder through a urethral catheter. As the bladder fills, x-ray films are taken. The catheter is then removed and additional films are taken as the patient voids. This test is often used to evaluate patients who suffer from chronic urinary tract infections.

Normal Values

Normal structure and function of the bladder and urethra

Possible Meanings of Abnormal Values

Neurogenic bladder
Prostatic enlargement
Ureterocele
Urethral diverticula
Urethral stricture

Urethral valve
Vesical diverticula
Vesicoureteral reflux

CONTRAINDICATIONS

- Pregnant women
  Caution: A woman in her childbearing years should undergo radiography only during her menses or 12 to 14 days after its onset to avoid any exposure to a fetus.
- Patients who are allergic to radiographic dye
- Patients with acute urinary tract infection
- Patient with urinary tract obstruction

Pre-Test Nursing Care

- Explain to the patient the purpose of the test and the procedure to be done. Explain that even though a catheter will be in place, the patient will fill the urge to void as the contrast medium fills the bladder.
- Obtain a signed informed consent.
- No fasting is required before the test.
- A Foley catheter is inserted into the bladder

Procedure

- The patient is assisted into the supine position.
- The contrast medium is instilled until the bladder is filled, then the catheter is clamped.
- X-ray films are taken with the patient in various positions.
- The catheter is removed, and the patient is assisted into the right oblique position.
- Additional films are taken as the patient voids.
- *Note*: Male patients are to have a lead shield in place over the testes to protect against radiation exposure. Protection is not feasible for female patients, in whom shielding of the ovaries would block radiographic visualization of the bladder.
- If the male patient is unable to void lying down, a standing position may be used.

Post-Test Nursing Care

Possible complication: Urinary tract infection

- Assess the patient for complaints of burning on urination, frequency of urination, and bladder spasms. Interventions should include:
  - Assessing vital signs (elevated temperature may indicate infection)
  - Encouraging the patient to increase fluid intake
  - Administering analgesics as ordered
  - Administering antibiotics as ordered
  - Suggesting warm tub baths
- Monitor intake and output for 24 hours. Observe urine for frank bleeding.
- Report abnormal findings to the primary care provider.

• • • • • • • • • • • • • • • • •

Cystourethroscopy
(Cystoscopy, Endourology, Urethroscopy)

Cystourethroscopy involves the insertion of a well-lubricated sheath into the urethra. During the procedure, a cystoscope is inserted through the sheath for direct visualization of the bladder. A urethroscope is used for examination of the bladder neck and the urethra. With the sheath in place, other instruments may be interchanged, allowing the physician to obtain tissue for biopsy, to resect lesions, to collect calculi, and to pass a ureteral catheter to the renal pelvis for pyelography.

Normal Values

Normal bladder and urethra

Possible Meanings of Abnormal Values

Calculi
Congenital anomalies
Diverticula
Polyps
Prostatic hypertrophy
Prostatitis
Tumors
Ulcers
Urethral stricture

CONTRAINDICATIONS

- Patients with acute cystitis, prostatitis, or urethritis

Pre-Test Nursing Care

- Explain to the patient the purpose of the test and the procedure to be done. If the patient is to have local anesthesia only, explain that a burning sensation may be felt as the sheath is inserted into the urethra and that the urge to void may be felt during the procedure.
- Obtain a signed informed consent.
- No fasting is required before the test if a local anesthetic is to be used. If a general anesthetic is planned, the patient must fast for 8 hours before the procedure.
- Instruct the patient to void before the procedure.
- Administer pre-procedure sedation, as ordered.

Procedure

- The patient is assisted into the lithotomy position with the feet supported in stirrups.
- The external genitalia are cleansed with antiseptic and draped.
- A local anesthetic is instilled into the urethra.
- The urethroscope is inserted into the well-lubricated sheath, and both are then inserted into the urethra.
- The urethroscope is then exchanged with the cystoscope to allow for examination of the bladder lining.

- A urine sample for routine analysis is obtained.
- The cystoscope is then replaced with the urethroscope to allow visualization of the urethra as the scope and the sheath are slowly removed.
- Gloves are worn throughout the procedure.

Post-Test Nursing Care

Possible complications:

Hematuria
Infection, leading to sepsis
Perforation of the bladder
Urinary retention

- Monitor the vital signs until stable. Note indications of infection and bladder perforation, such as elevated temperature, elevated pulse, and decreased blood pressure.
- Assess the patient for complaints of burning on urination, frequency of urination, and bladder spasms. Interventions should include:
  - Encouraging the patient to increase fluid intake
  - Administering analgesics as ordered (antispasmodic medication, such as B & O suppository, may also be ordered)
  - Administering antibiotics as ordered
  - Suggesting warm tub baths
- Monitor intake and output for 24 hours. Observe urine for frank bleeding.
- Report abnormal findings to the primary care provider.

• • • • • • • • • • • • • • • •

Cytomegalovirus
(CMV)

Cytomegalovirus (CMV) is a member of the herpesvirus family. It is a very common virus, in that it is estimated that, depending on the area, 40% to 100% of a population may be infected. In most people, the virus remains latent and causes no symptoms. In those who are immunocompromised, however, CMV can have devastating effects. In patients with the acquired immunodeficiency syndrome (AIDS), CMV infection can cause pneumonitis, esophagitis, colitis, encephalitis, hepatitis, and retinitis leading to blindness. In organ transplant patients, CMV is considered a major complication, often resulting in death. Infection with CMV during pregnancy can cause mental retardation and microencephaly in the newborn.

CMV is found in all body secretions. Pregnant health care workers should be cautioned about the potential risk of acquiring CMV. Because it is impossible to eliminate from a health care worker's caseload all patients who might be carrying CMV, it is essential that careful handwashing and strict adherence to universal precautions be a consistent part of patient care.

If the test is being used to diagnose acute infection with CMV, an initial blood sample, called the "acute titer" is obtained. A second sample, the "convalescent titer" is drawn 10 to 14 days later. A diagnosis of CMV is made when a fourfold increase between the acute titer and the convalescent titer occurs.

Normal Values

Negative or titer < 1:5:   no past infection

Abnormal Values

Positive for antibodies: past infection

Possible Meanings of Abnormal Values

Increased	Decreased
CMV infection	Susceptible to CMV

Contributing Factors to Abnormal Values

- False-positive results have occurred in individuals with rheumatoid factor present in their blood and in those exposed to Epstein-Barr virus.

Pre-Test Nursing Care

- Explain to the patient the purpose of the test and note that, depending on the purpose of the test, one or two blood samples will be drawn.
- No fasting is required before the test.

Procedure

- A 5-mL blood sample is drawn into a collection tube containing no additives.
- If the test is being done to determine presence of antibodies to CMV, only one sample is needed.
- Gloves are worn throughout the procedure.

Post-Test Nursing Care

- Apply pressure at venipuncture site. Apply dressing, periodically assessing for continued bleeding.
- Label the specimen and transport it to the laboratory.
- If a convalescent titer will be needed, remind the patient of the date to return for the blood to be drawn.
- Report abnormal findings to the primary care provider.
- Blood and organ transplants given to immunosuppressed patients who are found to have no antibodies to CMV should be from donors who are also seronegative.

D

Dexamethasone Suppression Test
(DST, ACTH Suppression Test, Cortisol Suppression Test)

In response to a stimulus such as stress, the hypothalamus secretes corticotropin-releasing hormone. This hormone stimulates the secretion of *adrenocorticotropic hormone* (ACTH) by the anterior pituitary gland. ACTH, in turn, causes the adrenal cortex to release the glucocorticoid hormone *cortisol*. As levels of cortisol in the blood rise, the pituitary gland is stimulated to decrease ACTH production by means of a negative feedback mechanism.

During the dexamethasone suppression test, a corticosteroid (dexamethasone) is given. Normally, this substance decreases the formation of ACTH owing to suppression of the pituitary gland. However, in patients with hyperfunctioning of the adrenal cortex (Cushing's syndrome), pituitary suppression does not prevent the hyperactive adrenal cortex from continuing to produce large amounts of cortisol. This test is used to diagnose Cushing's syndrome and to provide supportive data in cases of clinical depression.

Normal Values

< 5 µg/dL (140 nmol/L SI units)

Possible Meanings of Abnormal Values

Increased

Adrenal hyperfunction (Cushing's syndrome)
Clinical depression
Hyperthyroidism

Contributing Factors to Abnormal Values

- *False-positive* test results may occur with acute illnesses, alcoholism, anorexia nervosa, dehydration, diabetes mellitus, fever, malnutrition, nausea, obesity, pregnancy, severe stress, and with the following drugs: aldactone, barbiturates, caffeine, carbamazepine, diethylstilbestrol, estrogens, glutethimide, meprobamate, methyprylon, oral contraceptives, phenytoin, reserpine, tetracycline.
- *False-negative* test results may occur with Addison's disease, hypopituitarism, and with the following drugs: benzodiazepines, corticosteroids, cyproheptadine hydrochloride.

Pre-Test Nursing Care

- Explain to the patient the purpose of the test and the need for a blood sample to be drawn.
- No fasting is required before the test.
- The patient should avoid caffeine after midnight the night before the test.

Procedure

- Administer dexamethasone 1 mg orally at 11 PM.
- The next morning at 8 AM, a 5-mL blood sample is drawn in a collection tube containing either heparin or a silicone gel.
- Additional blood samples may be drawn at 4 PM and 11 PM.
- Gloves are worn throughout the procedure.

Post-Test Nursing Care

- Apply pressure at venipuncture site. Apply dressing, periodically assessing for continued bleeding.
- Label the specimen and transport it to the laboratory.
- Report abnormal findings to the primary care provider.

• • • • • • • • • • • • • • • • • •

D-Dimer Test
(Fibrin Degradation Fragment, Fragment D-Dimer)

During hemostasis, thrombin stimulates the formation of fibrin from fibrinogen. This fibrin, with the addition of fibrin stabilizing factor, forms a stable fibrin clot at the site of injury. Once the fibrin clot is no longer needed, it is dissolved by fibrinolytic agents such as plasmin, resulting in fibrin degradation products. The fragment D-Dimer is one of these degradation products. (See Coagulation Studies for a description of the process of hemostasis.)

Measurement of the fragment D-Dimer is used to evaluate thrombin and plasmin activity. It is very useful in testing for disseminated intravascular coagulation (DIC), especially when considered in conjunction with positive results of fibrin degradation products (FDPs). D-Dimer levels also increase during clot lysis caused by thrombolytic therapy.

Normal Values

< 0.5 µg/mL (< 0.5 mg/L SI units)

Possible Meanings of Abnormal Values

Increased

Arterial thrombosis
Disseminated intravascular coagulation (DIC)
Fibrinolysis
Late pregnancy
Malignancy
Postoperative period
Pulmonary embolism
Venous thrombosis

Contributing Factors to Abnormal Values

- Drugs that *increase* test results: thrombolytic agents.
- *False-positive* results may occur in the presence of high rheumatoid factor (RF) titers.

Pre-Test Nursing Care

- Explain to the patient the purpose of the test and the need for a blood sample to be drawn.
- No fasting is required before the test.

D

Procedure

- A 5-mL blood sample is drawn in a collection tube containing sodium citrate and citric acid.
- Gloves are worn throughout the procedure.

Post-Test Nursing Care

Possible complication: Hematoma at site due to prolonged bleeding time

- Apply pressure 3 to 5 minutes at venipuncture site. Apply dressing, periodically assessing for continued bleeding.
- Teach the patient to monitor the site. If the site begins to bleed, the patient should apply direct presure and, if unable to control the bleeding, return to the laboratory or notify the nurse.
- Report abnormal findings to the primary care provider.

• • • • • • • • • • • • • • • •

Digital Subtraction Angiography
(DSA, Transvenous–Digital Subtraction)

Angiography is a general term used to indicate visualization of any blood vessels, whether they be arteries or veins. With *digital subtraction angiography (DSA)*, images are taken both before and after injection of a contrast medium. A computer is used to select only certain parts of images to be displayed at one time. The first image is "subtracted" from the second, which eliminates bone and soft tissue from the final image. This results in a high-quality image of the vascular system. DSA reduces the risk of complications for the patient, because the vascular access for the test is venous, rather than arterial. The test is especially useful when studying the carotid and cerebral arteries.

Normal Values

Normal vasculature

Possible Meanings of Abnormal Values

Angiomas
Arteriosclerosis
Arteriovenous occlusion
Arteriovenous stenosis
Cerebral aneurysms
Cerebral embolism
Cerebral thrombosis
Intracranial tumor
Pheochromocytoma
Vascular malformation
Vasospasm

Contributing Factors to Abnormal Values

- Any movement by the patient, including swallowing, may alter quality of films taken.

CONTRAINDICATIONS

- Patients who are allergic to iodine, shellfish, or contrast medium dye
- Patients with bleeding disorders
- Pregnant women
  Caution: A woman in her childbearing years should undergo radiography only during her menses or 12 to 14 days after its onset to avoid any exposure to a fetus.
- Patients who are unable to cooperate owing to age, mental status, pain, or other factors
- Patients with renal failure or those susceptible to dye-induced renal failure (dehydrated patients)
- Patients who would refuse surgery if a surgically correctable problem was found during the procedure
- Patients with poor cardiac function
- Patients with diseases of the liver or thyroid, diabetes, or multiple myeloma

Pre-Test Nursing Care

- Explain to the patient the purpose of the test. Provide any written teaching materials available on the subject. Note that discomfort involved with this test is primarily due to lying on a hard table for an extended period of time and the needle puncture. Explain that an intense hot flushing may be experienced for 15 to 30 seconds when the dye is injected.
- Check for allergies to iodine, shellfish, or contrast medium dye. Inform the radiologist of such possible allergy and obtain an order for an antihistamine and a corticosteroid to be administered before the test.
- Patients receiving metformin (Glucophage) for non–insulin-dependent diabetes mellitus should discontinue the drug 2 days before elective surgery or angiographic examinations. This is due to the possible occurrence of lactic acidosis, a potentially fatal complication of biguanide therapy.
- Baseline laboratory data (CBC, PT, PTT) is obtained.
- Note any medications, such as anticoagulants or aspirin, that may prolong bleeding.
- Fasting for at least 4 hours is required before the test.
- Obtain a signed informed consent.
- Administer any pretest sedation after consent form is signed.
- Assess and document patient's peripheral pulses bilaterally before the test. Mark the location of the pulses with a marking pen.
- Perform and document a baseline neurologic assessment.

Procedure

- The patient is assisted to a supine position on the examination table.
- A maintenance intravenous line is initiated.
- The area of the puncture site is cleansed and anesthetized. A venous catheter is inserted.
- Contrast dye is injected through the catheter by a mechanized injector at a preset rate. Its flow is monitored by means of fluoroscopy. Once the vessel to be studied is visualized, the dye injection is discontinued.
- Radiographic films are taken.

- After films of satisfactory quality are obtained, the catheter is removed and pressure held on the puncture site for several minutes.
- Gloves are worn throughout the procedure.

Post-Test Nursing Care

Possible complications:
  Allergic reaction to dye
  Bleeding at puncture site
  Infection at the puncture site
  Renal failure
  Thrombosis

- Most allergic reactions to radiopaque dye occur within 30 minutes of administration of the contrast medium. Observe the patient closely for respiratory distress, hypotension, edema, hives, rash, tachycardia, and/or laryngeal stridor. Emergency resuscitation equipment must be readily accessible.
- A pressure dressing is applied to the puncture site. Check the dressing for bleeding and the area around the puncture site for swelling at frequent intervals.
- Assess peripheral pulses for adequacy.
- Monitor vital signs and neurologic status until stable.
- Bed rest is encouraged for 4 hours post procedure.
- Teach the patient to monitor the site and to notify the health care provider if signs or symptoms of infection occur, such as drainage, redness, warmth, edema, pain at the site or fever.
- Monitor urinary output.
- Encourage fluid intake to promote dye excretion.
- Renal function should be assessed before metformin is restarted.
- Report abnormal findings to the primary care provider.

• • • • • • • • • • • • • • • • •

2,3-Diphosphoglycerate
(2,3-DPG)

2,3-Diphosphoglycerate (2,3-DPG) is the most abundant intracellular organic phosphate in the red blood cells. It is involved with oxygen transport to the tissues and binds to specific amino acid sites on proteins. The oxygen affinity of red blood cells is inversely proportional to 2,3-DPG levels. When hemoglobin levels are decreased, as in anemia, 2,3-DPG levels increase and cause decreased oxygen binding of hemoglobin. This results in increased amounts of oxygen being released to the tissues at lower oxygen tensions. Deficiency of 2,3-DPG results in defects in the release of oxygen to the tissues.

Normal Values

Female:	4.5–6.1 µmol/mL of packed cells
	8.4–18.8 µmol/g of hemoglobin
Male:	4.2–5.4 µmol/mL of packed cells
	9.2–17.4 µmol/mL of hemoglobin

Possible Meanings of Abnormal Values

Increased	Decreased
Anemia	Acidosis
Cardiac disease	2,3-DPG deficiency
Chronic renal failure	Polycythemia
Cirrhosis	Respiratory distress syndrome
Cystic fibrosis	
Hyperthyroidism	
Lung disease	
Pyruvate kinase deficiency	
Thyrotoxicosis	
Uremia	

Contributing Factors to Abnormal Values

- Factors that may *increase* 2,3-DPG levels: high altitudes, strenuous exercise.
- Factors that may *decrease* 2,3-DPG levels: acidosis, receipt of banked blood.

Pre-Test Nursing Care

- Explain to the patient the purpose of the test and the need for a blood sample to be drawn.
- No fasting is required before the test.

Procedure

- A 5-mL blood sample is drawn in a collection tube containing a silicone gel.
- Gloves are worn throughout the procedure.

Post-Test Nursing Care

- Apply pressure at venipuncture site. Apply dressing, periodically assessing for continued bleeding.
- Label the specimen and transport it to the laboratory.
- Report abnormal findings to the primary care provider.

· · · · · · · · · · · · · · · · · ·

Disseminated Intravascular Coagulation Screening
(DIC Screening)

Disseminated intravascular coagulation (DIC) is a paradoxical, often fatal, condition in which both clotting and bleeding occur at abnormally high levels. DIC can be triggered by a variety of conditions, including amniotic fluid embolism, extensive surgery, hemolytic transfusion reactions, massive tissue trauma, metastatic malignancies, premature separation of the placenta in pregnancy, retained dead fetus, septicemia, severe burns, and shock. When triggered, widespread

TABLE 7
DIC Tests, Expected Results, and Reference Pages

Test	Result in DIC	Page No.
Most Sensitive and Specific Tests		
Fibrin degradation products	Increased	224
Fibrinogen	Decreased	225
D-Dimer	Increased	181
Less Sensitive and Specific Tests		
Prothrombin time	Prolonged	397
Partial thromboplastin time	Prolonged	348
Thrombin time	Increased	459
Platelet count	Decreased	364
Least Sensitive and Specific Tests		
Euglobulin clot lysis	Normal or prolonged	213
Factor assays	Deficiencies present	133
Peripheral blood smear examination	Damaged red blood cells and decreased platelets	80

clotting occurs in small vessels of the body, causing clotting factors and platelets to be used up. Thus, the patient develops a bleeding disorder with the following abnormal test results: low fibrinogen, prolonged prothrombin time, prolonged partial thromboplastin time, reduced platelet count, and elevated fibrin degradation products. Patients with DIC may exhibit bleeding ranging from minimal bleeding from venipuncture sites or mucous membranes to profuse hemorrhage from all orifices. Patients may develop organ dysfunction, such as renal failure and pulmonary and multifocal central nervous system (CNS) infarctions due to microvascular occlusion and anoxic injury in the affected organs.

Several tests are used in the diagnosis of DIC. Each of these tests, shown in Table 7, are described in detail elsewhere in this text.

• • • • • • • • • • • • • • • •

Doppler Studies
(Doppler Ultrasonography)

Ultrasonography is a noninvasive method of diagnostic testing in which ultrasound waves are sent into the body with a small transducer pressed against the skin. The transducer not only sends the sound waves into the body but also receives any returning sound waves, which are deflected back as they bounce off various structures. The transducer converts the returning sound waves into electric signals that are then transformed by a computer into audible sounds (Doppler method).

This particular form of ultrasonography is used to evaluate blood flow in the major veins and arteries of the arms, legs, and neck. The sound waves strike moving red blood cells and are reflected back to that transducer. The sound that is emitted by the transducer corresponds to the velocity of the blood flow through the vessel. This provides valuable information used in the diagnosis of chronic venous insufficiency, venous thromboses, peripheral artery disease, arterial occlusion, abnormalities of carotid artery blood flow, and arterial trauma. It can also be used to monitor patients after arterial reconstruction and bypass graft surgery.

Normal Values

Normal Doppler signal with no evidence of vessel occlusion

Possible Meanings of Abnormal Values

Arterial occlusion
Arterial stenosis
Arteriosclerosis
Cerebrovascular disease
Deep vein thrombosis
Peripheral arterial disease
Renal disease
Venous disease
Venous occlusion

Contributing Factors to Abnormal Values

- The transducer must be in good contact with the skin as it is being moved. A lubricant, such as mineral oil, glycerin, or a water-based jelly, is used to ensure good contact with the skin.

Pre-Test Nursing Care

- Explain to the patient the purpose of the test. Provide any written teaching materials available on the subject. Note that there is no discomfort involved with this test.
- Explain the importance of limiting movement during the test to ensure accurate measurements.
- No fasting is required before the test.

Procedure

- The patient is assisted to a supine position on the ultrasonography table.
- *For peripheral arterial studies:*
  - A blood pressure cuff is wrapped about the extremity, pressure readings are taken, and waveforms are recorded for the arteries distal to the cuff location. The cuff application sites and the arteries assessed include:
    - Calf: dorsalis pedis, posterior tibial arteries
    - Thigh: popliteal artery
    - Forearm: radial and ulnar arteries
    - Upper arm: brachial artery
- *For peripheral venous studies:*
  - The transducer is placed over the appropriate vein and waveforms are recorded. Variations in the waveforms due to respiratory influences are noted.

D

- Veins to be tested: popliteal, superficial femoral, common femoral, posterior tibial vein, brachial, axillary, subclavian, and jugular.
- *For other studies:*
  - Other test sites include the supraorbital, common carotid, external carotid, internal carotid, and vertebral arteries.
- A coupling agent, such as a water-based gel, is applied to the area to be evaluated.
- A transducer is placed on the skin and moved as needed to provide good visualization of the structures.
- The sound waves are transformed into a visual display of waveforms on the monitor. Printed copies of this display are made.

Post-Test Nursing Care

- Cleanse the patient's skin of remaining coupling agent.
- Report abnormal findings to the primary care provider.

• • • • • • • • • • • • • • • •

D-Xylose Absorption Test
(Xylose Tolerance Test)

D-Xylose is a monosaccharide that is normally absorbed in the small intestine and excreted by the kidneys. It is not metabolized by the body, meaning its serum levels are direct reflections of intestinal absorption of the substance. Adequate intestinal absorption is indicated by high serum and urinary levels of the substance. Malabsorptive disorders affecting the proximal small intestine, such as sprue and celiac disease, result in decreased levels of D-xylose in the blood and urine.

This test is used to differentiate between patients with diarrhea owing to maldigestion from pancreatic and biliary dysfunction and those with diarrhea due to malabsorption such as Crohn's disease. It involves ingestion of D-xylose and collection of both blood and urine samples.

Normal Values

Adult

Serum:	25–40 mg/dL (1.67–2.66 mmol/L SI units) 2 hours after D-xylose ingestion
Urine:	4 g of D-xylose excreted in 5 hours

Child

Serum:	> 30 mg/dL (> 2.01 mmol/L SI units)
Urine:	16%–33% excreted in 5 hours

Possible Meanings of Abnormal Values

Increased	Decreased
Disaccharidase deficiencies	Alcoholism
Hodgkin's disease	Amyloidosis
Scleroderma	Ascites
	Celiac disease
	Crohn's disease
	Cystic fibrosis
	Diarrhea
	Hookworm
	Myxedema
	Rheumatoid arthritis
	Severe congestive heart failure
	Sprue
	Viral gastroenteritis
	Whipple's disease

Contributing Factors to Abnormal Values

- Physical activity will alter test results.
- Drugs that will *decrease* test results: aspirin, atropine, indomethacin.

CONTRAINDICATIONS

- Patients who are dehydrated.
- Patients with kidney dysfunction.

Pre-Test Nursing Care

- Explain to the patient the purpose of the test and the need for collection of both blood and urine samples.
- Fasting overnight before the test and during the test is required.
- Withhold medications that may alter the test results.
- Explain 5-hour urine collection procedure to the patient.
- Stress the importance of saving *all* urine in the 5-hour period. Instruct the patient to avoid contaminating the urine with toilet paper or feces.
- Inform the patient of the presence of a preservative in the collection bottle.

Procedure

- Remind the patient to remain on bed rest and NPO throughout the testing period, with the exception of the D-xylose ingestion.
- A 10-mL blood sample is drawn in a collection tube containing no additives.
- Collect the first-voided morning urine specimen.
- Send both the blood sample and urine specimen to the laboratory immediately.
- Administer 25 g of D-xylose dissolved in 8 ounces of water, followed by an additional 8 ounces of water. (For child dosage, check with reference laboratory.)
- Drawn an additional blood sample in 2 hours in an adult patient; in 1 hour in a child. Use a 10-mL collection tube containing no additives.

- Obtain the proper container containing the appropriate preservative from the laboratory.
- *All* urine for the next 5 hours is collected in the container, which is to be kept refrigerated or on ice.
- Gloves are to be worn whenever dealing with the specimen collection.

Post-Test Nursing Care

Possible complication: D-xylose ingestion may cause abdominal discomfort or mild diarrhea.

- Apply pressure at venipuncture sites. Apply dressing, periodically assessing for continued bleeding.
- Label the blood specimen and transport it to the laboratory.
- Label the urine container and transport it on ice to the laboratory as soon as possible after the end of the 5-hour collection period.
- Resume diet and medications as taken before the test.
- Report abnormal findings to the primary care provider.

• • • • • • • • • • • • • • • • •

Echocardiography
(Echo, Heart Sonogram)

Ultrasonography is a noninvasive method of diagnostic testing in which ultrasound waves are sent into the body with a small transducer pressed against the skin. The transducer not only sends the sound waves into the body but also receives any returning sound waves, which are deflected back as they bounce off various structures. The transducer converts the returning sound waves into electric signals that are then transformed by a computer into a visual display on a monitor.

Echocardiography is a particular type of ultrasonography in which the transducer is placed at an area on the chest, where bone and lung tissue are absent, so that the sound waves can be directed toward cardiac structures. This is normally in the third or fourth intercostal space to the left of the sternum.

Two techniques are used in echocardiography. In M-mode, or motion-mode, echocardiography, a single ultrasound beam is used, which records the motion and dimensions of intracardiac structures in a linear tracing. In two-dimensional, or cross-sectional, echocardiography, the ultrasound beam sweeps through an arc, giving a cross-sectional view of the heart. This information is converted to images shown on the oscilloscope that are videotaped for review by a cardiologist.

Normal Values

No abnormalities of the heart chambers, valves, blood flow, or muscle

Possible Meanings of Abnormal Values

Aortic valve abnormalities
Atrial regurgitation
Atrial septal defect
Atrial stenosis

Atrial tumor
Cardiomyopathy
Congenital heart disease
Endocarditis
Marfan's syndrome
Mitral stenosis
Mitral valve prolapse and regurgitation
Myocardial infarction
Patent ductus arteriosus
Pericardial effusion
Pericarditis
Subacute bacterial endocarditis
Transposition of the great arteries
Tricuspid atresia
Ventricular septal defect

Contributing Factors to Abnormal Values

- The transducer must be in good contact with the skin as it is being moved. A lubricant, such as mineral oil, glycerin, or a water-based jelly, is used to ensure good contact with the skin.
- Quality of the test results may be hindered in the presence of patient movement, chest wall abnormalities, chronic obstructive lung disease, and obesity.

CONTRAINDICATIONS

- Patients who are unable to cooperate owing to age, mental status, pain, or other factors

Pre-Test Nursing Care

- Explain to the patient the purpose of the test. Provide any written teaching materials available on the subject. Note that there is no discomfort involved with this test.
- Explain the importance of limiting movement during the test to ensure accurate movements.
- No fasting is required before the test.

Procedure

- The patient is assisted to a supine position on the ultrasonography table.
- A coupling agent, such as a water-based gel, is applied to the chest wall.
- A transducer is placed on the skin and moved as needed to provide good visualization of the cardiac structures.
- The sound waves are transformed into a visual display on the monitor. Printed copies of this display are made.
- The patient may also be placed on the left side to obtain additional views of the heart.

Post-Test Nursing Care

- Cleanse the patient's skin of remaining coupling agent.
- Report abnormal findings to the primary care provider.

• • • • • • • • • • • • • • • • •

Electrocardiography
(ECG, EKG, Electrocardiogram)

Electrocardiography is the recording of the electrical current generated by the heart. Electrical impulses, generated by the heart during its depolarization and repolarization, are detected by monitoring electrodes placed on the body. The graphic depiction of this electrical activity is called an electrocardiogram (ECG or EKG). The standard type of electrocardiogram performed is the 12-lead EKG, which measures the electrical activity by way of 12 leads: three standard limb leads, three augmented limb leads, and six chest leads. The ECG is recorded on special paper on which each marking represents 0.04 second. This standardized marking allows measurement of the duration of the various ECG components.

The ECG is composed of several waveforms, including the P wave, the QRS complex, the T wave, the ST segment, the PR interval, and possibly a U wave. These waveforms are shown in Figure 5. Each of the waveforms represents different aspects of cardiac depolarization and repolarization.

The *P wave* represents atrial muscle depolarization. This wave is 0.11 second or less in duration. The *QRS complex,* which includes the time from the beginning of the Q wave to the end of the S wave, represents ventricular muscle depolarization. The QRS complex is 0.04 to 0.10 second in duration. The *T wave,* which follows the QRS complex, represents ventricular muscle repolarization. The *U wave* is occasionally seen in patients with hypokalemia. It follows the T wave and is sometimes mistaken for an extra P wave. The *PR interval,* measured from the beginning of the P wave to the beginning of the Q wave, represents the time required for atrial depolarization and the delay of the impulse in the atrioventricular node before ventricular depolarization. The PR interval usually lasts from 0.12 to 0.20 second. The *ST segment,* from the end of the S wave to the beginning of the T wave, represents early ventricular repolarization. The *QT interval,* measured from the beginning of the Q wave to the end of the T wave, represents the total time for ventricular depolarization and repolarization.

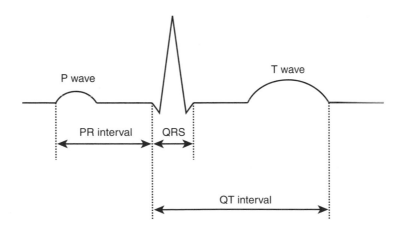

Figure 5 ECG waveforms. From Mudge, G.H. (1986). *Manual of electrocardiography* (2nd ed.). Boston: Little Brown. Reproduced by permission.

Normal Values

Normal rate, rhythm, and waveforms

Possible Meanings of Abnormal Values

Bundle branch blocks
Cardiac arrest
Conduction defects
Dysrhythmias
Electrolyte imbalances
Myocardial infarction
Myocardial ischemia
Pericarditis
Ventricular hypertrophy

Contributing Factors to Abnormal Values

- Interferences to the recording of the ECG are shown as artifacts. This may occur due to equipment failure, electrode adherence problems, electromagnetic interference, or patient movement.

Pre-Test Nursing Care

- Explain to the patient the purpose of the test and the need for electrodes to be attached to the chest and extremities. Note that the test causes no discomfort but that the patient will need to lie still and not speak during the procedure.
- No fasting is required before the test.

Procedure

- The patient is assisted to a supine position. The semi-Fowler's position may be used for patients with respiratory problems.
- Electrodes are applied:
  - one monitoring electrode is applied to the left arm, right arm, and left leg
  - a grounding electrode is placed on the right leg
  - a total of six electrode positions are used on the chest; the type of ECG machine used determines whether 1, 3, or all 6 of these are applied at one time.
- The electrodes used may be self-adhering disposable electrodes or reusable electrodes, which must be held in place with suction bulbs and with which electrode gel must be used.

Post-Test Nursing Care

- Remove the electrodes and cleanse the skin of any residual gel or adhesive.
- Report abnormal findings to the primary care provider.

• • • • • • • • • • • • • • • • •

Electroencephalography
(EEG)

In electroencephalography (EEG), the electrical activity of the brain is recorded. This is attainable by way of electrodes attached in several locations on the scalp that pick up electrical impulses from the superficial layers of the cerebral cortex and transmit them to an electroencephalograph for recording. The resultant waveforms are then analyzed. The test is used to diagnose epilepsy, intracranial abscesses, and tumors; to evaluate the brain's electrical activity in cases of possible cerebral damage such as that due to head injury or meningitis; and to confirm brain death, in which electrical activity of the brain is absent.

Normal Values

Normal brain waves

Possible Meanings of Abnormal Values

Brain death
Cerebral infarct
Encephalitis
Epilepsy
Increased intracranial pressure
Intracranial abscess
Intracranial hemorrhage
Intracranial tumor
Meningitis

Contributing Factors to Abnormal Values

- Drugs that may alter test results: anticonvulsants, barbiturates, caffeine, sedatives, tranquilizers.
- Hypoglycemia may affect the EEG results.
- Movement of the head, body, eyes, or tongue can cause changes in the brain wave patterns.

Pre-Test Nursing Care

- Explain to the patient the purpose of the test and the procedure to be done. Explain that there is no discomfort involved with this test. Note that no electricity enters the patient from the machine.
- No fasting is required before the test. However, no caffeine-containing drinks should be consumed within 8 hours of the test.
- Instruct the patient to shampoo the hair the night before the test to aid in securing the electrodes during the test.
- If a sleep-deprivation study is ordered in which the patient will need to fall asleep during the test, the patient should sleep as little as possible the night before the test.
- Medications that might influence test results should be withheld, if possible.

Procedure

- The procedure is usually conducted in an EEG laboratory. If testing for brain death, a portable EEG machine may be used at the bedside.
- The patient may either sit in a lounge chair or lie supine on a bed.
- Approximately 20 electrodes are applied to the scalp by the EEG technician in a standardized pattern using electrode paste. Grounding electrodes are applied to each ear.
- The patient is instructed to lie still with the eyes closed while the EEG recording is made. Any movements that might affect the EEG are documented.
- The recording is interrupted periodically to allow the patient to move into a more comfortable position.
- Additional components of the EEG that might be performed include:
  - *Hyperventilation:* The patient breathes rapidly for 3 minutes. The resulting alkalosis may elicit brain wave patterns associated with seizure disorders.
  - *Photostimulation:* A strobe light is flashed over the patient's face. This may elicit brain wave patterns characteristic of partial or generalized seizures.
  - *Sleep EEG:* The EEG is recorded while the patient is falling asleep, during sleep, and while the patient is waking. This is used to detect brain wave abnormalities that occur during sleep, such as those associated with frontal lobe epilepsy.

Post-Test Nursing Care

- Resume medications as taken before the test, with physician approval.
- Observe the patient for any seizure activity.
- After removal of the electrodes, the electrode paste is removed. Oil, acetone, or witch hazel may help to remove the paste; then the hair should be shampooed.
- Report abnormal findings to the primary care provider.

• • • • • • • • • • • • • • • •

Electrolytes

See:
Anion Gap
Calcium, Blood
Calcium, Urine
Chloride, Blood
Chloride, Urine
Magnesium
Phosphorus
Potassium, Blood
Potassium, Urine
Sodium, Blood
Sodium, Urine
Total Carbon Dioxide Content

• • • • • • • • • • • • • • • •

Electromyography
(EMG, Electromyelography)

E lectromyography (EMG) is the recording of electrical activity in skeletal muscle groups. The test involves insertion of needle electrodes into the muscle. The EMG then records the state of the muscle at rest and during voluntary contraction. The information assists in determining whether the cause of muscle weakness is due to *myopathy,* a disease of the striated muscle fibers or cell membranes, or due to *neuropathy,* a disease of the lower motor neuron.

Normal Values
Normal muscle electrical activity

Possible Meanings of Abnormal Values
Amyotrophic lateral sclerosis
Bell's palsy
Beriberi
Carpal tunnel syndrome
Dermatomyositis
Diabetic peripheral neuropathy
Eaton-Lambert syndrome
Motor neuron disease
Muscular dystrophy
Myasthenia gravis
Myopathy
Myositis
Poliomyelitis
Polymyositis
Radiculopathy

Contributing Factors to Abnormal Values
- Drugs that may interfere with test results: anticholinergics, cholinergics, skeletal muscle relaxants.

CONTRAINDICATIONS
- Patients with bleeding disorders

Pre-Test Nursing Care
- Explain to the patient the purpose of the test and the procedure to be performed. Note that discomfort involved with the test is due to the insertion of the needle electrodes. Muscle aching often occurs after the procedure.
- No fasting is required before the test.
- Caffeine and nicotine should be avoided for 3 hours before the test.
- Obtain a signed informed consent.

- The EMG may alter the results of enzyme tests, such as asparate aminotransferase, creatine kinase, or lactic dehydrogenase. If such tests are ordered, blood samples should be drawn before or 5 days after the EMG.

Procedure

- The skin is cleansed with alcohol.
- A needle that acts as a recording electrode is inserted into the muscle being studied.
- A reference electrode is placed nearby on the skin surface.
- While the muscle is at rest, the EMG display is observed for any evidence of spontaneous electrical activity.
- The patient is then asked to slowly contract the muscle.
- Recordings are made of the muscle activity at both rest and during muscle contraction.

Post-Test Nursing Care

- The needle is removed from the muscle and the site observed for bleeding.
- Mild analgesics may be needed to relieve muscle aching.
- Report abnormal findings to the primary care provider.

• • • • • • • • • • • • • • • •

Electroneurography
(ENG, Electromyoneurography)

Electroneurography (ENG) is the recording of nerve conduction velocity to assist in the evaluation of peripheral nerve disease or injury. An indication of the condition of the peripheral motor and sensory nerves is the nerve conduction velocity that occurs when a stimulus is applied through a surface electrode over a nerve. The test involves initiating an electrical impulse at a proximal site on a nerve and recording the time required for that impulse to reach a distal site on the same nerve. Nerve conduction velocities remain normal in the presence of muscle disease but are slowed in peripheral nerve diseases.

Normal Values

Normal nerve conduction velocity rates

Possible Meanings of Abnormal Values

Carpal tunnel syndrome
Diabetic peripheral neuropathy
Guillain-Barré syndrome
Muscular dystrophy
Myasthenia gravis
Peripheral nerve disease
Peripheral nerve injury

Contributing Factors to Abnormal Values
- Severe pain may cause inaccurate results.
- Nerve conduction velocity slows with age.

Pre-Test Nursing Care
- Explain to the patient the purpose of the test and the procedure to be performed. Note that discomfort involved with the test is due to minor electrical stimuli administered during the procedure.
- No fasting is required before the test.
- Obtain a signed informed consent.

Procedure
- The skin is cleansed with alcohol.
- A recording electrode is applied to the skin overlying a muscle innervated only by the nerve being tested.
- A reference electrode is placed nearby on the skin surface.
- The nerve is stimulated by a shock-emitting device at a nearby location.
- The time between the nerve impulse and muscle contraction is measured as the *distal latency*.
- The nerve is again stimulated, but at a location proximal to the area of suspected disease or injury.
- The time between the site of conduction and muscle contraction is measured as the *total latency*.
- The conduction velocity is calculated in meters per second by dividing the distance between the electrodes (in meters) by the difference between total latency and distal latency (in seconds).

Post-Test Nursing Care
- The electrodes and paste are removed, and the skin is cleansed.
- Mild analgesics may be needed to relieve muscle aching.
- Report abnormal findings to the primary care provider.

• • • • • • • • • • • • • • •

Electronystagmography
(ENG, Calibration Test, Caloric Testing, Gaze Nystagmus Test, Oculovestibular Reflex, Optokinetics Test, Pendulum Tracking, Positional Test)

Electronystagmography is the recording of eye movements in response to various stimuli. This test evaluates the oculovestibular reflex, which involves the interaction of the muscles controlling eye movement (ocular system) and the vestibular system. This reflex results in the appearance of involuntary back-and-forth eye movement, known as *nystagmus*. When the head is turned, the eyes normally deviate slowly in the opposite direction. On reaching the limit of their movement, they tend to quickly return to the center and the nystagmus ceases. Abnormal nystagmus involves the same type of movement, but it is prolonged. This can result from peripheral lesions, such as involvement of the vestibular portion of the eighth cranial nerve (acoustic nerve) or from cerebellar or brain stem involvement.

Because abnormal nystagmus is the primary sign of vestibular problems, electronystagmography can assist in identifying the cause of dizziness, vertigo, tinnitus, or hearing loss. The test is actually a set of tests, including the calibration test, the gaze nystagmus test, pendulum tracking, optokinetics tests, positional tests, and the caloric test. Recording of eye movement during each of these tests is accomplished through electrodes placed near the outer canthus of each eye (for detection of lateral nystagmus), electrodes placed above and below one eye (for detection of vertical nystagmus), and a ground electrode placed above the bridge of the nose.

Normal Values

Normal waveform patterns

Possible Meanings of Abnormal Values

Brain stem lesion
Cerebellum lesion
Cerebrum lesion
Cranial nerve VIII tumor
Congenital abnormalities
Hypothyroidism
Infection
Inflammation
Labyrinthitis
Meniere's disease
Multiple sclerosis
Ototoxicity

Contributing Factors to Abnormal Values

- Drugs that may alter test results: antivertigo drugs, CNS depressants, CNS stimulants.
- Blinking of the eyes, drowsiness, or improperly applied electrodes will alter test results.

 CONTRAINDICATIONS

- Patients with perforated eardrums
- Patients with pacemakers
- Patients unable to cooperate with the examination

Pre-Test Nursing Care

- Explain to the patient the purpose of the test and the procedures to be conducted.
- No fasting is required before the test.
- Alcohol, caffeine, and medications that may alter test results should be withheld for 24 to 48 hours before the test. Verify with the physician.
- Inspect the ear canals for intact tympanic membranes. Remove any excess wax from the canals.

E

Procedure

- Electrode paste is rubbed into the patient's skin for electrode placement at each of following five points: one lateral electrode at the outer canthus of each eye, one electrode above the left eye and one below the left eye for recording of vertical nystagmus, and one electrode in the center of the forehead.
- The contact on each electrode is cleansed with alcohol and allowed to dry.
- Electrodes are then placed at each of the five points, and an adhesive collar is used to hold each in place.
- During any of the subsequent testing, documentation is made of any complaints of dizziness by the patient.

Calibration Test

This test is used to calibrate the stylus for recording of each of the subsequent tests.

- The patient is assisted into a sitting position on the examination table.
- The patient looks straight ahead at a light. The light is moved 10 degrees to the right, back to center, and then 10 degrees to the left. The stylus is adjusted to correspond with these movements.

Gaze Nystagmus Test

- The patient may be seated or be in a supine position.
- Eye movement is recorded for 30 seconds while the patient's eyes are closed.
- To help the patient avoid thinking of the testing, provide an arithmetic problem for the patient to calculate during the testing period.

PendulumTracking

- The patient looks straight ahead and follows the movement of a pendulum for 20 seconds.
- This is followed by a 30-second recording while the patient looks straight ahead with the eyes closed.

Optokinetics Test

- The patient follows a target moving across the visual field from left to right. As one target leaves the visual field to the right, another target enters from the left. A 20-second recording is made, followed by a 30-second recording with the patient's eye closed.
- The procedure is repeated with the targets moving from right to left.

Positional Test

- A 5-second baseline recording of eye movement is made.
- With the patient's eyes closed, a 30-second recording is made after each of the following movements by the patient.
  - From a sitting position, the patient moves the head quickly to the right. After 30 seconds of recording, the patient slowly returns the head to the center.
  - From a sitting position, the patient moves the head quickly to the left. After 30 seconds of recording, the patient slowly returns the head to the center.
  - From a sitting position, the patient quickly assumes a supine position. A 30-second recording is made.
  - From a supine position, the patient quickly assumes a sitting position. A 30-second recording is made.
  - From a supine position, the patient quickly turns the entire body and head to the right. After 30 seconds of recording, the patient slowly returns to the supine position.

- From a supine position, the patient quickly turns the entire body and head to the left. After 30 seconds of recording, the patient slowly returns to the supine position.
- The patient is assisted to move on the table so that when a supine position is assumed, the head will hang over the end of the table. From a sitting position, the patient quickly lies down, allowing the head to hang over the edge. A 30-second recording is made.
- From a supine position with the head hanging over the edge of the table, the patient quickly sits up. A 30-second recording is made.
- From a sitting position, the patient quickly lies down while turning the head to the right and allows the head to hang over the edge. A 30-second recording is made.
- From a sitting position, the patient quickly lies down while turning the head to the left and allows the head to hang over the edge. A 30-second recording is made.

Caloric Test

- The patient is positioned with the head of the bed elevated 30 degrees.
- Protect the patient with towels and place an emesis basin under the ear being tested.
- The patient closes the eyes.
- Inform the patient that water is about to be introduced into the ear.
- Introduce the water so that it directly hits the tympanic membrane for 30 seconds.
- A 60-second recording of eye movement is made with the eyes closed, then 10 seconds with the eyes open and fixed straight ahead, then closed again until the nystagmus subsides or 3 minutes, whichever occurs first.
- This procedure is conducted a total of four times:
    - In the left ear, using water that is 86° F (30° C)
    - In the right ear, using water that is 86° F (30° C)
    - In the left ear, using water that is 111.2° F (44° C)
    - In the right ear, using water that is 111.2° F (44° C)
- *Note*: If patient has perforated tympanic membranes, this test is modified by using water-filled fingercots.

Post-Test Nursing Care

- Remove the electrodes and cleanse the patient's skin of any remaining paste.
- Assess the patient for weakness, dizziness, or nausea.
- Allow patient to rest as needed, and then assist with ambulation, if needed.
- Report abnormal findings to the primary care provider.

• • • • • • • • • • • • • • • • •

Electrophysiologic Study
(EPS, Bundle of His Procedure)

Electrophysiologic study (EPS) involves the introduction of an electrode catheter into the right atrium and the right ventricle. The catheter is usually inserted into a peripheral vein because of the greater risk for bleeding when using the arterial system for such testing. Once in place, the catheter is used to perform programmed electrical stimulation of the heart.

EPS is very useful in evaluating the conduction system of the heart. It is also used to attempt to induce any arrhythmia that may be affecting the patient. By stimulating the occurrence of the arrhythmia during EPS, the physician can, under controlled conditions, determine the appropriate treatment for the problem. It also provides information regarding how well antiarrhythmic drugs are working by noting how easily the arrhythmia is able to be induced.

Normal Values

Normal conduction intervals, refractory periods, and recovery times shown on EKG. No arrhythmias induced.

Possible Meanings of Abnormal Values

Atrioventricular node defects
Cardiac arrhythmias
Electroconduction defects
Heart blocks
Sinoatrial node defects

Contributing Factors to Abnormal Values

- Drugs that may alter test results: analgesics, antiarrhythmics, sedatives, tranquilizers.

CONTRAINDICATIONS

- Patients with acute myocardial infarction
- Patients who are unable to cooperate due to age, mental status, pain, or other factors

Pre-Test Nursing Care

- Explain to the patient the purpose of the test. Provide any written teaching materials available on the subject. Note that discomfort involved with this test is due to catheter insertion, but that it will be minimized by local anesthesia to the area. The patient may also experience flushing, anxiety, dizziness, and palpitations during the procedure.
- Fasting for at least 8 hours is required before the test.
- For an initial study, antiarrhythmic medications may be discontinued for several days before the test, if possible.
- Obtain a signed informed consent.

Procedure

- The patient is assisted to a supine position on the examination table in the cardiac catheterization laboratory.
- A maintenance intravenous line is initiated.
- Cardiac monitoring is initiated.
- Resuscitation and suctioning equipment should be readily available.
- The staff members should converse with the patient throughout the procedure to both allay patient fears, and to assess the patient's level of consciousness.
- The area of the puncture site, usually the femoral vein, is cleansed and then anesthetized.
- The needle puncture of the vein is made and the catheter is advanced to the heart. Positioning is monitored via fluoroscopy.
- Once the catheter is in the correct position, a baseline electrocardiagram is recorded.

- Pacing is then used to induce arrhythmias. Sustained arrhythmias are treated with pacing and, if unsuccessful, by cardioversion/defibrillation.
- When the procedure is completed, the catheter is removed and a pressure dressing is applied to the site.
- Gloves are worn throughout the procedure.

Post-Test Nursing Care

Possible complications:
> **Cardiac arrhythmias**
> **Catheter-induced embolic stroke or myocardial infarction**
> **Hemorrhage**
> **Peripheral vascular problems**
> **Phlebitis at catheter insertion site**

- Monitor vital signs and neurologic status every 15 minutes for 1 hour, then every 30 minutes for 2 hours, then every hour for 4 hours, and then every 4 hours.
- Assess the color, movement, temperature, and sensation (CMTS) and the pulse(s) of the affected extremity with each vital sign assessment. Compare with the other extremity.
- Check the dressing for bleeding and the area around the puncture site for swelling each time the vital signs are assessed.
- The patient is to remain on bed rest for at least 8 hours with the affected extremity immobilized.
- Resume medications as ordered.
- Report abnormal findings to the primary care provider.

• • • • • • • • • • • • • • • • •

Endoscopic Retrograde Cholangiopancreatography
(ERCP)

Endoscopic retrograde cholangiopancreatography (ERCP) is the radiographic viewing of the pancreatic ducts and the hepatobiliary tree through an endoscope. The procedure involves injection of a contrast medium through the ampulla of Vater. ERCP and percutaneous transhepatic cholangiography are the only procedures that allow direct visualization of the biliary and pancreatic ducts. Because of the comparatively low risk of complications, ERCP is the most commonly performed of these two procedures. The procedure is especially useful in the evaluation of patients with jaundice, because visualization of the biliary ducts can occur even when the patient's bilirubin level is high. Thus the test can provide information helpful in the diagnosis of obstructive jaundice and cancer of the duodenal papilla, pancreas, and biliary ducts, and in locating calculi and stenosis in the pancreatic ducts and hepatobiliary tree.

Normal Values

Normal size and patency of the biliary and bile ducts
Absence of calculi

Possible Meanings of Abnormal Values

Biliary cirrhosis
Carcinoma of the bile ducts
Carcinoma of the duodenal papilla
Carcinoma of the head of the pancreas
Chronic pancreatitis
Pancreatic cysts
Pancreatic fibrosis
Pancreatic tumor
Papillary stenosis
Pseudocysts
Sclerosing cholangitis
Stones of the bile or pancreatic ducts
Strictures of the bile or pancreatic ducts

Contributing Factors to Abnormal Values

- Retained barium from other examinations, vomiting, and diarrhea will affect test results.

CONTRAINDICATIONS

- Pregnant women
  Caution: A woman in her childbearing years should undergo radiography only during her menses or 12 to 14 days after its onset to avoid any exposure to a fetus.
- Patients with hypersensitivity to iodine, seafood, or contrast media
- Patients with known pancreatic and biliary problems: pancreatitis, pancreatic pseudocysts, stricture or obstruction of the esophagus or duodenum
- Patients with cardiac and respiratory disease.
- Patients who are unable to cooperate owing to age, mental status, pain, or other factors

Pre-Test Nursing Care

- *Note*: If a barium swallow or an upper gastrointestinal and small-bowel series test is ordered, these should be completed *after* the ERCP is performed. Otherwise the barium sulfate ingested during the other examinations may obscure the films made of the gallbladder.
- Explain to the patient the purpose of the test and the benefits and risks associated with the test. Provide any written teaching materials available on the subject.
- Obtain a signed informed consent from the patient.
- Inform the radiologist of any potential allergy to the contrast dye and obtain an order for an antihistamine and a corticosteroid to be given before the procedure.
- Patients receiving metformin (Glucophage) for non–insulin-dependent diabetes mellitus should discontinue the drug 2 days before elective surgery or angiographic examinations. This is due to the possible occurrence of lactic acidosis, a potentially fatal complication of biguanide therapy.
- The patient is to be NPO for 12 hours before the test.
- Instruct the patient to remove all objects containing metal, such as jewelry or undergarments, because these will show on the film.

Procedure

- An intravenous infusion of normal saline solution is started.
- A topical anesthetic is applied to the oropharyngeal area.
- The patient is placed in a left lateral position.
- A narcotic or sedative/hypnotic is administered.
- The endoscope is inserted through the mouth, esophagus, and stomach and then advanced to the duodenum.
- The patient is assisted to a prone position.
- An anticholinergic drug such as atropine or glucagon is given intravenously to reduce duodenal spasm and to relax the ampulla of Vater.
- A catheter is inserted through the ampulla and into the common bile or pancreatic ducts.
- The contrast medium is injected and several films are taken.

Post-Test Nursing Care

Possible complications:
> **Cholangitis**
> **Pancreatitis**
> **Perforation of ducts**
> **Urinary retention**

- Observe for indications of cholangitis (hyperbilirubinemia, fever, chills) and pancreatitis (upper left quadrant pain, tenderness, elevated serum amylase levels, and transient hyperbilirubinemia).
- Assess the patient's vital signs until stable.
- Withhold food and fluids until the gag reflex returns.
- Some abdominal discomfort may be present for several hours post procedure. However, prolonged, sharp abdominal pain, especially in conjunction with nausea or vomiting, is to be reported to the physician.
- Report abnormal findings to the primary care provider.

• • • • • • • • • • • • • • • • • •

Erythrocyte Sedimentation Rate
(ESR, Sedimentation Rate, Sed Rate, Westergren, Wintrobe)

The erythrocyte sedimentation rate (ESR) is a very nonspecific test for inflammatory and necrotic conditions. The ESR may also be increased in situations of physiologic stress, such as pregnancy. In these types of conditions, there is a change in blood proteins that leads to a clumping of red blood cells. The ESR measures the speed with which erythrocytes settle in a tube of blood that has been mixed with an anticoagulant. Cells that have clumped due to inflammatory and necrotic conditions settle more rapidly than single cells. Thus, the ESR (expressed in mm/h), would be increased in inflammatory and necrotic conditions.

There are several different methods available for testing the ESR. The simplest and most commonly used is the Westergren method. The Wintrobe method, although more complex, is considered more accurate. There is a direct relationship between the ESR and the course of disease. Thus, as the disease improves, owing to drug therapy, the ESR decreases.

Normal Values

Westergren Method

Female: 1–30 mm/h
Male: 1–13 mm/h

Wintrobe Method

Female: 1–20 mm/h
Male: 1–9 mm/h

Possible Meanings of Abnormal Values

Increased	Decreased
Anemia	Congestive heart failure
Coccidioidomycosis	Factor V deficiency
Crohn's disease	Hypoalbuminemia
Hemolytic anemia	Poikilocytosis
Infection	Polycythemia vera
Inflammatory process	Sickle cell anemia
Malignancies	
Myocardial infarction	
Osteomyelitis	
Pain	
Polymyalgia rheumatica	
Rheumatoid arthritis	
Systemic lupus erythematosus	
Temporal (giant cell) arteritis	
Tissue injury	

Contributing Factors to Abnormal Values

- The ESR may be increased during menstruation, after the 12th week of pregnancy, post partum, and in women older than the age of 70.
- The ESR may be decreased in the presence of elevated white blood cell count, albumin, and lipids.
- Drugs that may *increase* the ESR: dextran, heparin, oral contraceptives.
- Drugs that may *decrease* the ESR: albumin, aspirin, corticotropin, cortisone, lecithin, steroids.

Pre-Test Nursing Care

- Explain to the patient the purpose of the test and the need for a blood sample to be drawn.
- No fasting is required before the test.

Procedure

- A 5-mL blood sample is drawn in a collection tube containing EDTA.
- Gloves are worn throughout the procedure.

Post-Test Nursing Care

- Invert and gently mix the sample and the anticoagulant (EDTA).
- Apply pressure at venipuncture site. Apply dressing, periodically assessing for continued bleeding.
- Label the specimen and transport it to the laboratory immediately.
- Report abnormal findings to the primary care provider.

• • • • • • • • • • • • • • •

E

Esophageal Manometry
(Acid Reflux Test, Bernstein Test, Esophageal Function Studies)

Esophageal manometry is used to assess the esophagus for normal contractile activity. The lower esophageal sphincter (LES) pressure is measured, and recordings are made of the duration and sequence of peristaltic contractions. The test is conducted when the patient is experiencing difficulty in swallowing, heartburn, regurgitation, or vomiting or has chest pain for which no explanation has been found. The test involves placement of a manometric catheter at various levels in the esophagus. A pressure transducer in the catheter is used to obtain baseline pressure measurements. The patient is then asked to swallow, after which esophageal sphincter pressures are measured and peristaltic contractions are recorded. Two other aspects of the test involve testing for acid reflux and Bernstein (acid perfusion) testing.

Normal Values

Pressure at the lower esophageal sphincter: 10–22 mm Hg
Normal peristaltic waves present
pH in esophagus: > 5
Negative acid reflux and Bernstein tests

Possible Meanings of Abnormal Values

Achalasia
Diffuse spasm of the esophagus
Esophageal scleroderma
Gastric acid reflux
Reflux esophagitis

Contributing Factors to Abnormal Values

- Drugs that may *increase* esophageal pH: adrenergic blockers, alcohol, cholinergics, corticosteroids, reserpine.
- Drugs that may *decrease* esophageal pH: antacids, anticholinergics, histamine-2 blockers.

CONTRAINDICATIONS

- Patients who are unable to cooperate owing to age, mental status, pain, or other factors
- Patients with unstable vital signs

Pre-Test Nursing Care

- Explain to the patient the purpose of the test. Provide any written teaching materials available on the subject. Explain to the patient that the test involves the passage of small tubes into the esophagus, which may cause the throat to be sore for a short time after the procedure.
- Fasting for 8 hours is required before the test.
- Drugs that may alter test results are withheld before the test, if possible.
- Tobacco and alcohol are to be avoided for 24 hours before the test.

Procedure

- The patient is asked to swallow two or three very small tubes. Small holes along the sides of the tubes allow for pressure measurements to be made.
- The tubes are passed into the stomach and then pulled back up into the esophagus until a large change in pressure is noted. This is the location for the measurement of the lower esophageal sphincter (LES) pressure.
- The patient is then asked to swallow, during which recordings of the LES pressure and peristaltic contractions are made.
- For *acid reflux* testing, a 0.1 N hydrochloric acid solution is instilled in the stomach. The pH of the esophagus is then measured. If the pH decreases, gastroesophageal (acid) reflux is present.
- For *Bernstein* testing, normal saline is first infused into the esophagus as a control. Next, 0.1 N hydrochloric acid solution is instilled for 10 minutes. This is done as an attempt to reproduce symptoms of heartburn or chest discomfort. If the patient complains of discomfort during the acid instillation, the test is considered positive.

Post-Test Nursing Care

- Clamp the tubes and remove. Wear gloves during this activity.
- Encourage use of throat lozenges for sore throat, if needed.
- Resume medications as taken before the test.
- Report abnormal findings to the primary care provider.

● ● ● ● ● ● ● ● ● ● ● ● ● ● ● ● ●

Esophagogastroduodenoscopy
(EGD, Esophagoscopy, Gastroscopy, Upper Gastrointestinal Endoscopy)

Esophagogastroduodenoscopy (EGD) is the direct visualization of the esophagus, stomach, and upper duodenum through the use of a flexible fiberoptic endoscope. This endoscope is a multilumen instrument that allows viewing of the organ linings, insufflation of air, aspiration of fluid, removal of foreign objects, obtaining of tissue biopsy samples, and passage of a laser beam for obliteration of abnormal tissue or control of bleeding.

Normal Values

Normal esophagus, stomach, and duodenum

Possible Meanings of Abnormal Values

Diverticula
Duodenitis
Esophageal hiatal hernia
Esophageal stenosis
Esophagitis
Gastritis
Mallory-Weiss syndrome
Pyloric stenosis
Tumors
Ulcers
Varices

Contributing Factors to Abnormal Values

- Retention of barium after an upper gastrointestinal series hinders successful completion of this test.

CONTRAINDICATIONS

- Patients with large aortic aneurysm
- Patients with recent gastrointestinal surgery
- Patients with recent ulcer perforation
- Patients with Zenker's (esophageal) diverticulum
- Patients unable to cooperate with the examination

Pre-Test Nursing Care

- Explain to the patient the purpose of the test. Provide any written teaching materials available on the subject. Inform the patient that a topical anesthetic will be used on the throat to minimize discomfort during scope insertion. Explain that pressure in the stomach may be experienced during movement of the endoscope and during insufflation with air or carbon dioxide.
- Obtain a signed informed consent.
- Fasting for 8 to 12 hours is required before the test.
- Dentures are removed.
- Resuscitation and suctioning equipment should be readily available.
- Administer pre-procedure medications as ordered. An anticholinergic such as atropine may be used to decrease bronchial secretions. A medication such as meperidine, diazepam, or midazolam hydrochloride may be used for sedation and relief of anxiety.

Procedure

- The patient is assisted into the left lateral decubitus position on the endoscopy table.
- Baseline vital signs are obtained. Periodic vital sign assessment is performed during the procedure.

- A maintenance intravenous infusion is initiated.
- A topical anesthetic is sprayed into the throat.
- The endoscope is inserted into the mouth and passed through the esophagus and stomach and into the duodenum.
- The anatomy of the esophagus, stomach, and duodenum is inspected. Biopsy forceps may be used to remove a tissue specimen, or a cytology bronchial brush may be used to obtain cells from the surface of a lesion. Removal of foreign bodies is accomplished, if needed.
- Videotaping of the procedure is often done via a camera attached to the endoscope.
- Gloves are worn throughout the procedure.

Post-Test Nursing Care

Possible complications:

Aspiration of gastric contents
Bleeding
Perforation of esophagus, stomach, or duodenum
Oversedation

- Monitor vital signs every 15 minutes until stable.
- Observe the patient for indications of the following types of perforation: *esophageal perforation* (pain on swallowing and with neck movement), *thoracic perforation* (substernal or epigastric pain which increases with breathing or movement), *diaphragmatic perforation* (shoulder pain or dyspnea), and *gastric perforation* (abdominal or back pain, cyanosis, fever).
- Oversedation of the patient may require administration of a narcotic antagonist, such as naloxone.
- Withhold fluids and food until the gag reflex returns (approximately 2 hours).
- Provide an emesis basis for the patient. Instruct the patient to spit out saliva rather than swallow it until the gag reflex returns.
- Inform the patient that a bloated feeling is normal.
- Report abnormal findings to the primary care provider.

• • • • • • • • • • • • • • • •

Estradiol Receptor and Progesterone Receptor in Breast Cancer
(ER Assay, PR Assay)

Estradiol, which is produced primarily by the ovaries, and progesterone, which is produced by the corpus luteum of the ovary, may both create a hormonal environment suitable for growth of some types of breast cancer. In this test, estradiol and progesterone receptors in the cells of a sample of breast cancer tissue are measured to decide whether the tumor is likely to respond to treatments aimed at reducing the levels of the hormone. Approximately one half of the tumors found to be estradiol positive will respond to endocrine therapy, whereas estradiol-negative tumors rarely respond to such therapy.

Normal Values

Estradiol:	negative; < 3 fmol/mg of protein
Progesterone:	negative; < 5 fmol/mg of protein

Possible Meanings of Abnormal Values

Not applicable

Contributing Factors to Abnormal Values

- Antiestrogen drugs taken within the 2 months before the test may cause a *negative* estradiol receptor.

Pre-Test Nursing Care

- Explain to the patient the purpose of the test and the sampling procedure.
- No fasting is required before the test.

Procedure

- The skin is cleansed with an antiseptic and draped.
- A local anesthetic is usually administered.
- At least 1 g of breast tissue is removed by excision or needle biopsy.
- Gloves are worn throughout the procedure.

Post-Test Nursing Care

- The tissue sample is labeled and taken immediately to the laboratory to be frozen. If the sample is not frozen within 20 minutes, falsely low results will occur.
- At the conclusion of the procedure apply a dressing to the site, periodically assessing for continued bleeding.
- Administer pain medication as needed.
- Report abnormal findings to the primary care provider.

• • • • • • • • • • • • • • • •

Estrogen
(Estrogen Total, Estrogen Fractions, Estradiol, Estriol)

Estrogen is present in the body in several forms, including estradiol, estriol, and estrone. Because estrogen is produced by the adrenal cortex, the ovaries, and testes, determination of estrogen levels can be used in evaluation of all three glands. *Estradiol* is the most active of the estrogen forms, stimulating endometrial growth. It also suppresses the production of follicle-stimulating hormone (FSH) and stimulates production of luteinizing hormone (LH). *Estriol* is monitored during pregnancy to assess fetal and placental function. *Estrone* is converted from androstenedione in adipose tissue. Its function is not clearly understood, but increased estrone levels, when unopposed by progestone, have been associated with an increased risk of endometrial cancer.

Normal Values

Female:
  Premenopausal: 23–261 pg/mL (84–1325 pmol/L SI units)
  Postmenopausal: < 30 pg/mL (< 110 pmol/L SI units)
  Prepubertal: < 20 pg/mL (< 73 pmol/L SI units)
Male: < 50 pg/mL (< 184 pmol/L SI units)

Possible Meanings of Abnormal Values

Increased	Decreased
Adrenal hyperplasia	Amenorrhea
Adrenal tumor	Anorexia nervosa
Cirrhosis	Hypogonadism
Estrogen-secreting ovarian tumor	Hypopituitarism
Hepatic failure	Menopause
Klinefelter's syndrome	Ovarian failure
Precocious puberty	
Renal failure	
Stein-Leventhal syndrome	
Testicular tumor	

Contributing Factors to Abnormal Values

- Hemolysis of the blood sample may alter test results.
- Drugs that may *increase* estrogen levels: ampicillin, cascara, diethylstilbestrol, estrogens, hydrochlorothiazide, meprobamate, oral contraceptives, phenazopyridine hydrochloride, prochlorperazine, tetracycline.
- Drugs that may *decrease* estrogen levels: clomiphene citrate, dexamethasone, estrogen blockers.

Pre-Test Nursing Care

- Explain to the patient the purpose of the test and the need for a blood sample to be drawn.
- No fasting is required before the test.
- If possible, withhold drugs that may alter test results.

Procedure

- A 10-mL blood sample is drawn in a collection tube containing no additives.
- Gloves are worn throughout the procedure.

Post-Test Nursing Care

- Apply pressure at venipuncture site. Apply dressing, periodically assessing for continued bleeding.
- Label the specimen and transport it to the laboratory.
- Resume medications as taken before the test.
- Report abnormal findings to the primary care provider.

• • • • • • • • • • • • • • •

Euglobulin Lysis Time
(Euglobulin Clot Lysis, Fibrinolysis)

This test is used to evaluate systemic fibrinolysis, to monitor thrombolytic therapy in patients with acute myocardial infarction, and to differentiate between primary fibrinolysis and disseminated intravascular coagulation (DIC) so that correct pharmacologic therapy may be instituted.

During hemostasis, thrombin stimulates the formation of fibrin from fibrinogen. This fibrin, with the addition of fibrin stabilizing factor, forms a stable fibrin clot at the site of injury. Once the fibrin clot is no longer needed, it is dissolved by fibrinolytic agents such as plasmin, resulting in fibrin degradation products. (See Coagulation Studies for a description of the process of hemostasis.)

When the body's fibrinolytic system becomes overactive, any fibrin clot is dissolved as soon as it is formed, resulting in a bleeding disorder. This situation occurs with primary fibrinolysis caused by such things as cancer of the prostate, shock, and administration of thrombolytic agents such as streptokinase and urokinase. In cases of secondary fibrinolysis or DIC, the euglobulin lysis time is either normal or prolonged.

Normal Values

No lysis of plasma clot for 2 to 4 hours

Possible Meanings of Abnormal Values

Increased (Longer Lysis Time)	Decreased (Shorter Lysis Time)
Diabetes	Acute trauma
Disseminated intravascular coagulation	Amniotic embolism
	Antepartum hemorrhage
Pathologic fibrinolysis	Cirrhosis
Premature infants	Extracorporeal circulation
	Fetal death
	Hypoxia
	Incompatible blood transfusion
	Leukemia
	Pancreas cancer
	Postoperative period
	Prostate cancer
	Shock
	Thrombocytopenic purpura

Contributing Factors to Abnormal Values

- *Increased* fibrinolysis may occur with exercise, hyperventilation, and increasing age.
- *Decreased* fibrinolysis may occur in newborns, with obesity, and in postmenopausal women.
- Drugs that may *shorten* the lysis time (rapid fibrinolysis): asparaginase, clofibrate, corticotropin, dextran, steroids, streptokinase, tissue plasminogen activator (TPA), urokinase.

Pre-Test Nursing Care

- Explain to the patient the purpose of the test and the need for a blood sample to be drawn.
- No fasting is required before the test.

Procedure

- A 5-mL blood sample is drawn in a collection tube containing sodium citrate and citric acid.
- Gloves are worn throughout the procedure.

Post-Test Nursing Care

Possible complication: Hematoma at site due to prolonged bleeding time

- Apply pressure 3 to 5 minutes at venipuncture site. Apply dressing, periodically assessing for continued bleeding.
- Teach the patient to monitor the site. If the site begins to bleed, the patient should apply direct pressure and, if unable to control the bleeding, return to the laboratory or notify the nurse.
- Label the specimen, place it immediately in ice and transport it to the laboratory.
- Report abnormal findings to the primary care provider.

• • • • • • • • • • • • • • • •

Evoked Potential Studies
(EP Studies, Evoked Responses, Auditory Brain-Stem Evoked Potentials, Somatosensory Evoked Potentials, Visual Evoked Potentials)

Evoked potential studies measure the brain's electrical responses (evoked potentials, or responses) to stimulation of the sense organs or peripheral nerves. This aids in the diagnosis of lesions of the nervous system by evaluating the integrity of the visual, somatosensory, and auditory nerve pathways.

Somatosensory evoked potentials are used to assess patients with possible spinal cord lesions, stroke, and peripheral nerve disease, as suggested by patient complaints of numbness and weakness of the extremities. *Visual evoked potentials* are useful in the diagnosis of lesions involving the optic nerves and optic tracts, demyelinating diseases such as multiple sclerosis, and traumatic injury. *Auditory brain stem evoked potentials* are used to assess for lesions in the brain stem that involve the auditory pathway.

Normal Values

No neural conduction delay

Possible Meanings of Abnormal Values

Adrenoleukodystrophy
Amblyopia
Cervical spondylosis
Cochlear lesions

Guillain-Barré syndrome
Huntington's chorea
Intracerebral lesions
Multiple sclerosis
Optic chiasm lesion
Optic neuritis
Parkinson's disease
Retinopathy
Retrocochlear lesions
Sarcoidosis
Sensorimotor neuropathy
Spinal cord injury
Spinocerebellar degeneration
Transverse myelitis

Contributing Factors to Abnormal Values

- Improper placement of electrodes can alter test results.
- Inability of the patient to follow directions during the test will alter test results.

Pre-Test Nursing Care

- Explain to the patient the purpose of the test and the procedure to be done. Explain that there is no discomfort involved with this test.
- No fasting is required before the test.
- Instruct the patient to shampoo the hair the night before the test to aid in securing the electrodes during the test.
- Have the patient remove all jewelry before the test.

Procedure

- ### Somatosensory Evoked Potentials
  - The patient is placed in a comfortable position in either a lounge chair or on a bed.
  - Stimulating electrodes are applied over the peripheral nerves on the wrist, knee, and ankle.
  - Recording electrodes are placed on the scalp over the sensory cortex of the hemisphere opposite the limb to be stimulated.
  - Other stimulating electrodes may be placed over the second cervical vertebra and the lower lumbar vertebrae.
  - A painless electrical shock stimulus is delivered to the peripheral nerve through the stimulating electrode. The stimulus is enough to elicit a minor muscle response, such as a thumb twitch.
  - The rate at which the electric shock stimulus is delivered to the nerve electrodes and travels to the brain is measured and documented as waveforms that can then be analyzed.

- ### Visual Evoked Potentials
  - The patient is placed in a comfortable position in either a lounge chair or on a bed, 1 meter from the pattern-shift stimulator.
  - Electrodes are attached to the occipital, parietal, and vertex lobe areas.
  - A reference electrode is attached to the ear.

E

- One eye is covered, and the patient is instructed to fix the gaze on a dot in the center of the screen.
- A checkerboard pattern is projected and rapidly reversed.
- The computer interprets the brain's responses to the stimuli and records them in waveforms that can then be analyzed.
- The process is repeated with the other eye covered.

Auditory Evoked Potentials

- The patient is placed in a comfortable position in either a lounge chair or on a bed.
- Electrodes are positioned on the scalp at the vertex lobe area and on each earlobe.
- Earphones are placed in the patient's ears.
- A clicking noise stimulus is delivered into one ear while a continuous tone is delivered to the opposite ear.
- The responses to the stimuli are recorded as waveforms that can then be analyzed.

Post-Test Nursing Care

- After removal of the electrodes, the electrode paste is removed. Oil, acetone, or witch hazel may help remove the paste; then the hair should be shampooed.
- Report abnormal findings to the primary care provider.

• • • • • • • • • • • • • • • • •

Excretory Urography
(Intravenous Pyelography, IVP, Intravenous Urography)

Excretory urography uses radiopaque contrast dye to allow visualization of the kidneys, ureters, and bladder. This test was formerly known as intravenous pyelography (IVP); however, this name implied that only the kidneys were being studied. Excretory urography is performed in cases of suspected renal disease or urinary tract dysfunction. After injection of the dye, serial films are made as the dye filters through the kidneys and is excreted into the ureters and bladder. At the end of the procedure, a post-voiding film is also taken. This test provides a great deal of information regarding the structure of the kidneys and their ability to excrete the dye. It also is used for assessment of the ureters and bladder for obstruction, hematuria, stones, and trauma.

Normal Values

Normal size, shape, position, and functioning of kidneys, ureters, and bladder

Possible Meanings of Abnormal Values

Absence of one kidney
Bladder tumor
Chronic pyelonephritis
Congenital abnormalities
Glomerulonephritis
Hydronephrosis
Polycystic kidney disease

Prostatic enlargement
Renal calculi
Renal cysts
Renal tuberculosis
Renal tumor
Renovascular hypertension
Supernumerary kidney
Trauma
Ureteral calculi

Contributing Factors to Abnormal Values

- Retained barium, gas, or stool in the intestines may result in poor quality films.
- Any movement by the patient may alter quality of films taken.

CONTRAINDICATIONS

- Patients who are allergic to iodine, shellfish, or contrast medium dye
- Pregnant women
  Caution: A woman in her childbearing years should undergo radiography only during her menses or 12 to 14 days after its onset to avoid any exposure to a fetus.
- Patients who are unable to cooperate owing to age, mental status, pain, or other factors
- Patients with renal failure or those susceptible to dye-induced renal failure (dehydrated patients)

Pre-Test Nursing Care

- Explain to the patient the purpose of the test. Provide any written teaching materials available on the subject. Note that minimal discomfort during the test is due to the venipuncture and that during injection of the dye transient sensations including warmth, flushing, a salty taste, and nausea may be experienced.
- Check for allergies to iodine, shellfish, or contrast medium dye. Inform the radiologist of such possible allergy and obtain an order for an antihistamine and a corticosteroid to be administered before the test. A hypoallergenic nonionic contrast medium may be used for the test in allergic patients.
- Patients receiving metformin (Glucophage) for non–insulin-dependent diabetes mellitus should discontinue the drug 2 days before elective surgery or angiographic examinations. This is due to the possible occurrence of lactic acidosis, a potentially fatal complication of biguanide therapy.
- Fasting for 8 hours is required before the test. The patient should be well hydrated before the beginning of the fasting period.
- A laxative the night before the test or an enema or suppository the morning of the test may be ordered.
- If barium studies are also ordered, they are to be performed *after* this procedure has been successfully completed.
- Resuscitation and suctioning equipment should be readily available.

Procedure

- The patient is assisted to a supine position on the radiography table.
- A kidney, ureter, and bladder (KUB) film is taken to assess for gross abnormalities of the urinary tract.
- A maintenance intravenous line is initiated.
- The contrast dye is administered by intravenous injection.
- Serial films are made, usually at 1, 5, 10, 15, 20, and 30 minutes post injection.
- The patient is then asked to void, after which a post-voiding film is taken.
- Gloves are worn during the venipuncture.

Post-Test Nursing Care

Possible complication: Allergic reaction to dye

- Most allergic reactions to radiopaque dye occur within 30 minutes of administration of the contrast medium. Observe the patient closely for respiratory distress, hypotension, edema, hives, rash, tachycardia, and/or laryngeal stridor. Emergency resuscitation equipment must be readily accessible.
- Observe for allergic reaction to the dye for 24 hours.
- Apply pressure at venipuncture site. Apply dressing, periodically assessing for continued bleeding.
- Resume the patient's diet. Encourage fluid intake of at least three glasses of liquid to speed the excretion of the dye from the body.
- Report abnormal findings to the primary care provider.

• • • • • • • • • • • • • • • •

Exercise Electrocardiography
(Exercise ECG, Graded Exercise Tolerance Test, Stress Testing, Treadmill Test)

Exercise electrocardiography (stress testing) measures the efficiency of the heart during physical stress. Whereas a patient may have a normal resting electrocardiogram (ECG), the same patient may have an abnormal exercise ECG. This is due to the reaction of the heart to increased demand for oxygen. To simulate patient exercise in a controlled environment, the patient walks on a treadmill or pedals a stationary bicycle, while the ECG and blood pressure are monitored. The test continues until either the patient reaches the target heart rate or experiences chest pain or fatigue.

For patients unable or unwilling to exercise for the test, pharmacologic induction of myocardial ischemia can be done. Medications used to pharmacologically "stress" the heart include the vasodilators adenosine and dipyridamole and, more recently, the catecholamine dobutamine hydrochloride.

Normal Values

Negative: No symptoms or ECG abnormalities on attaining 85% of the maximum heart rate for the patient's age and sex

Possible Meanings of Abnormal Values

Coronary artery occlusive disease
Exercise-related hypertension
Intermittent claudication
Myocardial ischemia

Contributing Factors to Abnormal Values

- False-positive test results may occur with anemia, electrolyte imbalance, hypertension, hypoxia, left bundle branch block, left ventricular hypertrophy, valvular heart disease, Wolff-Parkinson-White syndrome.
- Drugs that may affect test results include beta-blockers, calcium channel blockers, digoxin, nitroglycerine.

CONTRAINDICATIONS

- Patients with active unstable angina
- Patients with acute myocardial infarction
- Patients with severe anemia, congestive heart failure, or coronary insufficiency
- Patients with cardiac inflammation (myocarditis, pericarditis)
- Patients with uncontrolled arrhythmias
- Patients with aortic dissection
- Patients with critical left ventricular outflow-tract obstruction
- Patients with critical aortic stenosis
- Patients with recent or active cerebral ischemia
- Patients with severe uncontrolled hypertension

Pre-Test Nursing Care

- Explain to the patient the purpose of the test and the need for electrodes to be attached to the chest. Note that the patient may become fatigued during the test and that he or she may ask for the test to be discontinued if fatigue or chest pain are experienced.
- Advise the patient to dress comfortably for the test.
- Intravenous access is established for emergency use, if needed.
- Baseline 12-lead ECG results should be obtained if not already available.
- Obtain a signed informed consent.
- Fasting for 3 hours is required before the test.
- Smoking should be avoided for 3 hours before the test.

Procedure

- The skin is cleansed with alcohol and abraded. Chest electrodes are applied, and the lead wires stabilized.
- A baseline ECG tracing and blood pressure are obtained.

Treadmill Test

- The patient is assisted to step onto the treadmill.
- Ensure patient safety through use of support railings to maintain balance.
- The treadmill is turned on to slow speed at first and increased in miles per hour and grade elevation of the treadmill.

Bicycle Test
- The patient pedals until reaching the desired speed.
- Throughout the testing, the ECG is monitored for changes. Blood pressure is also checked at pre-established intervals.
- If the ECG shows three consecutive premature ventricular contractions or significant increase in ectopy, the test is stopped immediately.

Post-Test Nursing Care
- Instruct the patient to continue walking as the treadmill speed slows.
- Monitor blood pressure and ECG for at least 15 minutes after the test is completed and the patient is resting.
- Remove the electrodes and cleanse the skin of any residual gel or adhesive.
- Report abnormal findings to the primary care provider.

• • • • • • • • • • • • • •

Febrile Agglutinins

Febrile agglutinins are those that are associated with diseases that cause fever. Such infectious diseases include brucellosis, rickettsial infections such as Rocky Mountain spotted fever and typhus, salmonellosis, and tularemia. To test for febrile agglutinins, a sample of the patient's serum is mixed with a few drops of prepared antigens on a slide. If agglutination occurs, antigen is added to serial dilutions of the patient's serum until agglutination is no longer noted.

Normal Values
Brucella antibody < 1:80
Rickettsia antibody < 1:40
Salmonella antibody < 1:80
Tularemia antibody < 1:40

Possible Meanings of Abnormal Values

Increased

Brucellosis
Rickettsial diseases
Rocky Mountain spotted fever
Salmonellosis
Tularemia
Typhus

Contributing Factors to Abnormal Values
- Hemolysis of the blood sample may alter test results.
- Drugs that may interfere with the development of febrile agglutinins: antibiotics.

Pre-Test Nursing Care

- Explain to the patient the purpose of the test and the need for a blood sample to be drawn. Inform the patient that additional blood samples may be needed every 3 to 5 days.
- No fasting is required before the test.

Procedure

- A 7-mL blood sample is drawn in a collection tube containing no additives.
- Gloves are worn throughout the procedure.

Post-Test Nursing Care

- Apply pressure at venipuncture site. Apply dressing, periodically assessing for continued bleeding.
- Label the specimen and transport it to the laboratory immediately.
- Report abnormal findings to the primary care provider.

• • • • • • • • • • • • • • • • • •

Fecal Fat

When a patient ingests a normal diet, the amount of fat excreted in the stool should account for no more than 20% of the total solids. A variety of fats, or lipids, are excreted in feces. They are composed of cells sloughed by the intestines, unabsorbed dietary lipids, and secretions from the gastrointestinal tract. In normal conditions, in which there are adequate biliary and pancreatic secretions, most dietary lipids are absorbed in the small intestine. However, if malabsorption occurs, the fecal fat is excreted in the stool. This is known as *steatorrhea*, which occurs in such conditions as Crohn's disease, cystic fibrosis, and Whipple's disease. Testing for fecal fat involves collection of all stool for 3 days.

Normal Values

1–7 g/d (3.5–25 mmol/d SI units)

Possible Meanings of Abnormal Values

Increased

Amyloidosis
Celiac disease
Crohn's disease
Cystic fibrosis
Diarrhea
Diverticulosis
Enteritis
Hepatobiliary disease
Lymphoma
Pancreatic disease

Post-bowel resection
Sprue
Whipple's disease

Contributing Factors to Abnormal Values
- Drugs that may alter test results: castor oil, mineral oil.

Pre-Test Nursing Care
- Explain to the patient the purpose of the test and the need for collection of stool.
- Instruct the patient to ingest a high-fat diet (approximately 100 g/d) for 3 days before the test and throughout the 3-day test period.
- Instruct the patient to collect every stool during the 3-day period so that all stool is sent to the laboratory. Tell the patient to avoid contaminating the stool with urine or toilet paper.
- Withhold the use of castor oil or mineral oil during the entire 6-day pre-test and testing period.

Procedure
- Each stool collected during the 72-hour period is sent to the laboratory immediately.
- Gloves are worn during any collection of the stool.

Post-Test Nursing Care
- Label the specimen and transport it to the laboratory.
- Resume diet and medications as taken before the test.
- Report abnormal findings to the primary care provider.

• • • • • • • • • • • • • • • • •

Ferritin

Ferritin is the primary protein in the body that stores iron. Thus, measurement of the ferritin level provides a good indication of the size of the iron storage compartment. This test, in conjunction with determination of the iron level and total iron-binding capacity, is used in the differential diagnosis of the various types of anemia.

Normal Values
Normal: > 20 ng/mL (> 20 µg/L SI units)
Elderly: Increased

Abnormal Values
Borderline deficient: 13–20 ng/mL (13–20 µg/L SI units)
Deficient: 0–12 ng/mL (0–12 µg/L SI units)
Excessive: > 400 ng/mL (> 400 µg/L SI units)

Possible Meanings of Abnormal Values

Increased	Decreased
Acute hepatitis	Gastrointestinal surgery
Acute myocardial infarction	Hemodialysis
Anemia other than	Inflammatory bowel disease
iron deficiency	Iron-deficiency anemia
Chronic inflammatory disease	Malnutrition
Chronic renal disease	Menstruation
Cirrhosis of the liver	Pregnancy
Hemochromatosis	
Hemosiderosis	
Hodgkin's disease	
Hyperthyroidism	
Infection	
Leukemia	
Malignancy	
Polycythemia	
Rheumatoid arthritis	
Thalassemia	

F

Contributing Factors to Abnormal Values

- Falsely increased levels of ferritin may occur with:
    - Intake of iron supplements and meals with a high-iron content
    - After blood transfusions
    - After receipt of radiopharmaceuticals used for nuclear scans

Pre-Test Nursing Care

- Explain to the patient the purpose of the test and the need for a blood sample to be drawn.
- No fasting is required before the test.

Procedure

- A 5-mL blood sample is drawn in a collection tube containing no additives.
- Gloves are worn throughout the procedure.

Post-Test Nursing Care

- Apply pressure at venipuncture site. Apply dressing, periodically assessing for continued bleeding.
- Label the specimen and transport it to the laboratory.
- Report abnormal findings to the primary care provider.

• • • • • • • • • • • • • • • •

Fibrin Degradation Products
(FDP, Fibrin Split Products [FSP], Fibrin Breakdown Products [FBP])

This test is used in the diagnosis of disseminated intravascular coagulation (DIC) and to monitor fibrinolytic therapy.

During hemostasis, fibrin, with the addition of fibrin stabilizing factor, forms a stable fibrin clot at the site of injury. Once the fibrin clot is no longer needed, it is dissolved by fibrinolytic agents such as plasmin, resulting in seven fibrin degradation products (FDPs), denoted as A, B, C, D, E, X, and Y. Their presence in the blood is indicative of recent clotting activity. (See Coagulation Studies for description of the process of hemostasis.)

The FDP test is conducted by mixing dilute serum with latex particles that carry antibodies to the D and E split products. If FDPs are present in the serum, there is clumping of the latex particles.

Normal Values

< 10 µg/mL (< 100 mg/L SI units)

Abnormal Values

FDP levels > 40 µg/mL are highly suggestive of DIC

Possible Meanings of Abnormal Values

Increased

Abruptio placentae
Acute leukemia
Autologous transfusions
Burns
Congenital heart disease
Disseminated intravascular coagulation
Heat stroke
Hypoxia
Infection
Intrauterine fetal death
Late pregnancy
Liver disease
Myocardial infarction
Portocaval shunt
Preeclampsia
Pulmonary emboli
Renal disease
Septicemia
Shock
Status post cardiopulmonary surgery
Transfusion reaction
Transplant rejection
Venous thrombosis

Contributing Factors to Abnormal Values

- Hemolysis of the blood sample may alter test results.
- Drugs that may *increase* FDP levels: barbiturates, heparin, streptokinase, urokinase.

Pre-Test Nursing Care

- Explain to the patient the purpose of the test and the need for a blood sample to be drawn.
- No fasting is required before the test.
- The blood sample is to be drawn before the initiation of heparin therapy.

Procedure

- A 5-mL blood sample is drawn into a special tube that contains bovine thrombin and an antifibrinolytic agent.
- Gloves are worn throughout the procedure.

Post-Test Nursing Care

Possible complication: Hematoma at site due to prolonged bleeding time

- Apply pressure 3 to 5 minutes at venipuncture site. Apply dressing, periodically assessing for continued bleeding.
- Teach the patient to monitor the site. If the site begins to bleed, the patient should apply direct pressure and, if unable to control the bleeding, return to the laboratory or notify the nurse.
- Label the specimen, place it on ice and transport it to the laboratory immediately.
- Report abnormal findings to the primary care provider.

* * * * * * * * * * * * * * * * *

Fibrinogen
(Factor I)

Measurement of fibrinogen levels is used when investigating suspected bleeding disorders, especially when other tests of coagulation, such as prothrombin time (PT), activated partial thromboplastin time (APTT), and thrombin clotting time (TCT) are abnormal. Fibrinogen is a polypeptide that is synthesized in the liver. During hemostasis, thrombin stimulates the formation of fibrin from fibrinogen. This fibrin, with the addition of fibrin stabilizing factor, forms a stable fibrin clot at the site of injury. (See Coagulation Studies for description of the process of hemostasis.)

Normal Values

200–400 mg/dL (2.0–4.0 g/L SI units)

Possible Meanings of Abnormal Values

Increased	Decreased
Acute infection	Abortion
Burns	Advanced cancer
Cancer	Amniotic fluid embolism
Glomerulonephritis	Anemia
Hepatitis	Cirrhosis
Inflammation	Disseminated intravascular
Late pregnancy	coagulation
Menstruation	Dysfibrinogenemia
Multiple myeloma	Eclampsia
Nephrosis	Fat embolism
Pneumonia	Fibrinolysis
Postoperative period	Hereditary afibrinogenemia
Rheumatic fever	Leukemia
Rheumatoid arthritis	Liver disease
Tissue damage/injury	Meconium embolism
Tuberculosis	Septicemia
Uremia	Shock
	Transfusion reaction

Contributing Factors to Abnormal Values

- Fibrinogen test results may be altered owing to hemolysis of the blood sample or if the patient has received a blood transfusion within 1 month before the test.
- Drugs that may *increase* fibrinogen levels: estrogens, oral contraceptives.
- Drugs that may *decrease* fibrinogen levels: anabolic steroids, androgens, asparaginase, phenobarbital, streptokinase, urokinase, valproic acid.

Pre-Test Nursing Care

- Explain to the patient the purpose of the test and the need for a blood sample to be drawn.
- No fasting is required before the test.

Procedure

- A 7-mL blood sample is drawn in a collection tube containing sodium citrate and citric acid.
- Gloves are worn throughout the procedure.

Post-Test Nursing Care

Possible complication: Hematoma at site due to prolonged bleeding time

- Apply pressure 3 to 5 minutes at venipuncture site. Apply dressing, periodically assessing for continued bleeding.
- Teach the patient to monitor the site. If the site begins to bleed, the patient should apply direct pressure and, if unable to control the bleeding, return to the laboratory or notify the nurse.
- Label the specimen and transport it to the laboratory immediately.
- Report abnormal findings to the primary care provider.

• • • • • • • • • • • • • • • •

Fibrinogen Uptake Test
(FUT)

Fibrinogen, an inactive polypeptide that circulates in the blood, is converted to fibrin after thrombin enzymatic action. Fibrin then combines with platelets to form blood clots. (See Co-agulation Studies for description of the process of hemostasis.) In this test, fibrinogen labeled with radioactive iodine (^{125}I) is injected intravenously. Once in the bloodstream, the radioactive fibrinogen moves to areas where clots are being formed. It is also found in the area of established clots. Thus, the test is useful in the diagnosis of deep venous thrombosis (DVT).

Although a useful test, the ^{125}I FUT has disadvantages as well. First, because of the high lev-els of fibrinogen normally found in the proximal thigh, the test cannot be used to detect DVT in that area. Second, at least 24 hours must elapse between administration of the ^{125}I and the scan-ning. This prevents the test from being used in emergency situations. Finally, the fibrinogen used for the test is garnered from donated blood, bringing with it the risks of blood transfusion.

Normal Values

No abnormal uptake of radionuclide in lower extremities

Abnormal Values

If the difference between the 10-minute and 24-hour post-injection values are at least 15 times greater, the test is considered positive for deep vein thrombosis.

Possible Meanings of Abnormal Values

Deep vein thrombosis
Thrombophlebitis
Thrombosis

Contributing Factors to Abnormal Values

- Any movement by the patient may alter quality of films taken.
- Other areas of inflammation within the extremity being tested and the presence of lym-phedema are both conditions in which there are increased levels of fibrinogen. Thus, test re-sults will be inaccurate.

CONTRAINDICATIONS

- Pregnant women
  Caution: A woman in her childbearing years should undergo radiography only during her menses or 12 to 14 days after its onset to avoid any exposure to a fetus.
- Patients who are lactating
- Patients who are allergic to iodine, shellfish, or contrast medium
- Patients who are unable to cooperate owing to age, mental status, pain, or other factors
- Patients who must be diagnosed for deep venous thrombosis in less than 24 hours

Pre-Test Nursing Care

- Explain to the patient the purpose of the test. Provide any written teaching materials avail-able on the subject. Note that discomfort involved with this test is primarily due to lying on a hard table for an extended period of time and the needle puncture. Reassure the patient that only trace amounts of the radionuclide are involved in the test.

- Check for allergies to iodine, shellfish, or contrast medium dye. Inform the radiologist of such possible allergy and obtain an order for an antihistamine and a corticosteroid to be administered before the test.
- The patient must remain still while the scan is being performed.
- No fasting is required before the test.
- Obtain a signed informed consent.
- Administer Lugol's solution or potassium iodine, as ordered, to block uptake of the radioactive iodine by the thyroid gland.

Procedure

- The patient is assisted to a supine position on the examination table.
- Areas of the lower extremities to be examined are marked.
- A radionuclide such as technetium-99m is administered by intravenous injection in a peripheral vein.
- A scintillation camera is positioned over the patient's lower extremities. This camera takes a radioactivity reading from the body. This information is transformed into a two-dimensional picture of the vessels.
- Readings are taken 10 minutes after the injection and again at 24 hours post injection.
- Gloves are worn during the radionuclide injection.

Post-Test Nursing Care

- Check the injection site for redness or swelling.
- If a woman who is lactating *must* have a nuclear scan, she should not breast feed the infant until the radionuclide has been eliminated, possibly for 3 days.
- Although the amount of diagnostic radionuclide excreted in the urine is low, the urine should not be used for any laboratory tests for the time period indicated by the nuclear medicine department. Clients should be told to flush the toilet three times after voiding.
- Gloves are worn whenever dealing with the urine.
- Encourage fluid intake by the patient to enhance excretion of the radionuclide.
- Report abnormal findings to the primary care provider.

• • • • • • • • • • • • • • • •

Folic Acid
(Folate)

Folic acid is a water-soluble vitamin formed by bacteria in the intestines and stored in the liver. It can also be found in such food sources as eggs, fruits, green leafy vegetables, liver, milk, orange juice, and yeast. This vitamin is necessary for normal functioning of red blood cells and white blood cells. It also plays a role in the metabolism of amino acids and nucleotides. An adequate folic acid level is essential for the pregnant woman to prevent neural tube defects in the developing fetus. Testing for folic acid is done in conjunction with testing for vitamin B_{12} in the diagnosis of macrocytic anemia. The body stores very little folic acid, so folic acid levels fall below normal 21 to 28 days after the beginning of the deficiency state.

Normal Values

Normal: > 3.2 ng/mL (> 7.3 nmol/L SI units)

Abnormal Values

Borderline deficient: 2.5–3.2 ng/mL (5.7–7.3 nmol/L SI units)
Deficient: < 2.5 ng/mL (< 5.7 nmol/L SI units)

Possible Meanings of Abnormal Values

Increased	Decreased
Blood transfusion	Alcoholism
Folic acid supplementation	Anorexia nervosa
Pernicious anemia	Cirrhosis
Vegetarianism	Diet (inadequate intake)
	Hemodialysis
	Hemolytic anemia
	Hyperthyroidism
	Inflammatory bowel disease
	Leukemia
	Macrocytic anemia due to pregnancy
	Malabsorption
	Megaloblastic anemia
	Neoplasia
	Pregnancy
	Sickle cell anemia
	Vitamin B_{12} deficiency

Contributing Factors to Abnormal Values

- Falsely increased results may occur due to hemolysis of sample.
- Falsely increased results may occur in patients with severe iron deficiency.
- Drugs that may *decrease* folic acid levels: alcohol, aminosalicylic acid, ampicillin, chloramphenicol, erythromycin, estrogens, lincomycin, methotrexate, oral contraceptives, penicillin, phenobarbital, phenytoin, tetracyclines, and trimethoprim.
- Drugs that *increase* folic acid levels: folic acid.

Pre-Test Nursing Care

- Explain to the patient the purpose of the test and the need for a blood sample to be drawn.
- Fasting is usually required for 8 hours before the test. Water intake is allowed. No alcohol is allowed before the test.

Procedure

- The 7-mL sample is drawn in a collection tube containing a silicone gel.
- Gloves are worn throughout the procedure.

Post-Test Nursing Care

- Apply pressure at venipuncture site. Apply dressing, periodically assessing for continued bleeding.
- Label the specimen and then protect it from light by inserting the tube into a paper bag.
- Transport the specimen to the laboratory as soon as possible. The sample must be kept refrigerated until tested.
- Report abnormal findings to the primary care provider.

• • • • • • • • • • • • • • • •

F Follicle-Stimulating Hormone
(FSH)

This test is used in the diagnosis of hypogonadism, infertility, menstrual disorders, and precocious puberty. Follicle-stimulating hormone (FSH) is secreted by the anterior pituitary gland. FSH promotes maturation of the ovarian follicle, which is needed for production of estrogen. As estrogen levels rise, luteinizing hormone (LH) is produced. FSH and LH are both needed for ovulation to occur in women. In addition, FSH controls the secretion of estrogen in women and stimulates the testes to produce sperm in men. FSH and LH are usually measured at the same time.

Normal Values

Female:

Premenopausal:	4–30 mIU/mL (4–30 IU/L SI units)
Midcycle peak:	10–90 mIU/mL (10–90 IU/L SI units)
Pregnancy:	low to undetectable
Postmenopausal:	40–250 mIU/mL (40–250 IU/L SI units)

Possible Meanings of Abnormal Values

Increased	Decreased
Acromegaly	Adrenal hyperplasia
Amenorrhea (primary)	Amenorrhea (secondary)
Anorchism	Anorexia nervosa
Castration	Delayed puberty
Gonadal failure	Hypogonadotropinism
Hyperpituitarism	Hypophysectomy
Hypogonadism	Hypothalamic dysfunction
Hypothalamic tumor	Neoplasm (adrenal, ovarian,
Hysterectomy	testicular)
Klinefelter's syndrome	Prepubertal child
Menopause	
Menstruation	
Orchiectomy	

Increased	Decreased
Ovarian failure	
Pituitary tumor	
Precocious puberty	
Stein-Leventhal syndrome	
Testicular failure	
Turner's syndrome	

Contributing Factors to Abnormal Values

- Hemolysis of the blood sample or having a radioactive scan within 1 week of the test may alter test results.
- Drugs that may *decrease* FSH levels: chlorpromazine, estrogens, oral contraceptives, progesterone, testosterone.

Pre-Test Nursing Care

- Explain to the patient the purpose of the test and the need for a blood sample to be drawn.
- No fasting is required before the test.
- If possible, withhold drugs that may alter test results for 48 hours before the test.

Procedure

- A 7-mL blood sample is drawn in a collection tube containing a silicone gel.
- Gloves are worn throughout the procedure.

Post-Test Nursing Care

- Apply pressure at venipuncture site. Apply dressing, periodically assessing for continued bleeding.
- Label the specimen and transport it to the laboratory.
- For female patients: on the laboratory slip, include the date on which the patient began her last menstrual period.
- Resume medications as taken before the test.
- Report abnormal findings to the primary care provider.

• • • • • • • • • • • • • • • • •

Free Erythrocyte Protoporphyrin
(FEP)

This test measures free erythrocyte protoporphyrin (FEP) as a method of detecting iron-deficiency anemia. As shown in the pathway of heme synthesis (see Aminolevulinic Acid), erythrocyte protoporphyrin is used in the final step of heme synthesis. A vital component needed to continue the synthesis is iron. If iron is not present, the protoporphyrin cannot be synthesized into hemoglobin. This substance is then known as free erythrocyte protoporphyrin.

Normal Values

< 35 µg/dl

Possible Meanings of Abnormal Values

Increased	Decreased
Hemolytic anemia	Megaloblastic anemia
Iron deficiency anemia	
Lead poisoning	
Thalassemia	

F

Contributing Factors to Abnormal Values

- Hemolysis of the blood sample may alter test results.

Pre-Test Nursing Care

- Explain to the patient the purpose of the test and the need for a blood sample to be drawn.
- No fasting is required before the test.

Procedure

- A 5-mL blood sample is drawn in a collection tube containing heparin.
- Gloves are worn throughout the procedure.

Post-Test Nursing Care

- Invert and gently mix the sample and the anticoagulant.
- Apply pressure at venipuncture site. Apply dressing, periodically assessing for continued bleeding.
- Label the specimen and transport it to the laboratory.
- Report abnormal findings to the primary care provider.

• • • • • • • • • • • • • • •

Fungal Antibody Tests

See:
Blastomycosis
Coccidioidomycosis
Cryptococcosis
Histoplasmosis Test

• • • • • • • • • • • • •

Galactose-1-Phosphate Uridyl Transferase
(Gal-1-PUT, Galactosemia Screening)

This test is used to detect the presence of the disease or carrier state of galactosemia, an inherited disorder transmitted as an autosomal recessive gene. In this disorder, galactose cannot be converted to glucose. Galactose is normally converted to glucose in the liver. For this conversion to occur, the enzyme galactose-1-phosphate uridyl transferase is required for conversion of galactose-1-phosphate into glucose-1-phosphate. When this enzyme is deficient, galactose-1-phosphate accumulates in the body, resulting in such problems as cataracts, liver disease, renal disease, and mental retardation.

Normal Values
18.5–28.5 U/g of hemoglobin

Abnormal Values
5–18.5 U/g of hemoglobin: may indicate the individual is a carrier of the disorder
< 5 U/g of hemoglobin: indicative of galactosemia

Possible Meanings of Abnormal Values
Decreased

Galactosemia

Pre-Test Nursing Care
- Explain to the patient the purpose of the test and the need for a blood sample to be drawn.
- No fasting is required before the test.

Procedure
- In an adult, a 5-mL blood sample is drawn in a collection tube containing heparin. For infants, a heel stick sample or umbilical blood may be used.
- Gloves are worn throughout the procedure.

Post-Test Nursing Care
- Apply pressure at venipuncture site. Apply dressing, periodically assessing for continued bleeding.
- The sample must immediately be placed on ice. Label the specimen and transport it to the laboratory.
- Report abnormal findings to the physician or nurse practitioner.
- If test results indicate the presence of galactosemia, instruct the patient (or parents) regarding the need to remove galactose-containing foods, especially milk, from the diet.

• • • • • • • • • • • • • • • • • •

Gallbladder Scan
(Hepatobiliary Imaging, HIDA Scan)

For a gallbladder scan, the patient is given a radionuclide compound, an iminodiacetic acid analogue labeled with technetium-99m (HIDA), by means of an intravenous injection. A scintillation camera is used to take a radioactivity reading from the body. These readings are fed into a computer, which translates these readings into a two-dimensional gray scale picture. These pictures are obtained at 15 to 30 minute intervals. If the biliary system has not visualized within 2 hours, the scan is repeated 2 to 4 hours later. This test is used in the diagnosis of cholecystitis. Delayed filling of the gallbladder is indicative of chronic or acalculus cholecystitis, whereas failure to visualize the gallbladder is diagnostic of an obstruction of the cystic duct, as in acute or calculus cholecystitis.

Normal Values

Negative (visualization of gallbladder within 1 hour after radionuclide injection)

Possible Meanings of Abnormal Values

Acalculus cholecystitis
Acute cholecystitis
Calculus cholecystitis
Chronic cholecystitis
Obstruction of common bile duct

Contributing Factors to Abnormal Values

- Any movement by the patient may alter quality of films taken.
- Retained barium from previous examinations may interfere with the test.

STOP CONTRAINDICATIONS

- Pregnant women
  Caution: A woman in her childbearing years should undergo radiography only during her menses or 12 to 14 days after its onset to avoid any exposure to a fetus.
- Patients who are lactating
- Patients who are unable to cooperate due to age, mental status, pain, or other factors

Pre-Test Nursing Care

- Explain to the patient the purpose of the test. Provide any written teaching materials available on the subject. Note that discomfort involved with this test is primarily due to lying on a hard table for an extended period of time and the needle puncture. Reassure the patient that only trace amounts of the radionuclide are involved in the test.
- The patient must remain still while the scan is being performed.
- Fasting for at least 2 hours is preferred before the test.
- Obtain a signed informed consent.

Procedure

- The technetium-99m–labeled IDA analog (HIDA) is administered by intravenous injection in a peripheral vein.
- The patient is assisted to a supine position on the examination table.
- A scintillation camera is positioned over the right upper quadrant of the patient's abdomen. This camera takes a radioactivity reading from the body. This information is transformed into a two-dimensional picture of the area.
- Scans are obtained at 15, 30, 60, and 90 minutes post injection.
- If the gallbladder does not visualize by 2 hours post injection, additional scans are conducted in 2 to 4 hours.
- Gloves are worn during the radionuclide injection.

Post-Test Nursing Care

- Check the injection site for redness or swelling.
- If a woman who is lactating *must* have a nuclear scan, she should not breast feed the infant until the radionuclide has been eliminated, possibly for 3 days.
- Although the amount of diagnostic radionuclide excreted in the urine is low, the urine should not be used for any laboratory tests for the time period indicated by the nuclear medicine department. Clients should be told to flush the toilet three times after voiding.
- Gloves are worn when dealing with the urine.
- Encourage fluid intake by the patient to enhance excretion of the radionuclide.
- Report abnormal findings to the primary care provider.

• • • • • • • • • • • • • • • •

G

Gallium Scan
(Body Scan)

The gallium scan is considered a total body scan. Although gallium can be used for scanning of individual organs, such as the liver or spleen, in this particular test, the entire body is scanned. The test is usually performed when the site of the disease, which may be malignancy, infection, or inflammation, has not been delineated. Although the liver, spleen, bones, and large bowel normally take up gallium, inflammatory and malignant processes also draw in gallium. Thus, the test is used to detect primary neoplasms, metastatic lesions, and inflammatory processes. The scan is performed 24 to 48 hours after radioactive gallium citrate has been injected. If needed, it can be performed only 4 to 6 hours after the injection, if the camera is moved slowly over the body.

Normal Values

Normal uptake of gallium in the liver, spleen, bones, and large bowel
No other areas of increased gallium uptake

Possible Meanings of Abnormal Values

Abscess
Infection
Inflammation
Malignancy

Contributing Factors to Abnormal Values

- Any movement by the patient may alter quality of films taken.
- Retained barium from previous examinations may interfere with the test.

CONTRAINDICATIONS

- Pregnant women
  Caution: A woman in her childbearing years should undergo radiography only during her menses or 12 to 14 days after its onset to avoid any exposure to a fetus.
- Patients who are lactating
- Patients who are unable to cooperate owing to age, mental status, pain, or other factors

Pre-Test Nursing Care

- Explain to the patient the purpose of the test. Provide any written teaching materials available on the subject. Note that discomfort involved with this test is primarily due to lying on a hard table for an extended period of time and the needle puncture. Reassure the patient that only trace amounts of the radionuclide are involved in the test.
- The patient must remain still while the scan is being performed.
- No fasting is required before the test.
- Obtain a signed informed consent.
- A laxative and/or cleansing enema may be ordered.

Procedure

- The radioactive gallium (^{67}Ga) citrate is administered by intravenous injection in a peripheral vein.
- At the designated time (4 to 6 hours or 24 hours post injection), the patient is taken to the nuclear medicine department.
- The patient is assisted to a supine position on the examination table.
- A scintillation camera is used to scan the entire body. This camera takes a radioactivity reading from the body. This information is transformed into a two-dimensional picture of the area.
- Scans are also made with the patient in the prone and lateral positions.
- Additional scans may be obtained at 48 and 72 hours post injection.
- Gloves are worn during the radionuclide injection.

Post-Test Nursing Care

- Check the injection site for redness or swelling.
- If a woman who is lactating *must* have a nuclear scan, she should not breast feed the infant until the radionuclide has been eliminated, possibly for 3 days.

- Although the amount of diagnostic radionuclide excreted in the urine is low, the urine should not be used for any laboratory tests for the time period indicated by the nuclear medicine department. Clients should be told to flush the toilet three times after voiding.
- Gloves are worn when dealing with the urine.
- Encourage fluid intake by the patient to enhance excretion of the radionuclide.
- Report abnormal findings to the primary care provider.

• • • • • • • • • • • • • • • •

Gamma-Glutamyl Transferase
(GGT, Gamma-Glutamyl Transpeptidase [GGTP])

Measurement of gamma-glutamyl transferase (GGT) assists in the diagnosis of liver problems. GGT is an enzyme found primarily in the liver, kidney, pancreas, prostate gland, and spleen. Its function is to assist in amino acid transport across cell membranes. GGT is often measured in conjunction with alkaline phosphatase (ALP) to determine whether the ALP is increased due to liver disease. Whereas ALP may be increased with either hepatobiliary or bone disorders, the GGT is more specific for hepatobiliary problems.

Normal Values

Female:	5–29 U/L
Male:	5–38 U/L
Child:	3–30 U/L
Newborn:	five times the child norms

Possible Meanings of Abnormal Values

Increased

Acute pancreatitis
Alcoholism
Biliary obstruction
Cholecystitis
Cholelithiasis
Cirrhosis
Congestive heart failure
Hepatitis
Liver disease
Liver metastases
Myocardial infarction
Pancreatic cancer
Renal cancer
Systemic lupus erythematosus

Contributing Factors to Abnormal Values

- Hemolysis of the blood sample will alter test results.
- Drugs that may *increase* GGT levels: alcohol, aminoglycosides, barbiturates, glutethimide, phenobarbital, phenytoin.
- Drugs that may *decrease* GGT levels: clofibrate, oral contraceptives.

Pre-Test Nursing Care

- Explain to the patient the purpose of the test and the need for a blood sample to be drawn.
- Fasting for 8 hours is required before the test.
- No alcohol is allowed for 24 hours before the test.

Procedure

- A 7-mL blood sample is drawn in a collection tube containing a silicone gel.
- Gloves are worn throughout the procedure.

Post-Test Nursing Care

Possible complication: With liver dysfunction, patient may have prolonged clotting time.

- Apply pressure 3 to 5 minutes at venipuncture site. Apply dressing, periodically assessing for continued bleeding.
- Teach the patient to monitor the site. If the site begins to bleed, the patient should apply direct pressure and, if unable to control the bleeding, return to the laboratory or notify the nurse.
- Label the specimen and transport it to the laboratory.
- Report abnormal findings to the primary care provider.

• • • • • • • • • • • • • • • •

Gastrin

Measurement of gastrin levels assists in the diagnosis of various gastric disorders. Gastrin is a polypeptide hormone produced and stored by the G cells of the antrum of the stomach and by the islets of Langerhans of the pancreas. Gastrin facilitates digestion by triggering gastric acid secretion in the following situations: presence of proteins, calcium, or alcohol in the stomach; vagal stimulation through chewing, tasting, or smelling of food; distention of the stomach antrum; or decreased stomach acidity. When the stomach's environment becomes acidic, the secretion of gastrin is inhibited. Gastrin also stimulates release of pancreatic enzymes, the gastric enzyme pepsin, the intrinsic factor, and bile from the liver and increases gastrointestinal motility. Abnormal gastrin secretion can occur when pathologic conditions exist. Such conditions include gastrinoma, the gastrin-secreting tumor in Zollinger-Ellison syndrome, gastric ulcers, duodenal ulcers, and pernicious anemia. Testing for gastrin provides information helpful in the diagnosis of these conditions. Provocative testing, such as through intravenous infusion of calcium gluconate, is used to distinguish ulcer disease from Zollinger-Ellison syndrome.

Normal Values

0–200 pg/mL (0–200 ng/L SI units)

Possible Meanings of Abnormal Values

Increased

Achlorhydria
Duodenal ulcer
Elderly
End-stage renal disease
Gastric ulcer
G-cell hyperplasia
Hyperparathyroidism
Peptic ulcer disease
Pernicious anemia
Postvagotomy
Pyloric obstruction
Stomach cancer
Uremia
Zollinger-Ellison syndrome

Contributing Factors to Abnormal Values

- Hemolysis of the sample may alter test results.
- Falsely increased results may occur with lipemic blood samples and intake of high-protein foods.
- Drugs that may *increase* gastrin levels: acetylcholine chloride, antacids, beta-blocking agents, calcium carbonate, calcium chloride, cholinergics, cimetidine, famotidine, insulin, nizatidine, ranitidine.
- Drugs that may *decrease* gastrin levels: adrenergic blockers, anticholinergics, caffeine, calcium salts, corticosteroids, ethanol, *Rauwolfia serpentia*, rescinnamine, reserpine, tricyclic antidepressants.

Pre-Test Nursing Care

- Explain to the patient the purpose of the test and the need for a blood sample to be drawn.
- Fasting for 12 hours is required before the test. Water is permitted.
- Alcohol is to be avoided for 24 hours before the test.

Procedure

- A 7-mL blood sample is drawn in a collection tube containing a silicone gel.
- Gloves are worn throughout the procedure.

Post-Test Nursing Care

- Apply pressure at venipuncture site. Apply dressing, periodically assessing for continued bleeding.
- Label the specimen and transport it to the laboratory.
- Report abnormal findings to the primary care provider.

• • • • • • • • • • • • • • • • •

Glucagon

Glucagon is a hormone secreted by the alpha cells of the pancreas. Its function is to elevate blood glucose levels by promoting the conversion of glycogen to glucose. Its secretion is stimulated by hypoglycemia and inhibited by the other pancreatic hormones, insulin and somatostatin. This test is used to determine the presence of a glucagonoma (alpha islet cell neoplasm), which causes increased glucagon levels, or hypoglycemia due to glucagon deficiency or pancreatic dysfunction, which results in decreased glucagon levels.

Normal Values

50–200 pg/mL (50–200 ng/L SI units)

Possible Meanings of Abnormal Values

Increased	Decreased
Acute pancreatitis	Chronic pancreatitis
Cirrhosis	Cystic fibrosis
Diabetes mellitus	Hypoglycemia
Glucagonoma	Idiopathic glucagon deficiency
Pheochromocytoma	Neoplastic replacement of
Postoperative period	the pancreas
Stress	Postpancreatectomy
Trauma	
Uremia	

Contributing Factors to Abnormal Values

- Hemolysis of the blood sample and having a radioactive scan within 48 hours before the test will alter test results.
- Strenuous exercise and stress may *increase* glucagon levels.
- Drugs that may *increase* glucagon levels: arginine hydrochloride, danazol, glucocorticoids, gastrin, insulin, nifedipine.
- Drugs that may *decrease* glucagon levels: atenolol, propranolol hydrochloride, secretin.

Pre-Test Nursing Care

- Explain to the patient the purpose of the test and the need for a blood sample to be drawn.
- Fasting for 10 to 12 hours is required before the test. Water is permitted.

Procedure

- A 7-mL blood sample is drawn in a chilled collection tube containing EDTA.
- Gloves are worn throughout the procedure.

Post-Test Nursing Care

- Apply pressure at venipuncture site. Apply dressing, periodically assessing for continued bleeding.
- Label the specimen, place it on ice, and transport it to the laboratory immediately.
- Report abnormal findings to the primary care provider.

• • • • • • • • • • • • • • • • •

Glucose, Blood
(Blood Sugar, Fasting Blood Sugar [FBS], Fasting Plasma Glucose [FPG])

Assessment of the blood glucose allows detection of problems with glucose metabolism. Glucose is normally formed in two ways: from the metabolism of ingested carbohydrates and from the conversion of glycogen to glucose in the liver. The maintenance of a normal blood glucose is dependent on proper functioning of two hormones. *Glucagon* causes the blood sugar to rise by speeding the breakdown of glycogen in the liver. *Insulin* allows glucose to pass into cells for use as energy, leading to a decrease in the blood glucose.

Although stressful conditions such as burns or trauma can increase the blood sugar, the most common cause of abnormal glucose metabolism is diabetes mellitus. The fasting blood sugar is an excellent screening tool for diabetes.

Normal Values

70–110 mg/dL (3.9–6.1 mmol/L SI units)

Possible Meanings of Abnormal Values

Increased (Hyperglycemia)	Decreased (Hypoglycemia)
Acromegaly	Addison's disease
Adenoma of pancreas	Anxiety
Brain trauma	Bacterial sepsis
Burns	Excessive exercise
Cushing's syndrome	Glycogen storage disease
Diabetes mellitus	Hepatic necrosis
Eclampsia	Hypothyroidism
Hyperlipoproteinemia	Islet cell carcinoma of the
Hyperthyroidism	pancreas
Liver disease	Malabsorption
Malnutrition	Pituitary hypofunction
Myocardial infarction	Postgastrectomy
Obesity	Reactive hypoglycemia due to
Pancreatitis	high carbohydrate intake
Pheochromocytoma	Stress

Increased (Hyperglycemia)	Decreased (Hypoglycemia)

Pituitary tumors
Prolonged inactivity
Shock
Trauma

Contributing Factors to Abnormal Values

- Drugs that may *increase* fasting blood glucose levels: anabolic steroids, androgens, arginine hydrochloride, ascorbic acid, asparaginase, aspirin, baclofen, benzodiazepines, chlorpromazine, chlorthalidone, cimetidine, clonidine hydrochloride, corticosteroids, corticotropin, dextran, dextrothyroxine, diazoxide, disopyramide phosphate, epinephrine, estrogens, ethacrynic acid, furosemide, glucose infusions, haloperidol, imipramine hydrochloride, isoproterenol, heparin, hydralazine hydrochloride, indomethacin, isoniazid, levodopa, lithium carbonate, mercaptopurine, methimazole, methyldopa, nalidixic acid, nicotine, oral contraceptives, oxazepam, para-aminosalicylic acid, phenolphthalein, phenytoin, progestins, promethazine hydrochloride, propranolol hydrochloride, propylthiouracil, reserpine, ritodrine hydrochloride, terbutaline sulfate, tetracyclines, thiazides, tolbutamide, triamterene.
- Drugs that may *decrease* fasting blood glucose levels: allopurinol, amphetamines, aspirin, beta-adrenergic blockers, caffeine, chlorpropamide, clofibrate, ethanol, guanethidine sulfate, isoniazid, insulin, isocarboxazid, marijuana, nitrazepam, oral hypoglycemic agents, para-aminosalicylic acid, phenazopyridine hydrochloride.

Pre-Test Nursing Care

- Explain to the patient the purpose of the test and the need for a blood sample to be drawn.
- Fasting of at least 8 hours is required before the test. Water is permitted.
- Insulin or oral hypoglycemic agents are to be withheld until after the blood sample is drawn.

Procedure

- A 5-mL blood sample is drawn in a collection tube containing either a silicone gel or a glycolytic inhibitor such as sodium fluoride.
- Gloves are worn throughout the procedure.

Post-Test Nursing Care

- Apply pressure at venipuncture site. Apply dressing, periodically assessing for continued bleeding.
- Label the specimen and transport it to the laboratory immediately. Blood glucose levels decrease when blood is left at room temperature.
- Report abnormal findings to the primary care provider.

• • • • • • • • • • • • • • • • •

Glucose-6-Phosphate Dehydrogenase
(G6PD)

This test measures glucose-6-phosphate dehydrogenase (G6PD), one of the many enzymes normally found in the red blood cells. This enzyme protects the cells from damage from oxidant chemicals. Genetic defects occur in which this enzyme is lacking. This is a sex-linked recessive trait carried on the X chromosome, so males are almost exclusively affected. When this deficiency of G6PD occurs, hemolysis of the red blood cells occurs, resulting in anemia. This genetic problem most frequently affects African-Americans, Greeks, Sardinians, and Sephardic Jews.

Conditions that may precipitate hemolytic episodes in individuals affected with G6PD deficiency include bacterial infection, diabetic acidosis, fava bean ingestion, septicemia, and viral infection. A variety of drugs may also cause hemolytic episodes in these patients. These drugs include analgesics, antimalarials, antipyretics, antipyrine, ascorbic acid, aspirin, chloramphenicol, doxorubicin hydrochloride, furazolidone, methylene blue, nalidixic acid, naphthalene, nitrofurantoin, phenazopyridine hydrochloride, primaquine, probenecid, quinacrine hydrochloride, quinidine, quinine sulfate, sulfamethoxazole, sulfonamides, tolbutamide, and large doses of vitamin K.

G

Normal Values

5–15 U/g of hemoglobin (quantitative test)
Negative (screening test)

Possible Meanings of Abnormal Values

Increased	Decreased
Chronic blood loss	Acidotic state
Hepatic coma	Congenital G6PD deficiency
Hyperthyroidism	Hemolytic anemia
Idiopathic thrombocytopenic purpura	Infection
Megaloblastic anemia	
Myocardial infarction	
Pernicious anemia	

Contributing Factors to Abnormal Values

- False-negative results may occur with hemolyzed samples and in patients who have had recent blood transfusions.
- Drugs that may *decrease* G6PD levels: aspirin and sulfas.

Pre-Test Nursing Care

- Explain to the patient the purpose of the test and the need for a blood sample to be drawn.
- No fasting is required before the test.

Procedure

- A 5-mL sample is drawn in a collection tube containing EDTA.
- Gloves are worn throughout the procedure.

Post-Test Nursing Care

- Apply pressure at venipuncture site. Apply dressing, periodically assessing for continued bleeding.
- Label the specimen and transport it to the laboratory.
- Report abnormal findings to the primary care provider.
- If a deficiency of G6PD is found, education of the patient is needed regarding the drugs and other conditions that may precipitate hemolysis. Caution must be exercised in the use of over-the-counter medications that might contain aspirin.

• • • • • • • • • • • • • • • •

Glucose, Postprandial
(2-Hour Postprandial Blood Sugar, 2-Hour PPBS, 2-Hour pc Glucose)

The postprandial glucose test is conducted to see how the body responds to the ingestion of a meal containing a standard amount of carbohydrates. In normal individuals, a fasting blood sugar drawn 2 hours after a meal ("postprandial") is rarely elevated. However, in diabetic patients, the postprandial value is significantly increased. Thus, the postprandial glucose test is used to confirm the diagnosis of diabetes in patients with abnormally high fasting blood sugar results. It can also be used to monitor the effectiveness of insulin therapy.

Normal Values

Normal: < 120 mg/dL (< 6.7 mmol/L SI units)
Note: Normal value increases 5 mg/dL for each decade of life.

Abnormal Values

Further study indicated:	120–200 mg/dL
Diabetes indicated:	> 200 mg/dL

Possible Meanings of Abnormal Values

Increased	Decreased
Acromegaly	Addison's disease
Advanced liver cirrhosis	Adrenal insufficiency
Anxiety	Anterior pituitary
Cerebral infarction	insufficiency
Cushing's syndrome	Functional hypoglycemia
Diabetes mellitus	Hyperinsulinism
Eclampsia	Islet cell adenoma
Hyperlipoproteinemias	Malabsorption

Increased	Decreased
Hyperthyroidism	Myxedema
Malignancies	Reactive hypoglycemia
Malnutrition	Steatorrhea
Myocardial infarction	
Pheochromocytoma	
Pregnancy	

Contributing Factors to Abnormal Values

- Smoking, caffeine intake, and stress may increase test results.
- Drugs that may *increase* postprandial blood glucose levels: anabolic steroids, androgens, arginine hydrochloride, ascorbic acid, asparaginase, aspirin, baclofen, benzodiazepines, chlorpromazine, chlorthalidone, cimetidine, clonidine hydrochloride, corticosteroids, corticotropin, dextran, dextrothyroxine, diazoxide, disopyramide phosphate, epinephrine, estrogens, ethacrynic acid, furosemide, glucose infusions, haloperidol, imipramine hydrochloride, isoproterenol, heparin, hydralazine hydrochloride, indomethacin, isoniazid, levodopa, lithium carbonate, mercaptopurine, methimazole, methyldopa, nalidixic acid, nicotine, oral contraceptives, oxazepam, para-aminosalicylic acid, phenolphthalein, phenytoin, progestins, promethazine hydrochloride, propranolol hydrochloride, propylthiouracil, reserpine, ritodrine hydrochloride, terbutaline sulfate, tetracyclines, thiazides, tolbutamide, triamterene.
- Drugs that may *decrease* postprandial blood glucose levels: allopurinol, amphetamines, aspirin, beta-adrenergic blockers, caffeine, chlorpropamide, clofibrate, ethanol, guanethidine sulfate, isoniazid, insulin, isocarboxazid, marijuana, nitrazepam, oral hypoglycemic agents, para-aminosalicylic acid, phenazopyridine hydrochloride.

Pre-Test Nursing Care

- Explain to the patient the purpose of the test and the need for a blood sample to be drawn.
- Depending on institutional policy, the patient will either receive a high-carbohydrate diet for 2 to 3 days before the test and a high carbohydrate breakfast the morning of the test or will receive a conventional diet.

Procedure

- Two hours after the patient finishes breakfast, a 5-mL blood sample is drawn in a collection tube containing a glycolytic inhibitor such as sodium fluoride.
- Gloves are worn throughout the procedure.

Post-Test Nursing Care

- Apply pressure at venipuncture site. Apply dressing, periodically assessing for continued bleeding.
- Label the specimen and transport it to the laboratory immediately. Blood glucose levels decrease when blood is left at room temperature.
- Report abnormal findings to the primary care provider.

• • • • • • • • • • • • • • • •

Glucose Tolerance Test
(GTT, Oral Glucose Tolerance Test [OGTT])

The glucose tolerance test is performed to rule out diabetes by evaluating the rate at which glucose is removed from the bloodstream. After administration of either an oral or intravenous glucose load, blood samples are drawn in ½, 1, 2, and 3 hours. The urine is also checked for any spilling of glucose into the urine during the testing period. For nondiabetic patients, the rise in blood glucose is relatively minor and no glucose appears in the urine. For diabetic patients, however, the glucose level shows a dramatic increase and remains greatly elevated for several hours. This test is also used in screening for gestational diabetes during pregnancy.

Normal Values

	Before Age 55	After Age 75	Pregnancy
Fasting	80–110 mg/dL	< 110 mg/dL	< 105 mg/dL
1 hour	120–160 mg/dL	< 200 mg/dL	< 190 mg/dL
2 hours	80–110 mg/dL	< 150 mg/dL	< 165 mg/dL
3 hours	80–110 mg/dL	< 140 mg/dL	< 145 mg/dL

Possible Meanings of Abnormal Values

Increased Tolerance	Decreased Tolerance
Addison's disease	Central nervous system lesions
Hypoparathyroidism	Cushing's syndrome
Hypothyroidism	Diabetes mellitus
Liver disease	Gastrectomy
Pancreatic islet cell hyperplasia	Gestational diabetes
Pancreatic islet cell tumor	Hemochromatosis
Reactive hypoglycemia	Hyperlipidemia
	Hyperthyroidism
	Severe liver damage

Contributing Factors to Abnormal Values

- Bed rest, infections, smoking, and stress may alter test results.
- Drugs that may *increase* glucose tolerance: allopurinol, amphetamines, aspirin, beta-adrenergic blockers, caffeine, chlorpropamide, clofibrate, ethanol, guanethidine sulfate, isoniazid, insulin, isocarboxazid, marijuana, nitrazepam, oral hypoglycemic agents, para-aminosalicylic acid, phenazopyridine hydrochloride.
- Drugs that may *decrease* glucose tolerance: anabolic steroids, androgens, arginine hydrochloride, ascorbic acid, asparaginase, aspirin, baclofen, benzodiazepines, chlorpromazine, chlorthalidone, cimetidine, clonidine hydrochloride, corticosteroids, corticotropin, dextran, dextrothyroxine, diazoxide, disopyramide phosphate, epinephrine, estrogens, ethacrynic acid, furosemide, glucose infusions, haloperidol, imipramine hydrochloride, isoproterenol, heparin, hydralazine hydrochloride, indomethacin, isoniazid, levodopa, lithium carbonate, mercaptopurine, methimazole, methyldopa, nalidixic acid, nicotine, oral contraceptives, ox-

azepam, para-aminosalicylic acid, phenolphthalein, phenytoin, progestins, promethazine hydrochloride, propranolol hydrochloride, propylthiouracil, reserpine, ritodrine hydrochloride, terbutaline sulfate, tetracyclines, thiazides, tolbutamide, triamterene.

CONTRAINDICATIONS

- Any conditions in which there is altered carbohydrate tolerance: endocrine disorders, myocardial infarction, postpartum, recent surgery, serious infections

Pre-Test Nursing Care

- Explain to the patient the purpose of the test and the need for multiple blood samples and urine samples to be collected.
- Fasting for 8 hours is required before the test. Water is permitted.
- No alcohol or coffee intake or excessive physical activity is allowed for 8 hours before the test.
- No smoking is allowed during the testing period.
- If possible, drugs that may influence test results are withheld for 3 days before the test.

G

Procedure

- A 7-mL blood sample is drawn in a collection tube containing a glycolytic inhibitor such as sodium fluoride.
- A urine sample is obtained and tested for glycosuria.
- The patient is given a glucose load:
  - Oral: 75–100 g of glucose dissolved in water or lemon juice (to improve taste of very sweet substance)
  - Intravenous: administer glucose load over 3 to 4 minutes.
- Additional blood samples are drawn at ½, 1, 2, and 3 hours. Urine samples are obtained at the same time intervals.
- If an intravenous glucose load was given, a sample is also drawn at 5 minutes, because the glucose is absorbed much more quickly when given intravenously.
- Water is permitted and encouraged during the testing period to ensure adequate urine output.
- The patient should rest quietly throughout the testing period.
- Gloves are worn throughout the procedure.

Post-Test Nursing Care
Possible complications:
    Hypoglycemia
    Hyperglycemia

- The patient should be observed for weakness, tremors, anxiety, sweating, or fainting. If symptoms occur, a blood sample is drawn and tested for glucose level. For hypoglycemia (low blood sugar), administer orange juice with sugar added or intravenous glucose. For hyperglycemia, insulin will be administered. In either case, the test is discontinued.
- Apply pressure at venipuncture site. Apply dressing, periodically assessing for continued bleeding.
- Label each specimen and transport to the laboratory immediately. Blood glucose levels decrease when blood is left at room temperature.
- Report abnormal values to the primary care provider.

• • • • • • • • • • • • • • • •

Glycosylated Hemoglobin
(G-Hb, Glycated Hgb, Glycohemoglobin, Hemoglobin A_{1c}, HbA_{1c}, $HgbA_{1c}$)

There are several forms of hemoglobin (Hgb), with Hgb A comprising 90% of the total. A portion of Hgb A, denoted as Hgb A_1, is glycolated, meaning it absorbs glucose. When blood glucose levels are above normal for an extended period of time, the hemoglobin of the red blood cells become saturated with glucose in the form of *glycohemoglobin*. This saturation is present for the 120-day life span of the red blood cell. By testing for glycosylated hemoglobin, the health care provider discovers what the average blood glucose level has been for the previous 2 to 3 months. This is especially valuable when monitoring diabetics whose blood sugar levels change dramatically from day to day and to monitor long-term diabetic control. Whereas a fasting blood sugar value may be influenced by the patient's recent adherence to the prescribed treatment regimen, the glycosylated hemoglobin is irreversible; it shows what type of diabetic control has occurred over several months. Because of this, the glycosylated hemoglobin test has become a valued component of diabetic care.

In reviewing test results, it is important to know what is being measured. Some laboratories report glycosylated Hgb as a whole, which includes A_{1a}, A_{1b}, and A_{1c}, whereas others report only Hgb A_{1c}, which can be 2% to 4% less than the value for glycosylated Hgb.

Normal Values

	Hgb A_{1c}	Glycosylated Hgb
Nondiabetic adult	2.2%–4.8%	
Nondiabetic child	1.8%–4.0%	

Abnormal Values

	Hgb A_{1c}	Glycosylated Hgb
Good diabetic control	2.5%–5.9%	7.5% or less
Fair diabetic control	6.0%–8.0%	7.6%–8.9%
Poor diabetic control	> 8.0%	9.0% or more

Possible Meanings of Abnormal Values

Increased	Decreased
Alcohol	Chronic loss of blood
Hyperglycemia	Chronic renal failure
Lead poisoning	Hemolytic anemia
Newly diagnosed diabetic	Pregnancy
Poor diabetic control	Sickle cell anemia
	Splenectomy
	Thalassemia

Pre-Test Nursing Care

- Explain to the patient the purpose of the test and the need for a blood sample to be drawn.
- No fasting is required before the test.
- This test is not affected by the time the blood sample is drawn, by food intake, by exercise, by stress, or by the prior administration of diabetic medications.

Procedure

- A 5-mL blood sample is drawn in a collection tube containing EDTA.
- Gloves are worn throughout the procedure.

Post-Test Nursing Care

- Apply pressure at venipuncture site. Apply dressing, periodically assessing for continued bleeding.
- Label the specimen and transport it to the laboratory.
- Report abnormal findings to the primary care provider.

• • • • • • • • • • • • • • • • • •

G

Gonorrhea Culture

Gonorrhea, the most common venereal disease, usually results from sexual transmission of *Neisseria gonorrhoeae*. This infection is responsible for approximately 50% of all cases of pelvic inflammatory disease in women. Cultures may be taken from the urethra in males and the endocervical canal in women. Other culture sites are the throat and rectum, if the person has had oral or anal sex.

Treatment is usually begun after a culture is found to be positive. However, if the patient is exhibiting symptoms or has had intercourse with an infected individual, treatment is begun once the specimen is obtained.

Normal Values

Negative

Possible Meanings of Abnormal Values

Positive

Gonorrhea

Contributing Factors to Abnormal Values

- Voiding by males within 1 hour of a urethral culture may make fewer organisms available for culture.
- Douching by females within 24 hours of a cervical culture may make fewer organisms available for culture.

Pre-Test Nursing Care

- Explain to the patient the purpose of the test and the type of specimen to be collected.
- No fasting is required before the test.

Procedure

- *For an endocervical culture:*
    - The female patient is assisted into the lithotomy position, draped, and encouraged to relax through deep breathing techniques.
    - A vaginal speculum lubricated with only warm water is inserted. (*Note*: The gonorrhea organism is sensitive to routinely used lubricants.)
    - Cervical mucus is removed using cotton balls held in ring forceps.
- A dry, sterile cotton swab is then inserted into the endocervical canal and rotated from side to side, remaining there for 10 to 30 seconds to allow absorption of organisms onto the swab.
- *For a urethral culture:*
    - The male patient is assisted into a supine position. This position is recommended to avoid falling if vasovagal syncope occurs during the procedure. Such a reaction would be characterized by profound hypotension, bradycardia, pallor, and diaphoresis.
    - The urethral meatus is cleansed with sterile gauze.
    - A calcium alginate swab or a sterile bacteriologic wire loop is inserted 2 to 3 cm into the urethra and rotated from side to side.
- *For a rectal culture:*
    - After the collection of an endocervical or urethral specimen, another sterile cotton swab is inserted approximately 1 inch into the anal canal and moved from side to side to obtain the specimen. If the swab becomes contaminated with stool, it is discarded and the specimen collection is repeated with a clean swab.
- *For a throat culture:*
    - The patient's head is tilted back. The posterior pharynx and tonsillar crypts are swabbed with the sterile swab, while avoiding any contact with the tongue or lips.
- Gloves are worn throughout any of the above procedures.

Post-Test Nursing Care

- After obtaining the specimen, roll the swab in a Z-pattern in a Thayer-Martin medium.
- Label and transport the specimen to the laboratory as soon as possible.
- Advise the patient to avoid all sexual contact until test results are available.
- Report abnormal findings to the primary care provider.
- Patients with positive test results should have their sexual partners examined.

• • • • • • • • • • • • • • • • •

Growth Hormone
(GH, Human Growth Hormone [hGH], Somatotropin, Somatotrophic Hormone [STH])

Growth hormone (GH) is a polypeptide produced by the anterior pituitary gland. Its primary function is to stimulate growth of the body. It also plays important roles in protein synthesis, fatty acid utilization, insulin mobilization, and RNA production. The synthesis and release of GH is regulated by the hypothalamus by growth hormone–releasing factor (GHRF) and growth hormone release–inhibiting factor (GHRIH, or somatostatin).

Hyposecretion of GH in children results in dwarfism, whereas hypersecretion of GH in children leads to gigantism and in adults, acromegaly. This test is used to determine hypofunctioning and hyperfunctioning of the pituitary gland, so that appropriate intervention can be initiated.

Normal Values

Adults: 2.0–6.0 ng/mL (2.0–6.0 µg/L SI units)
Children: < 10 ng/mL (< 10 µg/L SI units)

Possible Meanings of Abnormal Values

Increased	Decreased
Acromegaly	Dwarfism
Anorexia nervosa	Failure to thrive
Gigantism	Growth hormone deficiency
Hypoglycemia	Hyperglycemia
Hypothalamic tumor	Hypopituitarism
Hyperpituitarism	
Pituitary tumor	
Sleep (2 hours after)	
Starvation	
Surgery	

Contributing Factors to Abnormal Values

- Levels of growth hormone may vary with exercise, nutritional status, sleep, and stress.
- Testing for growth hormone should be scheduled no sooner than 48 hours after any diagnostic tests using radioactive materials.
- Drugs that may *increase* levels of growth hormone: arginine hydrochloride, estrogens, glucagon, levodopa, oral contraceptives.
- Drugs that may *decrease* levels of growth hormone: corticosteroids.

Pre-Test Nursing Care

- Explain to the patient the purpose of the test and the need for a blood sample to be drawn.
- Fasting for 8 hours is required before the test. Water is permitted.
- The patient should be at rest in a stress free environment for 30 minutes before the test.

Procedure

- A 5-mL blood sample is drawn in a collection tube containing a silicone gel.
- Gloves are worn throughout the procedure.

Post-Test Nursing Care

- Apply pressure at venipuncture site. Apply dressing, periodically assessing for continued bleeding.
- Label the specimen and transport it to the laboratory immediately.
- Report abnormal findings to the primary care provider.

• • • • • • • • • • • • • • • •

Growth Hormone Stimulation Test
(Arginine Test, GH Stimulation Test)

The growth hormone stimulation test is performed to diagnose growth hormone deficiency. Growth hormone (GH) is a polypeptide produced by the anterior pituitary gland. Its primary function is to stimulate growth of the body. It also plays important roles in protein synthesis, fatty acid utilization, insulin mobilization, and RNA production. The synthesis and release of GH is regulated by the hypothalamus by growth hormone–releasing factor (GHRF) and growth hormone release–inhibiting factor (GHRIH, or somatostatin).

A variety of methods are used to stimulate growth hormone secretion for this test. These include insulin-induced hypoglycemia, vigorous exercise, and drugs such as arginine hydrochloride, glucagon, levodopa, and clonidine hydrochloride.

Normal Values

> 10 ng/mL (> 10 µg/L SI units)

Possible Meanings of Abnormal Values

Decreased (Lack of GH Increase)

Growth hormone deficiency

Contributing Factors to Abnormal Values

- The growth hormone stimulation test should be scheduled no sooner than 48 hours after any diagnostic tests using radioactive materials.

CONTRAINDICATIONS

- Patients with cerebrovascular disease
- Patients with epilepsy
- Patients with low basal plasma cortisol levels
- Patients who have had a myocardial infarction

Pre-Test Nursing Care

- All steroid medications should be withheld before the test, if possible. If they must be given, record the drug name on the laboratory slip.
- Explain to the patient the purpose of the test and that the test will usually involve the intravenous infusion of a drug. Note that several blood samples will need to be drawn.
- Fasting for 8 to 10 hours is required before the test. Water is permitted.
- The patient should be at rest in a stress-free environment for 90 minutes before the test.

Procedure

- A baseline blood sample of 5 to 7-mL is drawn in a collection tube containing a silicone gel.
- Procedures will vary depending on the type of stimulator used. Check with reference laboratory for specific procedures.
  - For example, use of arginine, an amino acid, involves intravenous infusion of the drug over 30 minutes. Blood samples are then drawn 30, 60, and 90 minutes after the infusion is complete.
- Use of an intermittent infusion device, such as a saline lock, will allow drug administration and blood sampling without the need for numerous venipunctures.
- Gloves are worn throughout the procedure.

Post-Test Nursing Care

- Apply pressure at venipuncture site. Apply dressing, periodically assessing for continued bleeding.
- Carefully label any blood samples as to the time drawn. Samples must be taken to the laboratory immediately, because growth hormone has a half-life of only 20 to 25 minutes.
- Resume diet and medications as before the test.
- Report abnormal findings to the primary care provider.

•   •   •   •   •   •   •   •   •   •   •   •   •   •   •   •   •

Ham Test
(Acidified Serum Lysis Test)

The Ham test is conducted to identify paroxysmal nocturnal hemoglobinuria (PNH), a rare condition in which hemoglobin is found in the urine during and after sleep. This condition is thought to be related to the hypersensitivity of red blood cells to higher levels of carbon dioxide and the resulting decrease in blood pH. To perform the test, the patient's blood sample is mixed with ABO-compatible normal serum and acid, maintained at 37° C, and then examined for hemolysis. Normally, red blood cells do not undergo hemolysis. However, red blood cells from patients with PNH are especially susceptible to lysis under these conditions.

Normal Values

Negative: < 5% lysis

Possible Meanings of Abnormal Values

Increased

Aplastic anemia
Dyserythropoietic anemia
Leukemia
Paroxysmal nocturnal hemoglobinuria
Spherocytosis

Contributing Factors to Abnormal Values

- Hemolysis of the blood sample may alter test results.
- Transfusion of whole blood or packed cells within 3 weeks of this test may cause false-negative results.

CONTRAINDICATIONS

- Patients who have received a blood transfusion within 3 weeks before the test

Pre-Test Nursing Care

- Explain to the patient the purpose of the test and the need for a blood sample to be drawn.
- No fasting is required before the test.

Procedure

- A 7-mL blood sample is drawn in a collection tube containing EDTA.
- Gloves are worn throughout the procedure.

Post-Test Nursing Care

- Apply pressure at venipuncture site. Apply dressing, periodically assessing for continued bleeding.
- Label the specimen and transport it to the laboratory.
- Report abnormal findings to the primary care provider.

• • • • • • • • • • • • • • • •

Haptoglobin

Haptoglobin is an alpha$_2$-globulin protein produced in the liver. It combines with free hemoglobin that has been released due to red blood cell destruction. This action conserves the body's iron stores by preventing their excretion in the urine. Any condition that destroys red blood cells can thus deplete haptoglobin levels very rapidly, because it cannot be replaced quickly enough. Examples of such conditions are hemolytic anemia, mechanical disruption as from prosthetic heart valves, and antibodies, as seen in transfusion reactions.

Normal Values

13–163 mg/dL (0.13–1.63 g/L SI units)

Possible Meanings of Abnormal Values

Increased	Decreased
Acute infection	Autoimmune hemolytic anemia
Acute rheumatic disease	Congenital ahaptoglobinemia
Arterial disease	Erythroblastosis fetalis
Biliary obstruction	G6PD deficiency
Chronic infection	Hemolysis
Granulomatous disease	Hepatocellular disease
Inflammation	Hereditary spherocytosis
Malignant neoplasms	Hypertension
Peptic ulcer	Infectious mononucleosis
Pneumonia	Malarial infestation
Post-myocardial infarction	Paroxysmal nocturnal
Pregnancy	hemoglobinuria
Tissue necrosis	Prosthetic heart valves
Tuberculosis	Sickle cell disease
Ulcerative colitis	Systemic lupus erythematosus
	Thalassemia
	Thrombotic thrombocytopenic purpura
	Transfusion reaction
	Uremia

Contributing Factors to Abnormal Values

- Hemolysis of the blood sample will alter test results.
- Drugs that may *increase* haptoglobin levels: androgens, corticosteroids.
- Drugs that may *decrease* haptoglobin levels: chlorpromazine, diphenhydramine hydrochloride, estrogens, indomethacin, isoniazid, nitrofurantoin, oral contraceptives, quinidine, streptomycin.

Pre-Test Nursing Care

- Explain to the patient the purpose of the test and the need for a blood sample to be drawn.
- No fasting is required before the test.

Procedure

- A 7-mL blood sample is drawn in a collection tube containing no additives.
- Gloves are worn throughout the procedure.

Post-Test Nursing Care

- Apply pressure at venipuncture site. Apply dressing, periodically assessing for continued bleeding.
- Label the specimen and transport it to the laboratory immediately, taking care not to shake it, because this will cause unwanted hemolysis.
- Report abnormal findings to the primary care provider.

• • • • • • • • • • • • • • • • •

Heart Scan

(Cardiac Nuclear Scanning, MUGA Scan, Myocardial Scan, Nitroglycerin Scan, PYP Heart Scan, Thallium Scan, Thallium Stress Testing)

The heart scan is a noninvasive procedure that involves the intravenous injection of a radiopharmaceutical followed by nuclear imaging. There are four primary types of heart scan.

The *PYP scan* is also known as "hot spot myocardial imaging." It involves the injection of technetium-99m stannous pyrophosphate, which is thought to combine with calcium present in damaged myocardial cells. These hot spots appear within 12 hours of infarction and are most prominent 48 to 72 hours post infarction. This test is used to determine the occurrence, extent, and prognosis of myocardial infarction. The PYP scan is especially useful when the electrocardiogram and the cardiac enzyme studies are inconclusive.

The *thallium scan* involves the injection of thallium-201, which is absorbed in *healthy* tissue. Ischemic tissue eventually absorbs the radionuclide, but infarcted tissue never does. This results in what is known as "cold spots" on the scan. This scan is used to show myocardial perfusion, to demonstrate the location and extent of acute or chronic myocardial infarction, to diagnose coronary artery disease, and to monitor the effectiveness of angioplasty, coronary artery grafts, and antianginal therapy. In some patients, no evidence of myocardial ischemia occurs during a resting state. For this type of patient, the thallium is injected during exercise stress testing. The thallium accumulates in the myocardium in direct proportion to the perfusion to the area. Normal myocardial muscle will have a higher thallium concentration than ischemic heart muscle. This type of testing is know as *thallium stress testing*.

The *MUGA scan* stands for "multigated acquisition." This type of scan is similar to routine imaging of the heart, except that instead of one image, the scintillation events are distributed in multiple images. The camera records 14 to 64 points of a single cardiac cycle, resulting in sequential images that can be studied like motion picture films to show the left ventricular function and to determine the ejection fraction. This test also shows myocardial wall abnormalities.

The *nitroglycerin MUGA scan* is similar to the MUGA scan, except that the camera records points in the cardiac cycle after the sublingual administration of nitroglycerin. This assesses the effect of nitroglycerin on ventricular function.

Single-photon emission computed tomography (SPECT) is now being used to provide a three-dimensional image of the functioning heart. This test provides excellent resolution and allows areas of myocardial ischemia to be quantified. However, the cost of the equipment required for this testing is prohibitive for many institutions.

Normal Values

Normal ejection fraction, no evidence of myocardial ischemia or infarction

Possible Meanings of Abnormal Values

Aneurysm
Cardiomyopathy
Coronary artery disease
Myocardial infarction
Myocardial ischemia
Myocardial necrosis
Myocarditis

Contributing Factors to Abnormal Values

- Any movement by the patient may alter quality of films taken.
- Test results may be altered by myocardial trauma, recent nuclear scans, and drugs such as long-acting nitrates.

CONTRAINDICATIONS

- Pregnant women
  Caution: A woman in her childbearing years should undergo radiography only during her menses or 12 to 14 days after its onset to avoid any exposure to a fetus.
- Patients who are lactating
- Patients who are unable to cooperate owing to age, mental status, pain, or other factors

Pre-Test Nursing Care

- Explain to the patient the purpose of the test. Provide any written teaching materials available on the subject. Note that discomfort involved with this test is primarily due to lying on a hard table for an extended period of time and the venipuncture. Reassure the patient that only trace amounts of the radionuclide are involved in the test.
- The patient must remain still while the scan is being performed.
- Fasting for 4 hours before the test is required for the PYP and thallium scans.
- Obtain a signed informed consent form.
- Resuscitation and suctioning equipment should be readily available.

Procedure

- The selected radionuclide is administered by intravenous injection in a peripheral vein:
  - PYP scan: Injection 2 to 3 hours before the scan
  - Thallium scan: Scanning begins 5 minutes after injection
  - MUGA scan: Scanning begins 1 minute after injection
  - Nitroglycerin MUGA scan: Scan is done after each injection of nitroglycerin
- The patient is assisted to a supine position on the examination table.
- A scintillation camera is positioned over the patient's chest. This camera takes a radioactivity reading from the body. This information is transformed into a two-dimensional picture of the heart.
- Gloves are worn during the radionuclide injection.

Post-Test Nursing Care

- Check the injection site for redness or swelling.
- If a woman who is lactating *must* have a nuclear scan, she should not breast feed the infant until the radionuclide has been eliminated, possibly for 3 days.
- Although the amount of diagnostic radionuclide excreted in the urine is low, the urine should not be used for any laboratory tests for the time period indicated by the nuclear medicine department. Clients should be told to flush the toilet three times after voiding.
- Gloves are worn when dealing with the urine.
- No other radionuclide tests should be scheduled for 24 to 48 hours.
- Encourage fluid intake by the patient to enhance excretion of the radionuclide.
- Report abnormal findings to the primary care provider.

• • • • • • • • • • • • • • • • • •

Hematocrit
(Crit, Hct, Packed Cell Volume, PCV)

Hematocrit is defined as the proportion of red blood cells to plasma within a sample of blood. After collection of the sample, the specimen is centrifuged. Because of their weight, the red blood cells are forced to the bottom of the test tube. A determination of the percentage of these packed cells in comparison to the plasma is then made.

Hematocrit can be used to assess the extent of a patient's blood loss. A drop of 3% in hematocrit equals approximately one unit of blood loss. It is important to note, however, that the drop in hematocrit does not occur immediately. As a result of a large blood loss, there is a loss of equal proportions of red blood cells and plasma. Thus the hematocrit remains normal for a period of time. In an attempt to compensate for the blood loss and return the plasma volume to normal, the body shifts fluid from the intracellular and interstitial compartments to the intravascular compartment. Red blood cells, however, are not able to be replaced in such a short time. Thus, the relative percentage of red blood cells, as denoted by the hematocrit, will decrease.

Hematocrit is a useful measure only if the patient's hydration level is normal. When normal hydration is present and the total red blood cell count and hemoglobin are both normal, the hematocrit is approximately three times the hemoglobin result.

Normal Values

Female:	37%–48% (0.37–0.48 SI units)
Male:	42%–52% (0.42–0.52 SI units)
Pregnancy:	Decreased (dilutional)
Elderly:	Slightly decreased
Newborn:	Increased

Possible Meanings of Abnormal Values

Increased	Decreased
Any conditions that increase the red blood cell count (see Red Blood Cell Count)	Any conditions that decrease the red blood cell count (see Red Blood Cell Count)
Burns	Anemia
Dehydration (hemoconcentration)	Overhydration (hemodilution)
Shock	

Contributing Factors to Abnormal Values

- Tests results may be affected by problems with procedure technique:
    - Taking the sample from the arm in which an intravenous line is infusing results in hemodilution and a decreased hematocrit.
    - Leaving the tourniquet in place for more than 1 minute during the procedure will result in hemoconcentration. This can increase the hematocrit by 2.5%–5%.
- False increases may occur when the blood glucose level is greater than 400 mg/dL, when the patient is dehydrated, or in the presence of leukocytosis.

- Individuals living in high altitudes have increased hematocrit results.
- Hemolysis of the sample can alter test results.

Pre-Test Nursing Care

- Explain to the patient the purpose of the test and the need for a blood sample to be drawn.
- No fasting is required before the test.

Procedure

- Obtain the sample before the patient's bath, shower, or massage, because these activities can temporarily increase the hematocrit.
- The blood sample can be obtained in one of two ways:
  1. Hematocrit can be performed on capillary blood, so a finger stick (or heel stick for infants) may be used.
     a. After the puncture is made, discard the first drop of blood.
     b. Use a capillary tube for collection of a 0.5-mL sample.
     c. Do *not* squeeze the tissue to increase the bleeding, because this adds tissue fluids and causes dilution of the sample.
  2. Venipuncture may also be used. A 5-mL sample is drawn in a collection tube containing EDTA.
- Gloves are worn throughout the procedure.

Post-Test Nursing Care

- If venipuncture is used, invert the tube and gently mix the sample with the anticoagulant.
- Apply pressure at venipuncture or stick site. Apply dressing, periodically assessing for continued bleeding.
- Label the specimen and transport it to the laboratory. Note on the laboratory order slip if the stick method is used. Hematocrit results may be 5% to 10% higher when capillary blood is used rather than venous blood.
- Report abnormal findings to the primary care provider.

• • • • • • • • • • • • • • • •

Hemoglobin
(Hb, Hgb)

Hemoglobin is composed of the *heme* portion, which contains iron and the red pigment porphyrin, and the *globin* portion, which is a protein. By measuring the hemoglobin concentration of the blood, one is determining the oxygen-carrying capacity of the blood. This test is usually used to assess anemias. When the patient's hydration status is normal, the hemoglobin is approximately one third of the hematocrit value.

Normal Values

Female:	12–16 g/dL (7.4–9.9 mmol/L SI units)
Male:	13–18 g/dL (8.1–11.2 mmol/L SI units)
Pregnancy:	decreased (dilutional)
Elderly:	slightly decreased
Newborn:	increased

Possible Meanings of Abnormal Values

Increased	Decreased
Acquired hemolytic anemia	Blood loss
Burns	Bone marrow suppression
Chronic obstructive	Cancer
pulmonary disease	Cystic fibrosis
Congestive heart failure	Heavy menstrual flow
Dehydration	Hemodilution
Diarrhea	Hemoglobinopathies
Hemoconcentration	Hemolytic anemia
Intravascular hemolysis	Hodgkin's disease
Polycythemia vera	Hyperthyroidism
Sickle cell anemia	Iron-deficiency anemia
Thalassemia major	Kidney disease
	Leukemia
	Liver disease
	Sarcoidosis
	Systemic lupus erythematosus

Contributing Factors to the Abnormal Values

- Leaving the tourniquet in place for more than 1 minute during the procedure will result in hemoconcentration.
- False increases may occur with lipemic samples and when leukocytosis is present.
- Individuals living in high altitudes have increased hemoglobin results.
- Hemolysis of the sample can alter test results.
- Drugs that may *increase* hemoglobin level: gentamicin, methyldopa.
- Drugs that may *decrease* hemoglobin level: antibiotics, antineoplastic agents, apresoline, aspirin, indomethacin, MAO inhibitors, primaquine, rifampin, sulfonamides, trimethadione.

Pre-Test Nursing Care

- Explain to the patient the purpose of the test and the need for a blood sample to be drawn.
- No fasting is required before the test.

Procedure

- Obtain the sample before the patient's bath, shower, or massage, because these activities can temporarily increase the hematocrit.
- The blood sample can be obtained in one of two ways:

1. Hemoglobin can be performed on capillary blood, so a finger stick (or heel stick for infants) may be used.
   a. After the puncture is made, discard the first drop of blood.
   b. Use a capillary tube for collection of a 0.5-mL sample.
   c. Do *not* squeeze the tissue to increase the bleeding, because this adds tissue fluids and causes dilution of the sample.
2. Venipuncture may also be used. A 5-mL sample is drawn in a collection tube containing EDTA.
- Gloves are worn throughout the procedure.

Post-Test Nursing Care

- If venipuncture is used, invert the tube and gently mix the sample with the anticoagulant.
- Apply pressure at venipuncture site. Apply dressing, periodically assessing for continued bleeding.
- Label the specimen and transport it to the laboratory.
- Report abnormal findings to the primary care provider.

• • • • • • • • • • • • • • • • • •

Hemoglobin Electrophoresis
(Hgb Electrophoresis)

Hemoglobin electrophoresis is used to identify abnormal types or amounts of hemoglobin, the oxygen-carrying component of the blood. The hemoglobin molecules are placed in a solution through which an electrical current is sent. The various types of hemoglobin migrate through the solution at different rates, depending on the strength or weakness of their electrical charges. This movement allows a mapping of the types and relative percentages of hemoglobin present in the sample.

The types of hemoglobin that may be included in the electrophoresis are the following:

Hemoglobins Normally Found in the Body

Hemoglobin A: This is the major adult hemoglobin normally found in the body.
Hemoglobin A_2:   This is a minor hemoglobin normally found in the body.
Hemoglobin F: This hemoglobin, known as fetal hemoglobin, is normally found in the body in a very small quantity.

Hemoglobins Usually Absent from the Body

Hemoglobin C: This hemoglobin causes red blood cells to sickle.
Hemoglobins D/E: When these hemoglobins are present in a patient with sickle cell anemia or thalassemia, the disease tends to be of a more serious nature.
Hemoglobin H: This hemoglobin disrupts normal transport of oxygen to the tissues of the body. Hemoglobin H binds with the oxygen, which prevents it from being available to the tissues.
Hemoglobin S: This hemoglobin causes the red blood cells to distort into a sickle shape in response to decreased oxygen levels. Its presence is the basis for the diagnosis of *sickle cell trait,* which occurs in approximately 10% of African-Americans, and *sickle cell anemia,* which affects one in every 625 African-Americans.

Normal Values

Hgb A 95%–100%
Hgb A_2 2%–3%
Hgb F < 1%
Hgb C, D, E, and H: normally absent
Neonates: Hgb F > 50%

Possible Meanings of Abnormal Values

Hemoglobin C trait:	Hgb C = 45%
Hemoglobin C disease:	Hgb C > 90%
Hemolytic anemia:	Hgb D and Hgb E present
Sickle cell trait:	Hgb S 20%–40%
	Hgb A 60%–80%
	Hgb F < 2%
Sickle cell disease:	Hgb S 80%–100%
	Hgb F < 2%
	Hgb A is absent
Thalassemia minor:	Hgb F 2%–8%
	Hgb A_2 = 1%
Thalassemia major:	Hgb F 20%–90%
	Hgb A is decreased
	Hgb A_2 may be normal, low, or high

Contributing Factors to Abnormal Values

- Blood transfusions received in the past 3 to 4 months may alter test results.
- Hemolysis of the sample may alter test results.

Pre-Test Nursing Care

- Explain to the patient the purpose of the test and the need for a blood sample to be drawn.
- No fasting is required before the test.

Procedure

- The sample is drawn in a collection tube containing EDTA.
- Gloves are worn throughout the procedure.

Post-Test Nursing Care

- Invert and gently mix the sample and the anticoagulant.
- Apply pressure at venipuncture site. Apply dressing, periodically assessing for continued bleeding.
- Label the specimen and transport it to the laboratory.
- Report abnormal findings to the primary care provider.
- If sickle cell trait or sickle cell disease is found, genetic counseling should be offered.

• • • • • • • • • • • • • • • •

Hepatitis Antigens and Antibodies
(Hepatitis A, Hepatitis B, Hepatitis C, Delta Virus)

Hepatitis is inflammation of the liver that may be caused by a virus, bacteria, or a toxic substance. There are four major types of viral hepatitis that have been identified. Each is caused by a different virus and differs in its incubation period, mode of transmission, and severity.

Hepatitis A, formerly called infectious hepatitis, has an incubation period of 15 to 45 days and is primarily transmitted by the oral-fecal route. *Hepatitis B,* previously known as serum hepatitis, has an incubation period of 28 to 180 days. It is spread primarily by blood and body secretions. This form of hepatitis is more serious than hepatitis A. It is associated with the development of liver cancer and may be fatal.

Hepatitis C, was at one time called non-A, non-B hepatitis. It has an incubation period of 7 to 8 weeks. It is spread primarily by contact with blood and body fluids. Clinically, this form of hepatitis is similar to hepatitis B, but of less severity. It is also associated with development of liver cancer and frequently progresses to chronic hepatitis and cirrhosis of the liver. *Delta hepatitis* is caused by the delta virus, an RNA virus. This type of hepatitis seems to only infect people who already have hepatitis B.

There are numerous tests for the various forms of hepatitis.

Hepatitis A Antibody, IgM and IgG (HAV-Ab)

This test measures antibodies to the hepatitis A virus. If the antibodies are found to be of the IgM type, this is indicative of a current infection with hepatitis A. IgM antibodies appear 2 to 4 weeks after exposure to hepatitis and are detectable for only 4 to 8 weeks. If the antibodies are of the IgG type, this indicates a past infection with hepatitis A and probable immunity to the disease. IgG antibodies are the second type of immunoglobulins that appear in an immune response. These immunoglobulins are present for life, which provides immunity from reinfection with this type of hepatitis.

Hepatitis B Surface Antigen (HBsAg)

This test measures the surface antigen of the hepatitis B virus. It is used to screen potential blood donors and to diagnose hepatitis B virus. HBsAg is the earliest indicator of hepatitis B, often rising before clinical symptoms appear. This antigen usually appears 4 to 12 weeks after infection and is indicative of active hepatitis B. If the level of HBsAg continues above normal, the person is considered to be a carrier of hepatitis B.

Hepatitis B Surface Antibody (HBsAb, anti-HBs)

This test measures antibodies to the hepatitis B surface antigen. This antibody appears 2 to 16 weeks after the hepatitis B surface antigen has disappeared. The presence of this antibody demonstrates immunity to the hepatitis B virus, except for a few rare subtypes. This test is used to determine if a vaccine is needed for persons at risk for hepatitis B.

Hepatitis B Core Antigen (HBcAg)

This test measures a core antigen of the hepatitis B virus in liver cells. It is used only for research purposes.

Hepatitis B Core Antibody (HBcAb, anti-HBc)

This test measures antibodies to the core antigen of hepatitis B. This antibody appears in the serum 1 to 4 weeks after contraction of the hepatitis B virus, rises during the chronic phase of the illness, and remains present for the patient's lifetime. The HBcAb is elevated during the time between the disappearance of the surface antigen (HBsAg) and the appearance of the surface antibody (HBsAb). This time period is the "core window" phase. Thus, it is the most reliable test to determine the presence of hepatitis B infection when both the surface antibody and surface antigen are absent.

Hepatitis B e Antigen (HBeAg)

This test measures the e antigen of the hepatitis B virus. This antigen usually appears within 4 to 12 weeks of the infection and is present for only 3 to 6 weeks. The HBeAg level correlates with titers of the virus, so the test is used primarily to evaluate the degree of infectivity. If this antigen persists in the blood for more than 3 months, chronic liver disease is probable.

Hepatitis B e Antibody (HBeAb, anti-HBe)

This test measures antibodies to the e antigen of the hepatitis B virus. This antibody appears 8 to 16 weeks after the infection and usually indicates the acute infection is over. The presence of this antibody along with a positive result in testing for the hepatitis B surface antigen (HBsAg) usually indicates a carrier state.

Hepatitis C Antibody (Anti-HCV)

This test measures antibodies to the hepatitis C virus. Most cases of post-transfusion hepatitis are hepatitis C in nature.

Delta Hepatitis Antibody (Anti-HDV)

This test measures antibodies to the delta hepatitis virus. A positive test result suggests recent infection or carrier state for the virus, which only occurs in conjunction with the hepatitis B virus.

Normal Values

Negative

Possible Meanings of Abnormal Values

Positive

Hepatitis A antibody (HAV-ab)
Positive, IgM: acute hepatitis A infection
Positive, IgG: past exposure to hepatitis A, probable immunity
Hepatitis B surface antigen (HBsAG)
Either active hepatitis B or a carrier state
Hepatitis B surface antibody (HBsAB, anti-HBs)
Immunity to hepatitis B
Hepatitis B core antibody (HBcAb, anti-HBc)
Hepatitis B infection

Hepatitis B e antigen (HBeAg)
Hepatitis B infection
Hepatitis B e antibody (HBeAb, anti-HBe)
Hepatitis B infection or carrier state
Hepatitis C antibody (anti-HCV)
Hepatitis C
Delta hepatitis antibody (anti-HDV)
Hepatitis D

Contributing Factors to Abnormal Values

- Diagnostic testing in which radionuclides were used within 1 week before this test may falsely elevate test results.

Pre-Test Nursing Care

- Explain to the patient the purpose of the test and the need for a blood sample to be drawn.
- No fasting is required before the test.

Procedure

- A 7-mL blood sample is drawn in a collection tube containing a silicone gel.
- Gloves are worn throughout the procedure.

Post-Test Nursing Care

- Apply pressure at venipuncture site. Apply dressing, periodically assessing for continued bleeding.
- Label the specimen and transport it to the laboratory.
- Report abnormal findings to the primary care provider.

• • • • • • • • • • • • • • • •

Herpes Simplex Antibody
(Herpes Genitalis, Herpes Simplex Virus [HSV], Herpesvirus)

This test measures antibodies to the herpes simplex virus. Herpes simplex is a common viral infection transmitted through contact with mucous membrane secretions. Herpes simplex 1 (HSV-1) is caused by the human herpesvirus 1 and is usually found in the respiratory tract, eyes, or mouth (cold sores). Herpes simplex 2 (HSV-2) is caused by the human herpesvirus 2 and is generally found in the genitourinary tract. HSV-2 is also known as genital herpes (herpes genitalis). The common pattern of infection with the herpesvirus is primary infection, latency, and reactivation (secondary infection). A newborn may become infected (neonatal herpes) during vaginal delivery if the mother is currently infected with genital herpes. Should a woman acquire the herpes virus during pregnancy, the fetus may have congenital herpes, resulting in disorders of the central nervous system and brain damage.

Normal Values

Negative or titer < 1:10:   no infection

Abnormal Values

Titer of 1:10–1:100:   infection within 7 days
Titer of 1:100–1:500:   current to late infection
Titer of > 1:500:   established latent infection

Possible Meanings of Abnormal Values

Increased

HSV infection

Contributing Factors to Abnormal Values

- Hemolysis of the sample will alter test results.

Pre-Test Nursing Care

- Explain to the patient the purpose of the test and the need for a blood sample to be drawn.
- No fasting is required before the test.

Procedure

- A 5-mL blood sample is drawn into a collection tube containing no additives.
- Gloves are worn throughout the procedure.
- A culture of any lesions may also be obtained to isolate the type of HSV.

Post-Test Nursing Care

- Apply pressure at venipuncture site. Apply dressing, periodically assessing for continued bleeding.
- Label the specimen and transport it to the laboratory as soon as possible.
- Report abnormal findings to the primary care provider.
- Explain to the pregnant patient that, should genital herpes be present at the time of delivery, cesarean section may be necessary.
- Sexual partners of patients testing positive for HSV–2 should also be tested.

High-Density Lipoprotein
(HDL)

Cholesterol is synthesized in the liver from dietary fats. It is transported in the blood by the low-density lipoproteins (LDLs, or "bad" cholesterol) and high-density lipoproteins (HDLs, or "good" cholesterol). HDLs carry excess cholesterol back to the liver for removal from the body. Thus, higher levels of HDL are desired because they seem to be associated with a decreased risk for coronary heart disease.

The high-density lipoprotein (HDL) level is measured as part of the lipid profile. Using the information from the lipid profile, another parameter that is analyzed is the cholesterol/HDL ratio. The greater this ratio, the greater the risk for developing atherosclerosis. For men, the average ratio is approximately 5; for women, 4.4.

Normal Values

Risk factor for coronary heart disease (CHD):
  Negative: > 60 mg/dL (> 1.55 mmol/L SI units)

Abnormal Values

Risk factor for coronary heart disease (CHD):
  Positive: < 35 mg/dL (< 0.91 mmol/L SI units)

Possible Meanings of Abnormal Values

Increased	Decreased
Alcoholism	Chronic inactivity
Chronic liver disease	Diabetes mellitus
Decreased risk for CHD	End-stage liver disease
Long-term aerobic exercises	Hyperthyroidism
	Hypertriglyceridemia
	Increased risk of CHD
	Obesity
	Smoking

Contributing Factors to Abnormal Values

- Radiologic contrast agents and recent weight changes may alter test results.
- Drugs that may *increase* HDL levels: aspirin, cimetidine, estrogens, ethanol, lovastatin, nicotinic acid, oral contraceptives, phenothiazines, phenytoin, steroids, sulfonamides, terbutaline sulfate.
- Drugs that may *decrease* HDL levels: androgens, beta-blockers.

Pre-Test Nursing Care

- Explain to the patient the purpose of the test and the need for a blood sample to be drawn.
- Fasting for 12 hours is required before the test. Water is permitted.

Procedure

- A 7-mL blood sample is drawn in a collection tube containing EDTA.
- Gloves are worn throughout the procedure.

Post-Test Nursing Care

- Apply pressure at venipuncture site. Apply dressing, periodically assessing for continued bleeding.
- Label the specimen and transport it to the laboratory.
- Report abnormal findings to the primary care provider.

Histoplasmosis Test

This test assesses for the presence of antibodies to histoplasmosis, the most common systemic fungal infection. This disease is caused by *Histoplasma capsulatum*, an organism that lives in moist soil, the floors of chicken houses, and bird droppings, especially those of blackbirds and starlings. The fungus is endemic to the central and eastern portions of North America. It is most often found in the states of Ohio and Missouri and the valleys of the Mississippi River. The disease is usually localized as a pulmonary disorder, often resembling tuberculosis. Those individuals with debilitating or chronic diseases, such as the acquired immunodeficiency syndrome (AIDS) or diabetes, and those receiving certain types of drug therapy that may alter the immune system, such as steroids and antineoplastic agents, are considered more highly susceptible to this disease.

Normal Values

Immunodiffusion: negative
Complement-fixation titer: < 1:8

Abnormal Values

Titers of 1:8 to 1:16 indicate infection.
Titers > 1:32 indicate active disease.

Possible Meanings of Abnormal Values

Increased

Histoplasmosis

Contributing Factors to Abnormal Values

- Antibodies may be found normally in people who live where the fungus is considered endemic.
- There may be a cross-reaction with blastomycosis, resulting in falsely high titers.
- Skin tests can cause a serologic test to become positive. Thus, skin tests should be withheld until after the blood sample is drawn.
- Many mycoses cause immunosuppression, leading to low titers, or false-negative test results.
- Contamination of the blood sample will alter test results.
- Hemolysis of the sample due to excessive agitation may alter results.
- Antibodies may appear early in the disease and then disappear.

Pre-Test Nursing Care

- Obtain a travel and work history from the patient.
- Explain to the patient the purpose of the test, noting that it involves drawing a blood sample.
- The patient is to be NPO for 12 hours before the test.

Procedure

- The test should be conducted 2 to 4 weeks after exposure to the organism.
- A 7-mL blood sample is drawn in a collection tube containing no additives.
- Gloves are worn throughout the procedure.

Post-Test Nursing Care

- Apply pressure at venipuncture site. Apply dressing, periodically assessing for continued bleeding.
- Label the specimen and transport it immediately to the laboratory, taking care to avoid excessive agitation of the sample.
- Advise the patient that other procedures to test for this fungus may be done. Such testing might include sputum cultures and skin testing.
- Report abnormal findings to the primary care provider.

● ● ● ● ● ● ● ● ● ● ● ● ● ● ● ● ● ●

HIV Testing
(Acquired Immunodeficiency Syndrome Tests, AIDS Serology, ELISA for HIV and Antibody, Human Immunodeficiency Virus (HIV) Antibody Test, Western Blot for HIV and Antibody)

Human immunodeficiency virus (HIV) is the virus that causes acquired immunodeficiency syndrome (AIDS). The HIV virus attacks the body's helper T cells, which are important components of cell-mediated immunity. This results in immunosuppression and susceptibility to opportunistic infections such as *Pneumocystis carinii* and *Candida albicans*. Modes of transmission of the virus include direct contact between the blood of the infected person with that of an uninfected person and through sexual and body fluid transmission. Thus, individuals at high risk for AIDS include sexually active homosexuals, individuals with multiple sexual partners, intravenous drug users who have shared needles, persons who have received numerous transfusions of blood products (such as hemophiliacs), and newborns of infected women.

Multiple tests are available for HIV testing. The most common is the enzyme-linked immunosorbent assay or ELISA. This test is used to screen for HIV but is not considered to be a confirmatory test. This is because of false-negative and false-positive test results that are possible with this testing method. ELISA detects antibodies to HIV, not the HIV antigens. Therefore, a positive ELISA will not occur until antibodies have had time to form. If the ELISA is positive, the test is repeated using the same blood sample. If the test is again positive, the Western blot is performed. The Western blot test uses electrophoresis techniques to separate out component proteins of HIV, thus allowing detection of HIV antibodies. Should the Western blot test also be positive, the person is considered to have serologic evidence of HIV infection. It is important to note, and inform the patient, that this means there has been exposure to the virus and the virus is present in the body, but this does not necessarily indicate the occurrence of clinical AIDS.

Normal Values

Negative for antibodies to HIV

Possible Meanings of Abnormal Values

Positive

AIDS
HIV exposure

Contributing Factors to Abnormal Values

- Antibody results may be negative for up to 35 months after infection with HIV. This is due to the latency period of the virus. During this period of time, known as the "window phase," the patient shows no symptoms of the infection. However, the patient may pass on the infection to others during this phase.

Pre-Test Nursing Care

- Explain to the patient the purpose of the test and the need for a blood sample to be drawn.
- An informed written consent is required.
- No fasting is required before the test.

Procedure

- A 10-mL blood sample is drawn in a collection tube containing a silicone gel.
- Gloves are worn throughout the procedure.

Post-Test Nursing Care

Possible complication: Infection at venipuncture site due to immunocompromised state

- Apply pressure at venipuncture site. Apply dressing, periodically assessing for continued bleeding.
- Teach the patient to monitor the site and to notify the health care provider if signs or symptoms of infection occur, such as drainage, redness, warmth, edema, pain at the site, or fever.
- Label the specimen, following institutional policy regarding maintaining confidentiality of patient's identity and test results. Transport the specimen to the laboratory.
- Report abnormal findings to the primary care provider.
- Provide to the patient emotional support, counseling, and education regarding the transmission of AIDS.

• • • • • • • • • • • • • • • •

Human Leukocyte Antigen Test
(HLA Test, HLA Typing, Tissue Typing)

Human leukocyte antigen (HLAs) are glycoproteins found on many types of tissue cells, leukocytes, and platelets. The HLA test is done to determine what leukocyte antigens are present on the surface of the cells. This information is crucial when organ transplantation is being considered, because histocompatibility (tissue compatibility) *must* be present to minimize the chance for organ rejection.

Another use of HLA typing is paternity testing. In this situation, the HLAs of a child are compared with those of the potential father. If the HLA typing does not match, it disqualifies the man from being the father. However, if the HLA typing does match, it indicates that man *might* be the father.

There are many HLA antigens. However, some specific antigens have been found to be associated with certain diseases. The most common example of this is HLA-B27, which has been found in patients with ankylosing spondylitis, Reiter's syndrome, and rheumatoid arthritis.

Normal Values

Requires interpretation of HLA antigen combination

Possible Meanings of Abnormal Values

Positive for HLA-B27

Ankylosing spondylitis
Reiter's syndrome
Rheumatoid arthritis

Contributing Factors to Abnormal Values

- Hemolysis of the blood sample may alter test results.
- Receipt of a blood transfusion within 72 hours before the test will alter test results.

Pre-Test Nursing Care

- Explain to the patient the purpose of the test and the need for a blood sample to be drawn.
- No fasting is required before the test.

Procedure

- A 7-mL blood sample is drawn in a collection tube containing heparin.
- Gloves are worn throughout the procedure.

Post-Test Nursing Care

- Apply pressure at venipuncture site. Apply dressing, periodically assessing for continued bleeding.
- Label the specimen and transport it to the laboratory.
- Report abnormal findings to the primary care provider.

● ● ● ● ● ● ● ● ● ● ● ● ● ● ●

Human Placental Lactogen
(HPL, Human Chorionic Somatomammotropic [HCS])

This test is used to evaluate placental functioning. Human placental lactogen (HPL) is a protein hormone produced by the placenta. In pregnancy, HPL promotes increased blood glucose levels. The level of HPL slowly increases throughout pregnancy, reaching a level of 7 µg/mL at term, and dropping abruptly to zero after delivery. Low HPL values during pregnancy may indicate fetal distress and warrant further assessment of fetal viability with nonstress testing and amniocentesis.

Normal Values

Value rises during pregnancy:

5th–27th week:	< 4.6 µg/mL
28th–31st week:	2.4–6.1 µg/mL
32nd–35th week:	3.7–7.7 µg/mL
36th week to term:	5–8.6 µg/mL

Possible Meanings of Abnormal Values

Increased	Decreased
Maternal diabetes mellitus	Choriocarcinoma
Maternal liver disease	Fetal distress
Maternal sickle cell disease	Hydatidiform mole
Multiple pregnancies	Intrauterine growth
Rh isoimmunization	retardation
	Postmaturity syndrome
	Threatened abortion
	Toxemia of pregnancy

Contributing Factors to Abnormal Values
- Hemolysis of the blood sample and recent radioactive scans may alter test results.

Pre-Test Nursing Care
- Explain to the patient the purpose of the test and the need for a blood sample to be drawn.
- No fasting is required before the test.

Procedure
- A 7-mL blood sample is drawn in a collection tube containing no additives.
- Gloves are worn throughout the procedure.

Post-Test Nursing Care

- Apply pressure at venipuncture site. Apply dressing, periodically assessing for continued bleeding.
- Label the specimen and transport it to the laboratory.
- Report abnormal findings to the primary care provider.

• • • • • • • • • • • • • • • •

Human T-Cell Lymphotrophic I/II Antibody
(HTLV-I, HTLV-II)

Human T-cell lymphotrophic virus is the name for several different retroviruses. HTLV-III is the former name of the human immunodeficiency virus (HIV) known to cause acquired immunodeficiency syndrome (AIDS). HTLV-I and HTLV-II do not cause AIDS. They are, however, associated with other types of diseases. HTLV-I is linked with adult T-cell leukemia. HTLV-II is associated with adult hairy-cell leukemia. However, presence of the antibody to these viruses in the blood does not necessarily mean the person will develop the disease.

H

Normal Values

Negative

Possible Meanings of Abnormal Values

Positive

Acute HTLV infection
Adult T-cell leukemia
Adult hairy-cell leukemia
Demyelinating neurologic disorders
Tropical spastic paraparesis

Pre-Test Nursing Care

- Explain to the patient the purpose of the test and the need for a blood sample to be drawn.
- No fasting is required before the test.

Procedure

- A 7-mL blood sample is drawn in a collection tube containing a silicone gel.
- Gloves are worn throughout the procedure.

Post-Test Nursing Care

- Apply pressure at venipuncture site. Apply dressing, periodically assessing for continued bleeding.
- Label the specimen and transport it to the laboratory.
- Report abnormal findings to the primary care provider.

• • • • • • • • • • • • • • • •

17-Hydroxycorticosteroids
(17-OHCS, Porter–Silber Test)

The adrenal cortex secretes three types of hormones: the glucocorticoids (primarily cortisol), the mineralocorticoids (aldosterone), and the sex hormones (androgens, estrogen, progesterone). The test for 17-hydroxycorticosteroids (17-OHCS) measures the metabolites, or products, of the breakdown of the glucocorticoids known as cortisone and hydrocortisone. It is thus a test of adrenal cortical function. This test has been used in the differential diagnosis of Cushing's syndrome and Addison's disease. Urinary cortisol levels and plasma cortisol levels are more sensitive tests and are replacing this test.

Normal Values
Female: 2.0–6.0 mg/d (5.5–17 μmol/day SI units)
Male: 3.0–10.0 mg/d (8–28 μmol/day SI units)

Possible Meanings of Abnormal Values

Increased	Decreased
Acetonuria	Addison's disease
Acromegaly	Adrenal infarction
Acute illness	Adrenal hemorrhage
Adrenal hyperplasia	Anorexia nervosa
Adrenal tumor	Congenital adrenal hyperplasia
Cushing's syndrome	Hypopituitarism
Ectopic ACTH-producing tumor	Hypothyroidism
Fructosuria	
Glucosuria	
Hirsutism	
Hypertension (severe)	
Insomnia	
Obesity	
Pituitary tumor	
Pregnancy	
Stress	
Thyrotoxicosis	
Virilism	

Contributing Factors to Abnormal Values
- Drugs that may *increase* 17-OHCS levels: acetazolamide, ascorbic acid, cephalothin, cefoxitin, chloral hydrate, chlordiazepoxide, chlorpromazine, colchicine, corticotropin, cortisone acetate, digitalis glycosides, erythromycin, glutethimide, gonadotropins, hydrocortisone, hydroxyzine hydrochloride, iodides, meprobamate, methenamine mandelate, methicillin sodium, methyprylon, paraldehyde, quinidine, quinine sulfate, spironolactone, troleandomycin.

- Drugs that may *decrease* 17-OHCS levels: apresoline, carbamazepine, corticosteroids, dextropropoxyphene, estrogens, medroxyprogesterone acetate, meperidine hydrochloride, morphine, oral contraceptives, pentazocine, phenothiazines, phenytoin, promethazine hydrochloride, reserpine, salicylates, thiazides.

Pre-Test Nursing Care

- Explain 24-hour urine collection procedure to the patient.
- Stress the importance of saving *all* urine in the 24-hour period. Instruct the patient to avoid contaminating the urine with toilet paper or feces.
- Inform the patient of the presence of a preservative in the collection bottle.
- If possible, withhold any drugs that may interfere with test results.

Procedure

- Obtain the proper container containing the appropriate preservative from the laboratory.
- Begin the testing period in the morning after the patient's first voiding, which is discarded.
- Timing of the 24-hour period begins at the time the first voiding is discarded.
- *All* urine for the next 24 hours is collected in the container that is to be kept refrigerated or on ice.
- If any urine is accidentally discarded during the 24-hour period, the test must be discontinued and a new test begun.
- The ending time of the 24-hour collection period should be posted in the patient's room.
- Gloves are to be worn when dealing with the specimen collection.

Post-Test Nursing Care

- Label the container and transport it on ice to the laboratory as soon as possible after the end of the 24-hour collection period.
- Resume medications as taken before the test.
- Report abnormal findings to the primary care provider.

• • • • • • • • • • • • • • • •

5-Hydroxyindoleacetic Acid
(5 HIAA)

Serotonin is produced by argentaffin cells in the gastrointestinal tract. Functions of serotonin include vasoconstriction and regulation of smooth muscle contraction, such as that occurring during peristalsis. Serotonin is metabolized in the liver, resulting in the production of 5-hydroxyindoleacetic acid (5-HIAA), which is excreted in the urine. Argentaffinomas, early carcinoid tumors of the intestine, secrete abnormal amounts of serotonin. This abnormal secretion, which can reach as high as 300 to 1,000 mg/24 h, can be found through measurement of 5-HIAA in the urine.

Normal Values

Qualitative random sample: Negative
Quantitative: 2–9 mg/24 h (10–47 µmol/d SI units)
     Lower in women than in men

Possible Meanings of Abnormal Values

Increased

Benign or malignant carcinoid tumors of the intestine
Intake of foods high in serotonin (see Contributing Factors to Abnormal Values)
Tumors in other organs

Contributing Factors to Abnormal Values

- Test results may be altered by improper 24-hour urine collection technique, severe diarrhea, or ingestion of foods containing large amounts of serotonin, such as avocados, bananas, eggplants, pineapples, red plums, tomatoes, and walnuts.
- Drugs that may *increase* 5-HIAA levels: glyceryl guaiacolate, methocarbamol, reserpine.
- Drugs that may *decrease* 5-HIAA levels: chlorpromazine, imipramine hydrochloride, isoniazid, MAO inhibitors, methenamine mandelate, methyldopa, phenothiazines, promazine hydrochloride, promethazine hydrochloride.

Pre-Test Nursing Care

- Explain 24-hour urine collection procedure to the patient.
- Stress the importance of saving *all* urine in the 24-hour period. Instruct the patient to avoid contaminating the urine with toilet paper or feces.
- Maintain a diet low in serotonin (see Contributing Factors to Abnormal Values) for 4 days before the test.
- Inform the patient of the presence of an acid solution in the collection bottle.
- Check with the laboratory regarding any questionable medications that the patient may be taking to determine the need to hold any medications before the test.
- Notify the physician of the patient's medications that may alter the test results.

Procedure

- Obtain the proper container containing an acidic preservative such as hydrochloric acid or boric acid from the laboratory.
- Begin the testing period in the morning after the patient's first voiding, which is discarded.
- Timing of the 24-hour period begins at the time the first voiding is discarded.
- *All* urine for the next 24 hours is collected in the container, which is to be kept refrigerated or on ice.
- If any urine is accidentally discarded during the 24-hour period, the test must be discontinued and a new test begun.
- The ending time of the 24-hour collection period should be posted in the patient's room.
- Gloves are worn when dealing with the specimen collection.

H

Post-Test Nursing Care

- Label the container and transport it on ice to the laboratory as soon as possible after the end of the 24-hour collection period.
- Resume the patient's usual diet and medications after test completion.
- Report abnormal findings to the primary care provider.

• • • • • • • • • • • • • • • • • •

Hysterosalpingography
(Uterosalpingography)

Hysterosalpingography is used to detect blocked fallopian tubes. It can also confirm the presence of uterine abnormalities. A cannula is inserted into the cervix through which contrast medium is injected. This allows for viewing of the uterus and the fallopian tubes by fluoroscopy. The incidence of allergic reaction to the dye is reduced, because the dye is usually not absorbed when administered in this way. Radiographic films are taken throughout the procedure.

H

Normal Values

Normal size, shape, position of uterus and fallopian tubes
Patent fallopian tubes

Possible Meanings of Abnormal Values

Intrauterine adhesions
Intrauterine fibroids
Intrauterine foreign body
Partial or complete blockage of fallopian tube(s)
Uterine fistula

Contributing Factors to Abnormal Values

- Retained barium, gas, or stool in the intestines may result in poor quality films.
- Tubal spasm or excess traction may cause false-positive test results owing to the appearance of a stricture in normal fallopian tubes.
- Excessive traction can cause false-negative test results owing to displacement of adhesions, making the fallopian tubes appear normal.

CONTRAINDICATIONS

- Patients who are allergic to iodine, shellfish, or contrast medium dye
- Patients who are pregnant or suspected of being pregnant
- Patients who are in their menses
- Patients with undiagnosed vaginal bleeding
- Patients with pelvic inflammatory disease

Pre-Test Nursing Care

- Explain to the patient the purpose of the test. Provide any written teaching materials available on the subject. Note that discomfort during this test is due to menstrual-like cramping and shoulder pain owing to injection of the dye and its normal leakage in the peritoneal cavity.
- Check for allergies to iodine, shellfish, or contrast medium dye. Inform the radiologist of such possible allergy.
- Patients receiving metformin (Glucophage) for non–insulin-dependent diabetes mellitus should discontinue the drug 2 days before elective surgery or angiographic examinations. This is due to the possible occurrence of lactic acidosis, a potentially fatal complication of biguanide therapy.
- Obtain a signed informed consent.
- No fasting is required before the test.
- A laxative the night before the test or an enema or suppository the morning of the test may be ordered.
- Pre-procedure sedation may be ordered.

Procedure

- The patient is placed in the lithotomy position.
- A plain abdominal x-ray film is taken to check for absence of retained barium, gas, or stool in the intestine.
- A speculum is inserted into the vagina.
- The cervix is cleansed, and a cannula is inserted into the cervix.
- Contrast medium is injected through the cannula.
- The flow of the dye is followed fluoroscopically through the uterus and fallopian tubes.
- Films are taken throughout the procedure.
- Gloves are worn throughout the procedure.

Post-Test Nursing Care

Possible complications:

   Allergic reaction to dye
   Infection of the endometrium or fallopian tubes
   Uterine perforation

- Most allergic reactions to radiopaque dye occur within 30 minutes of administration of the contrast medium. Observe the patient closely for respiratory distress, hypotension, edema, hives, rash, tachycardia, and/or laryngeal stridor. Emergency resuscitation equipment must be readily accessible.
- Observe for allergic reaction to the dye for 24 hours.
- A perineal pad is applied. Inform the patient that a bloody vaginal discharge may be present for 1 to 2 days after the procedure.
- Monitor vital signs at least every 4 hours for 24 hours.
- Observe for indications of infection, including elevated temperature, chills, flushing, tachycardia, and abdominal pain.
- Renal function should be assessed before metformin is restarted.
- Report abnormal findings to the primary care provider.

• • • • • • • • • • • • • • • •

Immunoelectrophoresis
(Antibodies, Gamma Globulins, Immunoglobulins, IgA, IgD, IgE, IgG, IgM)

The total blood protein consists of albumin and globulin, which is further divided into the alpha, beta, and gamma globulins. The gamma globulins are called *immunoglobulins*, because, as components of antibodies, they play a vital role in the immune process. Five types of immunoglobulins are measured during electrophoresis: IgA, IgD, IgE, IgG, and IgM.

Immunoglobulin G (IgG) is the most abundant of the gamma globulins, accounting for approximately 75% of the total. IgG provides protection against viruses, bacteria, and toxins and is the only immunoglobulin that crosses the placenta. IgG is particularly important in the secondary response of the immune system. When the immune system is confronted with an antigen for the first time, the *primary* response is made by IgM and is soon followed by an elevation of the IgG level. IgG retains memory of the antigen, so that the next time the immune system is challenged by the antigen, IgG is ready to immediately respond.

Immunoglobulin A (IgA), which makes up 10% to 15% of the total gamma globulins, is the second most abundant gamma globulin. IgA is present in several body fluids, including colostrum, saliva, and tears. This immunoglobulin is considered the first line of defense against organisms attempting to invade the respiratory, gastrointestinal, and urinary tracts.

Immunoglobulin M (IgM) accounts for 7% to 10% of the gamma globulins. It is the first immunoglobulin to respond to an antigen coming in contact with the immune system for the first time. Thus, because the IgM level is the first to increase in the primary response, the IgM level is an indicator of an acute infection. IgM is also responsible for the formation of natural antibodies, such as the ABO blood groups.

Immunoglobulin E (IgE) is present in very small amounts. It plays a role in allergic responses, such as hypersensitivity and anaphylactic reactions. Its level also increases in parasitic infestations.

Immunoglobulin D (IgD) is also present in very small amounts. Its function is unknown.

To conduct *immunoelectrophoresis*, an electrical current is passed through the blood serum, causing the various immunoglobulins to separate according to their electrical charge. Each immunoglobulin forms a band that has a characteristic appearance. This appearance is altered when an abnormality of a particular immunoglobulin is present.

Normal Values

Adult

IgG: 639–1,349 mg/dL (6.39–13.49 g/L SI units)
IgA: 70–312 mg/dL (0.70–3.12 g/L SI units)
IgM: 56–352 mg/dL (0.56–3.52 g/L SI units)
IgD: 0.5–3 mg/dL (0.005-0.03 g/L SI units)
IgE: 0.01-0.04 mg/dL (0.0001-0.0004 g/L SI units)

Newborn

IgG: 640–1,250 mg/dL (6.40–12.50 g/L SI units)
IgA: 0–11 mg/dL (0-0.11 g/L SI units)
IgM: 5–30 mg/dL (.05-0.30 g/L SI units)
IgD and IgE: negligible

Possible Meanings of Abnormal Values

IgG

Increased	Decreased
IgG myeloma	Acquired immunodeficiency syndrome (AIDS)
Infectious disease	Agammaglobulinemia
Liver disease	Bacterial infections
Lymphomas	Humoral immune deficiency
Multiple sclerosis	IgA myeloma
Neurosyphilis	Leukemia
Parasitic disease	Lymphoid aplasia
Rheumatic fever	Preeclampsia
Rheumatoid arthritis	
Sarcoidosis	
Severe malnutrition	
Sjögren's syndrome	
Systemic lupus erythematosus	

IgA

Increased	Decreased
Alcoholism	Agammaglobulinemia
Carcinoma	Chronic sinopulmonary disease
Cirrhosis	Hereditary ataxia-
Chronic infections	telangiectasia
Dysproteinemia	Humoral immune deficiency
Exercise	Hypogammaglobulinemia
Liver disease	Inflammatory bowel disease
Multiple myeloma	Late pregnancy
Obstructive jaundice	Leukemia
Rheumatoid arthritis	Nephrotic syndrome
Sinusitis	

IgM

Increased	Decreased
Actinomycosis	Agammaglobulinemia
Bartonellosis	Amyloidosis
Fungal infections	Humoral immune deficiency
Infectious mononucleosis	Hypogammaglobulinemia
Malaria	IgG and IgA myeloma
Rheumatoid arthritis	Inflammatory bowel disease
Systemic lupus erythematosus	Leukemia
Trypanosomiasis	Lymphoid aplasia
Waldenström's macroglobulinemia	Nephrotic syndrome

IgE

Increased	Decreased
Asthma	Acquired immunodeficiency syndrome (AIDS)
Dermatitis	Advanced carcinoma
Eczema	Agammaglobulinemia
Food and drug allergies	Ataxia-telangiectasia
Hay fever	IgE deficiency
IgE myeloma	Non–IgE myeloma
Pemphigoid	
Periarteritis nodosa	
Rhinitis	
Sinusitis	
Wiskott-Aldrich syndrome	

IgD

Increased	Decreased
Autoimmune disease	Acquired immunodeficiency syndrome (AIDS)
Chronic infections	Non–IgD myeloma
Dysproteinemia	
IgD myeloma	

Contributing Factors to Abnormal Values

- Drugs that may *increase* IgA: asparaginase.
- Drugs that may *decrease* IgA: carbamazepine, dextran, estrogens, gold, immunosuppressive drugs, methylprednisolone, oral contraceptives, penicillamine, phenytoin, valproic acid.
- Drugs that may *increase* IgM: chlorpromazine.
- Drugs that may *decrease* IgM: carbamazepine, dextran.
- Drugs that may *increase* IgE: gold compounds.
- Drugs that may *decrease* IgE: phenytoin.
- Drugs that may *decrease* IgD: phenytoin.

Pre-Test Nursing Care

- Explain to the patient the purpose of the test and the need for a blood sample to be drawn.
- No fasting is required before the test.

Procedure

- A 7-mL blood sample is drawn in a collection tube containing no additives.
- Gloves are worn throughout the procedure.

Post-Test Nursing Care

- Apply pressure at venipuncture site. Apply dressing, periodically assessing for continued bleeding.
- Label the specimen and transport it to the laboratory.
- Report abnormal findings to the primary care provider.

• • • • • • • • • • • • • • •

Immunoglobulin Light Chains
(Bence Jones Protein)

Patients with such conditions as multiple myeloma and amyloidosis often have an increased production of a single homogeneous immunoglobulin or immunoglobulin fragment (i.e., kappa or lambda light chains). These immunoglobulin light chains, called Bence Jones proteins, are small and easily cleared by the kidney. Hence, they will be present in the urine and are usually absent in the plasma. Historically, the detection of light chains in urine was based on their unique solubility characteristics related to temperature. On heating a urine sample, these proteins will precipitate out of solution when at 40° C to 60° C, redissolve at 100° C, and reappear on cooling. This "heat precipitation test" is insensitive and nonspecific. Today, sensitive and specific detection of immunoglobulin light chains (i.e., Bence Jones protein) is obtained using immunoelectrophoresis.

Normal Values

Absence of immunoglobulin light chains in the urine

Possible Meanings of Abnormal Values

Increased

Adult Fanconi's syndrome
Amyloidosis
Benign monoclonal gammopathy
Chronic lymphocytic leukemia
Chronic renal insufficiency
Cryoglobulinemia
Hyperparathyroidism
Malignant lymphoma
Metastases
Multiple myeloma
Primary amyloidosis
Rheumatoid arthritis
Systemic lupus erythematosus
Waldenström's macroglobulinemia

Contributing Factors to Abnormal Values

- False-negative test results may occur with dilute urine or in the presence of severe urinary tract infection.

Pre-Test Nursing Care

- Explain the procedure to the patient, stressing the importance of not contaminating the specimen.

Procedure

- A minimum of 50 mL of urine is needed for the test. Collection of an early morning specimen is best.
- Use of clean-catch midstream technique is recommended to prevent contamination of the specimen.
  - A clean-catch kit containing cleansing materials and a sterile specimen container is given to the patient.
  - Male patients should cleanse the urinary meatus with the materials provided or with soap and water, void a small amount of urine into the toilet, and then void directly into the specimen container.
  - Female patients should cleanse the labia minora and urinary meatus, cleansing from front to back. While keeping the labia separated, the female should void a small amount into the toilet and then void directly into the specimen container.
  - Instruct patients to avoid touching the inside of the specimen container and lid.
- A 24-hour urine collection may be needed to detect trace amounts of protein. If so, refrigerate specimen throughout the collection.
- Gloves are to be worn by the health care worker when dealing with the specimen.

Post-Test Nursing Care

- Label the specimen. The specimen must be taken to the laboratory immediately or refrigerated to prevent bacterial growth that can lead to a breakdown of proteins.
- Report abnormal findings to the primary care provider.

• • • • • • • • • • • • • • • • • •

Immunoscintigraphy

Immunoscintigraphy is based on the use of monoclonal antibody technology. In this type of testing, radioactive antibodies travel to specific sites within the body for the detection of certain malignancies. Although in the future more types of cancer will be able to be tested for in this way, the current testing is limited to detecting recurrent metastatic colorectal or ovarian cancer. The monoclonal antibodies for this test have the radionuclide indium chloride-111 attached to them. After the antibodies are injected and locate on cancer cells, the radionuclide is able to be detected through scanning.

Normal Values

No areas of increased radionuclide uptake in the body

Possible Meanings of Abnormal Values

Ovarian cancer
Recurrent colorectal cancer

Contributing Factors to Abnormal Values

- Any movement by the patient may alter quality of films taken.
- *False-positive* results can occur owing to uptake of the radionuclide in degenerative joint disease, abdominal aortic aneurysm, and inflammatory gastrointestinal diseases.

 ## CONTRAINDICATIONS

- Pregnant women
  Caution: A woman in her childbearing years should undergo radiography only during her menses or 12 to 14 days after its onset to avoid any exposure to a fetus.
- Patients who are lactating
- Patients who are unable to cooperate owing to age, mental status, pain, or other factors

Pre-Test Nursing Care

- Explain to the patient the purpose of the test. Provide any written teaching materials available on the subject. Note that discomfort involved with this test is limited to the venipuncture. Reassure the patient that only trace amounts of the radionuclide are involved in the test.
- The patient must remain still while the scan is being performed.
- No fasting is required before the test.
- Obtain a signed informed consent.

Procedure

- The radiolabeled monoclonal antibody is administered by intravenous injection in a peripheral vein.
- At the designated time (48 to 72 hours post injection), the patient is taken to the nuclear medicine department.
- The patient is assisted to a supine position on the examination table.
- Scans are made of the anterior and posterior chest, abdomen, and pelvis.
- Gloves are worn during the radionuclide injection.

Post-Test Nursing Care

- Check the injection site for redness or swelling.
- If a woman who is lactating *must* have a nuclear scan, she should not breast feed the infant until the radionuclide has been eliminated, possibly for 3 days.
- Although the amount of diagnostic radionuclide excreted in the urine is low, the urine should not be used for any laboratory tests for the time period indicated by the nuclear medicine department. Clients should be told to flush the toilet three times after voiding.
- Gloves are worn when dealing with the urine.
- Encourage fluid intake by the patient to enhance excretion of the radionuclide.
- Report abnormal findings to the primary care provider.

· · · · · · · · · · · · · · ·

Insulin
(Insulin Assay, Serum Insulin)

This test measures the level of insulin in the serum. Insulin is a hormone secreted by the beta cells of the islets of Langerhans. It regulates the metabolism and transport of carbohydrates, amino acids, proteins, and lipids. Insulin secretion occurs when the plasma level of glucose increases. As the plasma glucose level decreases, secretion of insulin ceases. Measurement of the serum insulin level is used to assist in the diagnosis of hypoglycemic states and diabetes mellitus.

Normal Values

0–29 μ/mL   (0–208 pmol/L SI units)

Possible Meanings of Abnormal Values

Increased	Decreased
Acromegaly	Hyperglycemia
Cushing's syndrome	Hypopituitarism
Dystrophia myotonia	Insulin-dependent diabetes mellitus
Fructose intolerance	
Galactose intolerance	
Hyperinsulinism	
Hypoglycemia	
Insulinoma	
Liver disease	
Non–insulin-dependent diabetes mellitus	
Obesity	
Pancreatic islet cell lesion	

Contributing Factors to Abnormal Values

- Radioactive scans within 7 days before the test will alter test results.
- Hemodialysis destroys insulin.
- Drugs that may *increase* insulin levels: albuterol, calcium gluconate in the newborn, epinephrine, fructose, glucagon, glucose, levodopa, medroxyprogesterone acetate, oral contraceptives, prednisolone, quinidine, spironolactone, sucrose, terbutaline sulfate, thyroid hormones, tolazamide, tolbutamide.
- Drugs that may *decrease* insulin levels: beta-adrenergic blockers, asparaginase, calcitonin, cimetidine, diazoxide, ethacrynic acid, ethanol, ether, furosemide, metformin, nifedipine, phenobarbital, phenytoin, thiazide diuretics.

Pre-Test Nursing Care

- Explain to the patient the purpose of the test and the need for a blood sample to be drawn.
- Fasting for 8 hours is required before the test. Water is permitted.
- Insulin should be withheld before the test.

Procedure

- A 7-mL blood sample is drawn in a collection tube containing no additives.
- Gloves are worn throughout the procedure.

Post-Test Nursing Care

- Apply pressure at venipuncture site. Apply dressing, periodically assessing for continued bleeding.
- Label the specimen, place it in ice, and transport it to the laboratory immediately.
- Resume medications as taken before the test.
- Report abnormal findings to the primary care provider.

• • • • • • • • • • • • • • • • • •

Insulin Antibody Test
(Anti-Insulin Antibody)

Most insulin preparations are derived from beef and pork pancreases and contain insulin-related peptides. IgG antibodies, known as anti-insulin AB, form in response to these peptides. With subsequent insulin injections, these antibodies join and neutralize the insulin so that it is no longer able to function appropriately. Larger doses of insulin are then required to attempt to meet the patient's needs. The insulin antibody test is performed to help determine the cause of the allergy to the insulin and the most appropriate therapeutic agent for the patient.

Normal Values

Undetectable for bovine or porcine insulin

Possible Meanings of Abnormal Values

Positive	Negative
Allergy to insulin	Insulinoma
Factitious hypoglycemia	
Insulin resistance	

Contributing Factors to Abnormal Values

- Radioactive scans within 7 days before the test will alter test results.

Pre-Test Nursing Care

- Explain to the patient the purpose of the test and the need for a blood sample to be drawn.
- No fasting is required before the test.

Procedure

- A 7-mL blood sample is drawn in a collection tube containing no additives.
- Gloves are worn throughout the procedure.

Post-Test Nursing Care
- Apply pressure at venipuncture site. Apply dressing, periodically assessing for continued bleeding.
- Label the specimen and transport it to the laboratory.
- Report abnormal findings to the primary care provider.

• • • • • • • • • • • • • • • • • •

Iron
(Fe)

Iron is a mineral of the body that is found primarily in the hemoglobin. Its function is to carry oxygen to the tissues, and it indirectly assists in returning carbon dioxide to the lungs. Measurement of iron levels assists in the diagnosis of anemia. Iron levels vary throughout the day; therefore, laboratories usually specify the time the blood sample should be drawn.

Normal Values
50–150 µg/dL (9.0–26.9 µmol/L SI units)
Elderly: decreased

Possible Meanings of Abnormal Values

Increased	Decreased
Acute liver damage	Blood loss
Aplastic anemia	Burns
Hemochromatosis	Cancer
Hemolytic anemia	Infection
Hemosiderosis of excessive iron intake	Inflammation
	Myocardial infarction
Lead poisoning	Nephrosis
Nephritis	Pregnancy
Pernicious anemia	Rheumatoid arthritis
Polycythemia	Uremia
Thalassemia	

Contributing Factors to Abnormal Values
- Falsely increased iron levels may occur owing to intake of vitamin B_{12} within 48 hours before testing the iron level or hemolysis of the sample
- Iron levels may be up to ten times higher in the morning as at night.
- Falsely decreased iron levels may occur owing to a lipemic specimen or in the presence of inflammatory states.
- Drugs that may *increase* the iron level: dextran, iron supplements, and oral contraceptives.
- Drugs that may *decrease* the iron level: chloramphenicol and corticotropin.

Pre-Test Nursing Care

- Explain to the patient the purpose of the test and the need for a blood sample to be drawn.
- Fasting is required for 12 hours before the test. Water intake is allowed.
- No iron supplements are to be taken within 24 to 48 hours before the test.

Procedure

- Obtain the blood sample in the morning, usually after 10 AM.
- A 5-mL blood sample is obtained in a collection tube containing a silicone gel.
- Gloves are worn throughout the procedure.

Post-Test Nursing Care

- Apply pressure at venipuncture site. Apply dressing, periodically assessing for continued bleeding.
- Label the specimen and transport it to the laboratory.
- Report abnormal findings to the primary care provider.
- Should the iron level be found to be low, provide the patient with information regarding dietary sources of iron, such as dried fruits, eggs, and organ meats.

• • • • • • • • • • • • • • • • •

K Iron Tests

See:
Ferritin
Iron
Total Iron-Binding Capacity
Transferrin
Transferrin Saturation

• • • • • • • • • • • • • • • •

17-Ketosteroids (17-KS)

This test provides an indication of adrenal function. The adrenal cortex secretes three types of hormones: the glucocorticoids (primarily cortisol), the mineralocorticoids (aldosterone), and the sex hormones (androgens, estrogen, progesterone). The test for 17-ketosteroids (17-KS) measures the adrenal hormones and metabolites of testicular androgens. All 17-ketosteroids are not androgens, but they do produce androgenic effects. Testosterone, which is the most potent androgen, is not measured by this test in that testosterone is not a 17-ketosteroid. Thus this test is but an approximation of androgenic activity. To provide a more complete representation of androgenic activity, plasma testosterone levels should also be measured.

Normal Values

Female > 15 years:	5.0–15.0 mg/d (17.3–52.0 µmol/d SI units)
Male > 15 years:	9.0–22.0 mg/d (31.2–76.3 µmol/d SI units)
11–14 years:	2.0–7.0 mg/d (6.9–24.2 µmol/d SI units)
Birth 10 years:	0.1–3.0 mg/d (0.4–10.4 µmol/d SI units)

Possible Meanings of Abnormal Values

Increased	Decreased
Adrenal hyperplasia	Addison's disease
Adrenocortical tumors	Castration
Adrenogenital syndrome	Chronic illness
Cushing's syndrome	Gout
Hirsutism	Hypogonadism
Hyperpituitarism	Hypopituitarism
Infection (severe)	Klinefelter's syndrome
Obesity	Myxedema
Ovarian luteal cell tumors	Menopause
Pregnancy	Nephrosis
Premature infants	Thyrotoxicosis
Stein-Leventhal syndrome	
Stress	
Testicular interstitial cell tumors	

Contributing Factors to Abnormal Values

- Stress and exercise may alter test results.
- Drugs that may *increase* 17-KS levels: ampicillin, ascorbic acid, cephalothin, chloramphenicol, chlordiazepoxide, chlorpromazine, cloxacillin sodium, corticotropin, cortisone, dexamethasone, digitoxin, erythromycin, ethinamate, hydralazine hydrochloride, meprobamate, methicillin sodium, methyprylon, morphine, nalidixic acid, oxacillin sodium, penicillin, phenazopyridine hydrochloride, phenothiazines, piperidine, pyridium, quinidine, quinine sulfate, salicylates, secobarbital, spironolactone, testosterone, troleandomycin.
- Drugs that may *decrease* 17-KS levels: aminoglutethimide, chlordiazepoxide, chlorpromazine, corticosteroids, dexamethasone, digoxin, estrogens, glucose, meprobamate, metyrapone, oral contraceptives, paraldehyde, penicillin, phenytoin, probenecid, promazine hydrochloride, propoxyphene hydrochloride, pyrazinamide, quinine sulfate, quinidine, reserpine, salicylates, secobarbital, spironolactone.

Pre-Test Nursing Care

- Explain 24-hour urine collection procedure to the patient.
- Stress the importance of saving *all* urine in the 24-hour period. Instruct the patient to avoid contaminating the urine with toilet paper or feces.
- Inform the patient of the presence of a preservative in the collection bottle.
- Encourage the patient to avoid excessive physical activity and stress during the testing period.
- If possible, withhold medications that may alter test results.

Procedure

- Obtain the proper container containing the appropriate preservative from the laboratory.
- Begin the testing period in the morning after the patient's first voiding, which is discarded.
- Timing of the 24-hour period begins at the time the first voiding is discarded.
- *All* urine for the next 24 hours is collected in the container, which is to be kept refrigerated or on ice.
- If any urine is accidentally discarded during the 24-hour period, the test must be discontinued and a new test begun.
- The ending time of the 24-hour collection period should be posted in the patient's room.
- Gloves are to be worn when dealing with the specimen collection.

Post-Test Nursing Care

- Label the container and transport it on ice to the laboratory as soon as possible after the end of the 24-hour collection period.
- Resume medications as taken before the test.
- Report abnormal findings to the primary care provider.

• • • • • • • • • • • • • • • •

Kidney Sonogram
(Renal Ultrasonography)

Ultrasonography is a noninvasive method of diagnostic testing in which ultrasound waves are sent into the body with a small transducer pressed against the skin. The transducer not only sends the sound waves into the body but also receives any returning sound waves, which are deflected back as they bounce off various structures. The transducer converts the returning sound waves into electric signals, which are then transformed by a computer into a visual display on a monitor.

In renal ultrasonography, the transducer is passed over the flank area. This allows visualization of the kidneys and the perirenal tissues. This test is especially valuable for use in patients who are unable to have other renal examinations because of hypersensitivity to contrast media or pregnancy. It can also be used for post-transplant evaluation and guidance for biopsy, aspiration, or nephrostomy tube insertion.

Normal Values

Normal size, shape, and location of kidneys
Absence of calculi, cysts, hydronephrosis, obstruction, or tumor

Possible Meanings of Abnormal Values

Hydronephrosis
Perirenal hematoma
Renal calculi

Renal cyst
Renal tumor
Ureteral obstruction

Contributing Factors to Abnormal Values

- The transducer must be in good contact with the skin as it is being moved. A lubricant, such as mineral oil, glycerin, or a water-based jelly, is used to ensure good contact with the skin.
- Retained barium from previous tests may hinder testing.
- Obesity may interfere with the clarity of the images.

Pre-Test Nursing Care

- Explain to the patient the purpose of the test. Provide any written teaching materials available on the subject. Note that there is no discomfort involved with this test.
- No fasting is required before the test.

Procedure

- The patient is assisted to a prone position on the ultrasonography table.
- A coupling agent, such as a water-based gel, is applied to the flank area.
- A transducer is placed on the skin and moved as needed to provide good visualization of the kidneys.
- The sound waves are transformed into a visual display on the monitor. Printed copies of this display are made.

Post-Test Nursing Care

- Cleanse the patient's skin of remaining coupling agent.
- Report abnormal findings to the primary care provider.

• • • • • • • • • • • • • • • •

K

Kidney, Ureter, and Bladder Radiography
(KUB, Flat Plate X-ray of the Abdomen, Scout Film)

Kidney, ureter, and bladder radiography, better known as the KUB, provides an overall view of the lower abdomen that shows the position of the kidneys, ureters, and bladder. The ureters are not normally visible on the KUB unless abnormal, as when calculi are present. The test is a simple x-ray film with the patient in a supine position. It requires no physical preparation of the patient. Renal enlargement, renal displacement, congenital anomalies, and renal or ureteral calculi are just a few of the abnormalities that may be seen as a result of this test. In addition to abnormalities of the urinary tract, the KUB may be used to assess for the presence of ascites and for gas within the intestines.

Normal Values

Normal size, shape, and location of kidneys. Ureters not seen. Bladder shown as shadow.

Possible Meanings of Abnormal Values

Accumulation of gas in intestine
Ascites
Calculi
Congenital abnormalities
Cysts
Hydronephrosis
Intestinal obstruction
Paralytic ileus
Renal trauma
Tumor
Vascular calcification

Contributing Factors to Abnormal Values

- Any movement by the patient may alter quality of films taken.
- Retained barium, gas, or stool in the intestines may alter the test results.

CONTRAINDICATIONS

- Pregnant women
  Caution: A woman in her childbearing years should undergo radiography only during her menses or 12 to 14 days after its onset to avoid any exposure to a fetus.

Pre-Test Nursing Care

- Explain to the patient the purpose of the test. Provide any written teaching materials available on the subject. Note that the test involves no discomfort.
- No fasting is required before the test.
- The test should be completed before the patient has any diagnostic tests involving barium.

Procedure

- The patient is assisted to a supine position on the radiography table.
- The patient's arms are extended overhead.
- Films are taken of the patient's abdomen.

Post-Test Nursing Care

- Schedule any additional testing for differential diagnosis as ordered.
- Report abnormal findings to the primary care provider.

• • • • • • • • • • • • • • •

Lactic Acid
(Blood Lactate)

Lactic acid is produced by anaerobic glycolysis. In other words, lactic acid is produced as a result of carbohydrate metabolism in an environment in which the cells do not have enough oxygen to allow for conversion of fuel to carbon dioxide and water. An example of this type of situation is strenuous exercise. Lactic acid is used for muscle contraction when energy needs exceed the supply of oxygen. Lactic acid accumulates in situations where there is an excess production of lactate and removal of the lactic acid from the blood by the liver is decreased, as can occur in liver disease.

Normal Values

0.5–2.2 mEq/L (0.5–2.2 mmol/L, SI units)

Possible Meanings of Abnormal Values

Increased	Decreased
Alcoholism	Hypothermia
Cardiac arrest	
Dehydration	
Diabetes mellitus	
Hemorrhage	
Hepatic coma	
Hyperthermia	
Hypoxia	
Lactic acidosis	
Liver disease	
Malignancy	
Peritonitis	
Renal failure	
Shock	
Strenuous exercise	

Contributing Factors to Abnormal Values
- Hemolysis of the blood sample may alter test results.
- Lactic acid levels may be falsely low in the presence of high LDH levels.
- Drugs that may *increase* lactic acid levels: alcohol, epinephrine, glucose, sodium bicarbonate.

Pre-Test Nursing Care
- Explain to the patient the purpose of the test and the need for a blood sample to be drawn.
- No fasting is required before the test.

L

Procedure

- A 7-mL blood sample is drawn in a collection tube containing a glycolytic inhibitor, such as sodium fluoride, avoiding use of a tourniquet and clenching of the patient's hand when possible.
- Gloves are worn throughout the procedure.

Post-Test Nursing Care

- Apply pressure at venipuncture site. Apply dressing, periodically assessing for continued bleeding.
- Label the specimen and transport it to the laboratory.
- Report abnormal findings to the primary care provider.

• • • • • • • • • • • • • • • • •

Lactic Dehydrogenase and Isoenzymes
(Lactate Dehydrogenase, LDH, LD)

Lactic dehydrogenase (LDH) is an intracellular enzyme found primarily in the heart, liver, skeletal muscles, and the erythrocytes. It is present in smaller amounts in the brain, kidneys, lungs, pancreas, and spleen. LDH is released after damage has occurred to the tissue.

LDH can be measured as the total enzyme in the serum, or each of its five isoenzymes may be measured. The isoenzymes and their primary sources include:

LDH_1:   Heart muscle and erythrocytes
LDH_2:   Reticuloendothelial system (normally in serum)
LDH_3:   Lungs
LDH_4:   Kidneys, pancreas, and placenta
LDH_5:   Liver and skeletal muscle

LDH, along with asparate aminotransferase (AST) and creatine kinase (CK), is assessed in the case of suspected myocardial infarction (MI). It typically appears in the bloodstream within 12 hours of the tissue injury, with peak values occurring 24 to 48 hours post-injury. The peak value may reach 300–800 IU/L following an MI. LDH levels are usually elevated for approximately 10 days. Thus, LDH becomes elevated after CK following an MI. In diagnosing a suspected MI, the total LDH, along with LDH_1 and LDH_2, is usually evaluated, with LDH_1 being greater than LDH_2. Isolated increases of LDH may occur in the absence of physical problems.

Normal Values

Total LDH: 110–210 IU/L (1.83–3.50 µkat/L SI units)
Isoenzymes: LDH_1:   17%–27%
                LDH_2:   28%–38%
                LDH_3:   17%–28%
                LDH_4:   5%–15%
                LDH_5:   5%–15%

Possible Meanings of Abnormal Values

Increased	Decreased
Abruptio placenta	Radiation therapy
Biliary obstruction	
Bone metastases	
Cancer of prostate	
Eclampsia	
Fractures	
Hemolytic anemia	
Hepatitis	
Infectious mononucleosis	
Leukemia	
Liver cancer	
Liver damage	
Macrocytic anemias	
Malignant tumors	
Muscular dystrophy	
Myocardial infarction	
Pancreatitis	
Pneumonia (*Pneumocystis carinii*)	
Pulmonary infarction	
Shock	
Trauma	

Contributing Factors to Abnormal Values

- Hemolysis of the blood sample and strenuous exercise prior to the test will alter test results.
- Drugs that may *increase* LDH levels: alcohol, anabolic steroids, anesthetics, aspirin, bismuth salts, carbenicillin, chlorpromazine, clindamycin, clofibrate, codeine, dicumarol, floxuridine, fluorides, halothane, imipramine hydrochloride, levodopa, lithium, lorazepam, meperidine hydrochloride, methotrexate, methyltestosterone, metoprolol tartrate, mithramycin, morphine, niacin, nifedipine, nitrofurantoin, norethindrone, procainamide hydrochloride, propoxyphene hydrochloride, propranolol hydrochloride, quinidine, sulfamethoxazole, thyroid hormone.
- Drugs that may *decrease* LDH levels: ascorbic acid, oxalates.

Pre-Test Nursing Care

- Explain to the patient the purpose of the test and the need for a blood sample to be drawn.
- No fasting is required before the test.

Procedure

- A 5-mL blood sample is drawn in a collection tube containing a silicone gel.
- Gloves are worn throughout the procedure.

L

Post-Test Nursing Care

- Apply pressure at venipuncture site. Apply dressing, periodically assessing for continued bleeding.
- Label the specimen and transport it to the laboratory.
- Report abnormal findings to the primary care provider.

• • • • • • • • • • • • • • • • • •

Lactose Tolerance Test

Lactase is an enzyme found in the small intestine. Its function is the digestion of lactose, a sugar found in milk. In some people, especially African American and Asian people, there is a deficiency of lactase. When individuals who are lactase deficient ingest milk, the lactose builds up in the intestine, where it is metabolized by the bacteria normally found there. This results in abdominal cramping, bloating, and diarrhea.

This test is used to test for lactose intolerance. After the patient receives a lactose solution, blood samples are drawn at several designated time intervals to monitor the blood glucose level. At the same time, the patient is observed for any of the physical symptoms associated with lactose intolerance. If the gastrointestinal symptoms appear and the blood glucose level increases by less than 20 mg/dL, lactase insufficiency is indicated.

Normal Values

A rise in plasma glucose levels of >20 mg/dL and no abdominal symptoms (abdominal pain, bloating, flatus, diarrhea).

Possible Meanings of Abnormal Values

Decreased

Enterogenous diarrhea
Lactase insufficiency

Contributing Factors to Abnormal Values

- Strenuous exercise and smoking may alter the test results.
- Drugs that may alter test results: benzodiazepines, insulin, oral contraceptives, propranolol hydrochloride, thiazide diuretics.

Pre-Test Nursing Care

- Explain to the patient the purpose of the test and the need for multiple blood samples to be drawn.
- Fasting and avoidance of strenuous exercise for 8 hours are required before the test.
- No smoking is allowed during the test.

Procedure

- A 7-mL fasting blood sample is drawn in a collection tube containing a glycolytic inhibitor such as sodium fluoride.

- The adult patient is given 50 to 100 g of lactose in 200 mL of water. (*Note:* The dose for a child is based on body weight.)
- Additional blood samples are drawn at 30 minutes, 1 hour, and 2 hours after lactose ingestion.
- Gloves are worn throughout the procedure.

Post-Test Nursing Care

- Apply pressure at venipuncture site. Apply dressing, periodically assessing for continued bleeding.
- Label the specimen and transport it to the laboratory.
- Report abnormal findings to the primary care provider.
- Patients with abnormal test results will require additional testing for other types of sugar intolerance, such as glucose or galactose.

• • • • • • • • • • • • • • • • •

Laparoscopy
(Gynecologic Laparoscopy, Pelvic Endoscopy, Pelviscopy, Peritoneoscopy)

This procedure is used to evaluate patients complaining of pelvic pain, for detecting carcinoma, ectopic pregnancy, endometriosis, pelvic inflammatory disease, and pelvic masses, and to view the fallopian tubes as part of an infertility workup. Laparoscopy is also used to perform such procedures as lysis of adhesions, ovarian biopsy, and tubal ligation. Laparoscopic surgery can also be used for other types of surgery such as cholecystectomy. Laparoscopy is the direct visualization of the peritoneal cavity via a laparoscope inserted through the anterior abdominal wall. During the procedure, one or two small incisions are made to allow insertion of the laparoscope and other instruments. The limited incisional size is advantageous in shortening the surgical time and recovery time from this procedure.

Normal Values

Normal uterus, fallopian tubes, and ovaries.

Possible Meanings of Abnormal Values

Abdominal organ abnormalities
Adhesions
Ascites
Ectopic pregnancy
Endometriosis
Hydrosalpinx
Ovarian cyst
Ovarian tumor
Pelvic inflammatory disease
Salpingitis
Uterine fibroids

CONTRAINDICATIONS

- Patients with advanced abdominal wall malignancy.
- Patients with advanced respiratory or cardiovascular disease.
- Patients with intestinal obstruction, abdominal mass, or abdominal hernia.
- Patients with chronic tuberculosis.
- Patients with history of peritonitis.
- Patients with possible adhesions resulting from multiple previous surgical procedures.
- Patients with suspected intra-abdominal hemorrhage.

Pre-Test Nursing Care

- Explain to the patient the purpose of the test and the procedure to be done. Note that some abdominal and shoulder pain will be felt for 24 to 36 hours after the procedure, but that aspirin or other mild analgesic will control it. Shoulder pain results from pressure on the diaphragm by carbon dioxide used during the procedure.
- Fasting for 8 hours is required before the test.
- Obtain a signed written consent.
- An enema before the procedure is sometimes ordered.
- Ask the patient to void before the procedure.
- The patient's abdomen is shaved as ordered.

Procedure

- This sterile procedure is usually conducted in the operating room.
- The patient is given a general anesthetic and is then placed in the lithotomy position with her legs supported in the stirrups. A Trendelenburg position may be used to move the intestines away from the pelvic organs.
- The bladder may be catheterized and a bimanual examination of the pelvis performed to detect abnormalities.
- A uterine manipulator is inserted through the vagina and cervix and into the uterus to permit the pelvic organs to be moved for better visualization.
- The abdomen is cleansed and draped.
- A small incision is made in the subumbilical area into the peritoneal cavity.
- The Veres (pneumoperitoneum) needle is inserted into the incision and used to fill the peritoneal cavity with approximately 3 L of carbon dioxide. This gas lifts the abdominal wall from the intra-abdominal viscera.
- The needle is removed and a trocar and sheath are inserted into the peritoneal cavity.
- The trocar is removed and replaced with the laparoscope.
- When visual examination and any other planned procedures, such as tubal ligation, are completed, the laparoscope is removed, the carbon dioxide is evacuated, and the sheath is removed.
- The incision is closed with sutures, clips, or Steri-strips, and a dressing is applied.
- The uterine manipulator is removed and a perineal pad is applied.
- Videotaping of the procedure is usually done via a camera attached to the laparoscope.

Post-Test Nursing Care

Possible complications:

- **Hemorrhage**
- **Punctured visceral organ, such as the intestine**

- Remind the patient that abdominal and shoulder discomfort is not unusual following the procedure. Aspirin may be taken.
- Instruct the patient to immediately report any excessive pain.
- Monitor vital signs and urinary output until stable.
- Resume diet as taken prior to the procedure.
- Instruct the patient to restrict activity for 2 to 7 days.
- Report abnormal findings to the primary care provider.

• • • • • • • • • • • • • • • • •

Lead

Lead is a heavy metal used in paint, leaded gasoline, insecticides, and pottery glaze. Because of its presence in paint, lead is a hazard in older homes with peeling paint easily accessible to young children. Lead poisoning is considered a public health problem. It leads to neurologic dysfunction and possible permanent brain damage.

Normal Values

<20 mcg/dL (<0.95 micromol/L, SI units)

Possible Meanings of Abnormal Values

Increased

Ataxia
Metal poisoning
Microcytic anemia from lead poisoning
Neuropathy

Pre-Test Nursing Care

- Explain to the patient the purpose of the test and the need for a blood sample to be drawn.
- No fasting is required before the test.

Procedure

- A 3-mL blood sample is drawn in a lead-free collection tube containing heparin.
- Gloves are worn throughout the procedure.

Post-Test Nursing Care

- Apply pressure at venipuncture site. Apply dressing, periodically assessing for continued bleeding.
- Label the specimen and transport it to the laboratory.
- Report abnormal findings to the primary care provider.

• • • • • • • • • • • • • • • • •

Legionnaire's Disease Antibody Test

Legionnaire's disease is a type of atypical pneumonia caused by *Legionella pneumophila*. It is characterized by flu-like symptoms, including high fever, mental confusion, headache, pleuritic pain, myalgia, dyspnea, productive cough, and hemoptysis. It occurs most often among middle-aged and older men, smokers, and individuals with chronic diseases or those receiving immunosuppressive therapy. The organism has been isolated from soil; those working with or living near soil excavations are at risk of contracting the disease.

Diagnosis of Legionnaire's disease is made through determination of the presence of *Legionella* antibodies. Antibody titers are low during the first week, rise the second and third weeks, peak at 5 weeks, and then drop slowly over several years. One antibody titer is performed within the first week of the illness (acute phase) and a second is done 3 to 6 weeks after the fever begins (convalescent phase). A fourfold rise in titer >1:128 between these two antibody assessments is diagnostic of the disease. A single titer of at least 1:256 indicates a previous infection with *Legionella*. Once the disease has been diagnosed, treatment can begin. Such treatment includes administration of erythromycin and rifampin.

Normal Values

Negative

Possible Meanings of Abnormal Values

Increased

Legionnaire's disease

Contributing Factors to Abnormal Values

- Hemolysis of the blood sample will alter test results.

Pre-Test Nursing Care

- Explain to the patient the purpose of the test and the need for a blood sample to be drawn.
- No fasting is required before the test.

Procedure

- A 7 mL blood sample is drawn in a collection tube containing a silicone gel.
- Gloves are worn throughout the procedure.

Post-Test Nursing Care

- Apply pressure at venipuncture site. Apply dressing, periodically assessing for continued bleeding.
- Label the specimen and transport it to the laboratory.
- Report abnormal findings to the primary care provider.

• • • • • • • • • • • • • • • •

Leucine Aminopeptidase
(LAP)

Leucine aminopeptidase (LAP) is an enzyme produced by the liver and present in the blood, bile, and urine. This test is useful in diagnosis of conditions when the alkaline phosphatase is elevated. LAP changes parallel those of alkaline phosphatase except that LAP is usually normal in bone diseases or malabsorption problems. LAP is a more sensitive indicator of choledocholithiasis and liver metastases. It is quickly excreted by the kidneys; when serum LAP is increased, urinary LAP is usually increased as well. However, when urine LAP is increased, serum LAP may have already returned to normal.

Normal Values

Female:	75–185 U/mL
Male:	80–200 U/mL

Possible Meanings of Abnormal Values

Increased
Cholelithiasis
Cirrhosis
Hepatitis
Jaundice
Liver cancer
Liver dysfunction
Pancreatic cancer
Pancreatitis
Pregnancy

Contributing Factors to Abnormal Values

- Drugs that may *increase* LAP levels: estrogens, hepatotoxic drugs, oral contraceptives, progesterone.

Pre-Test Nursing Care

- Explain to the patient the purpose of the test and the need for a blood sample to be drawn.
- No fasting is usually required before the test. Some laboratories may require an 8-hour fast.

Procedure

- A 7-mL blood sample is drawn in a collection tube containing no additives.
- Gloves are worn throughout the procedure.

L

Post-Test Nursing Care

Possible complication:

Prolonged bleeding at site because of vitamin K deficiency caused by liver dysfunction.

- Apply pressure 3 to 5 minutes at venipuncture site. Apply dressing, periodically assessing for continued bleeding.
- Teach the patient to monitor the site. If the site begins to bleed, the patient should apply direct pressure and, if unable to control the bleeding, return to the laboratory or notify the nurse.
- Label the specimen and transport it to the laboratory.
- Report abnormal findings to the primary care provider.

• • • • • • • • • • • • • • • •

Lipase

Lipase is an enzyme produced by the pancreas that converts fats and triglycerides into fatty acids and glycerol. Measurement of this enzyme is done to distinguish abdominal pain owing to acute pancreatitis from that owing to other causes that might benefit from surgical intervention. Lipase is usually evaluated in conjunction with serum amylase. Lipase increases in the blood within 24 to 36 hours after the onset of acute pancreatitis, which is after amylase increases. Lipase remains elevated up to 14 days longer than amylase.

Normal Values

0–160 U/L or 4–24 U/dL (0.67–4.00 µkat/L, SI units)

Possible Meanings of Abnormal Values

Increased

Acute cholecystitis
Acute pancreatitis
Biliary obstruction
Chronic relapsing pancreatitis
Cirrhosis
Intestinal obstruction
Pancreatic cancer

Contributing Factors to Abnormal Values

- Hemolysis of the blood sample may alter test results.
- Drugs that may *increase* lipase levels: aminosalicylic acid, azathioprine, bethanecol chloride, cholinergics, codeine, corticosteroids, corticotropin, dexamethasone, ethacrynic acid, ethanol, furosemide, heparin, indomethacin, meperidine hydrochloride, mercaptopurine, methacholine chloride, morphine, phenformin, triamcinolone.
- Drugs that may *decrease* lipase levels: calcium ions.

Pre-Test Nursing Care

- Explain to the patient the purpose of the test and the need for a blood sample to be drawn.
- Fasting for 8 to 12 hours is required before the test. Water is permitted.

Procedure

- A 7-mL blood sample is drawn in a collection tube containing a silicone gel.
- Gloves are worn throughout the procedure.

Post-Test Nursing Care

- Apply pressure at venipuncture site. Apply dressing, periodically assessing for continued bleeding.
- Label the specimen and transport it to the laboratory.
- Report abnormal findings to the primary care provider.

• • • • • • • • • • • • • • • • •

Lipid Profile

See:
Cholesterol
High-density Lipoprotein
Low-density Lipoprotein
Triglycerides

• • • • • • • • • • • • • • • • •

Liver Biopsy
(Percutaneous Liver Biopsy, Percutaneous Needle Biopsy of the Liver)

A percutaneous needle biopsy of the liver is considered a closed procedure and can be performed at the bedside. Indications for the test include:

Suspected disease of the liver, such as tumors, cysts, or cirrhosis;
Infiltrative diseases, such as sarcoidosis or amyloidosis;
Persistently elevated liver enzymes;
Jaundice of unknown etiology;
Hepatomegaly of unknown etiology; and
Possible rejection of a transplanted liver.

A 14 to 18 gauge needle is inserted directly through the skin into the liver, either blindly or guided through the concurrent use of ultrasonography, and a sample of liver tissue is aspirated. An open procedure, where the biopsy is performed through a surgical incision, is an alternate method. Regardless of the type of biopsy procedure used, the biopsied tissue is placed in a collection container and covered with an appropriate solution (e.g., 10% formalin, Ringer's solution). The laboratory will appropriately fix, prepare, and stain the tissue for microscopic examination by a pathologist.

Normal Values

Absence of abnormal cells and tissue.

Possible Meanings of Abnormal Values

Abscess
Amyloidosis
Benign tumor
Cirrhosis
Cyst
Hemochromatosis
Hemosiderosis
Hepatitis
Malignant tumor (primary or metastatic)
Metabolic disorders
Sarcoidosis
Schistosomiasis
Weil's disease
Wilson's disease

CONTRAINDICATIONS

- Patients with bleeding disorders.
- Patients with prothrombin times in the anticoagulant range (two to three times the control value).
- Patients with decreased platelet count (<50,000/mm^3).
- Patients in whom there is difficulty in determining liver location, as in presence of ascites.
- Patients with extrahepatic obstruction.
- Patients with infection (subdiaphragmatic, right hemithoracic, or biliary tract).
- Patients with suspected vascular tumor (hemangioma) of the liver.
- Patients who are unable to cooperate during the procedure (anyone unable to remain still or unable to hold his or her breath following exhalation).

Pre-Test Nursing Care

- Explain the procedure to the patient. Have the patient practice holding breath after exhalation. Explain that the patient may feel discomfort in right shoulder or the biopsy site during the procedure.
- Instruct the patient to remain NPO for at least 6 hours before the test.
- Obtain signed informed consent.
- Assess for coagulation deficiencies. Monitor prothrombin time (PT), partial thromboplastin time (PTT), and platelet count. Treatment regimen to reverse coagulopathies may include administration of vitamin K, fresh frozen plasma transfusion, or platelet transfusion.
- Obtain baseline hematocrit.
- Administer sedation, if ordered.

Procedure

- The procedure is usually performed at the bedside by the physician.
- Baseline vital signs are taken and recorded. Vital signs are also taken periodically during the procedure.

- The patient is placed in the supine or left lateral position. The patient's right hand should be under the head, and the head turned to the left.
- A local anesthetic is administered.
- The patient is instructed to inhale and exhale deeply several times and then to hold the breath following a full expiration. This maintains the diaphragm in its highest position to minimize chance of puncture during the procedure.
- The needle is inserted in the right midaxillary line at the 6–7th or 8–9th intercostal space, depending on the level of maximal liver dullness.
- The tissue sample is aspirated, and the needle is quickly removed.
- Once the needle is removed, the patient is allowed to breath normally.
- The tissue sample is placed in a specimen bottle containing a 10% formalin solution and sent to pathology.
- A pressure dressing is applied to the site.
- The entire procedure usually takes approximately 10 to 15 minutes.
- Gloves are worn throughout the procedure.

Post-Test Nursing Care

Possible complications:
- **Bile peritonitis**
- **Hemorrhage**
- **Perforation of an abdominal organ**
- **Pneumothorax**
- **Shock**

- Monitor vital signs frequently, following the institution's policy for postoperative care. Assess for signs of hemorrhage (elevated pulse, decreasing blood pressure) and peritonitis (elevated temperature).
- Assess rate, rhythm, and depth of respirations. Assess breath sounds. Assess for dyspnea, pleuritic chest pain, cyanosis, hypotension, and restlessness.
- Assess for hemorrhage by observing dressing for bleeding. **Do not** remove pressure dressing to look for bleeding. Obtain hematocrit 6 to 8 hours after the test. Report any drop from pretest level immediately.
- Observe for pain.
  - Right upper quadrant pain may result from subscapular accumulation of blood or bile.
  - Right shoulder pain may result from blood on the undersurface of the diaphragm.
- Maintain pressure on the biopsy site by turning patient on right side for 1 to 4 hours, placing a rolled towel or small towel under the costal margin, and maintaining bedrest for 24 hours.
- Instruct the patient to avoid coughing or straining, which increases intra abdominal pressure. Strenuous activities or heavy lifting are to be avoided for 1 to 2 weeks.
- Report abnormal findings to the primary care provider.

• • • • • • • • • • • • • • •

Liver Function Tests

See:
Alanine Aminotransferase (ALT) (formerly, SGPT: serum glutamic-pyruvic transaminase)
Alkaline Phosphatase (ALP)
Ammonia
Asparate Aminotransferase (AST) (formerly, SGOT: serum glutamic-oxaloacetic transaminase)
Bilirubin
Gamma-Glutamyl Transferase (GGT)
5'-Nucleotidase
Urobilinogen

• • • • • • • • • • • • • •

Liver and Pancreatobiliary System Ultrasonography
(Gallbladder and Biliary System Sonogram, Liver Sonogram, Pancreas Sonogram)

Ultrasonography is a noninvasive method of diagnostic testing in which ultrasound waves are sent into the body with a small transducer pressed against the skin. The transducer not only sends the sound waves into the body but also receives any returning sound waves, which are deflected back as they bounce off various structures. The transducer converts the returning sound waves into electric signals that are then transformed by a computer into a visual display on a monitor.

In this particular type of ultrasonography, the areas evaluated include the gallbladder, biliary system, liver, and pancreas. This procedure is now used much more frequently than oral cholecystography, since ultrasonography involves no radiation exposure for the patient. This test is used for evaluating jaundice, hepatomegaly, and abdominal trauma, and in the diagnosis of acute cholecystitis, suspected metastatic tumors of the liver, and suspected pancreatic carcinoma. It can also be used to guide the insertion of a biopsy needle.

Normal Values
Normal gallbladder, bile ducts, liver, and pancreas.

Possible Meanings of Abnormal Values
Acute cholecystitis
Biliary obstruction
Cholelithiasis
Dilation of the bile ducts
Gallbladder carcinoma
Gallbladder polyps
Hematoma

Hepatic abscess
Hepatocellular disease
Liver cyst
Liver metastases
Pancreatic carcinoma
Pancreatitis
Primary hepatic tumor
Pseudocyst of the pancreas
Subphrenic abscesses

Contributing Factors to Abnormal Values

- The transducer must be in good contact with the skin as it is being moved. A lubricant, such as mineral oil, glycerin, or a water-based jelly, is used to ensure good contact with the skin.
- Test results are hindered by the presence of bowel gas, retained barium, or dehydration.

Pre-Test Nursing Care

- Explain to the patient the purpose of the test. Provide any written teaching materials available on the subject. Note that there is no discomfort involved with this test.
- The patient is to eat a fat-free meal in the evening and then fast for 8 to 12 hours before the test. This promotes accumulation of bile in the gallbladder, resulting in better visualization during ultrasonography.

Procedure

- The patient is assisted to a supine position on the ultrasonography table.
- A coupling agent, such as a water-based gel, is applied to the area to be evaluated.
- A transducer is placed on the skin and moved as needed to provide good visualization of the structures.
- The sound waves are transformed into a visual display on the monitor. Printed copies of this display are made.

Post-Test Nursing Care

- Cleanse the patient's skin of remaining coupling agent.
- Report abnormal findings to the primary care provider.

• • • • • • • • • • • • • • • • •

Liver/Spleen Scan
(Liver Scan)

For a liver/spleen gallbladder scan, the patient is given a radionuclide compound, usually a gallium-67 citrate, technetium-99m, or iodine-131 radiopharmaceutical via an intravenous injection. A scintillation camera is used to take a radioactivity reading from the body. These readings are fed into a computer, which translates these readings into a two-dimensional gray scale picture. These pictures are obtained 30 minutes following the injection. This test is used in the diagnosis of abscesses, hematomas, tumors, and infiltrative processes of the liver and/or spleen, and to evaluate jaundice.

Normal Values

Normal size, shape, and position of liver and spleen.

Possible Meanings of Abnormal Values

Abscesses of the liver/spleen
Amyloidosis of the liver/spleen
Cirrhosis
Granulomas of the liver/spleen
Hematomas of the liver/spleen
Hepatic cysts
Portal hypertension
Sarcoidosis of the liver/spleen
Tumors of the liver/spleen

Contributing Factors to Abnormal Values

- Any movement by the patient may alter quality of films taken.
- Retained barium from previous examinations may interfere with the test.

CONTRAINDICATIONS

- Pregnant women (*Caution:* A woman in her childbearing years should undergo radiography only during her menses or 12–14 days after its onset to avoid any exposure to a fetus.).
- Patients who are lactating.
- Patients who are unable to cooperate owing to age, mental status, pain, or other factors.

Pre-Test Nursing Care

- Explain to the patient the purpose of the test. Provide any written teaching materials available on the subject. Note that discomfort involved with this test is primarily owing to lying on a hard table for an extended period of time and the needle puncture. Reassure the patient that only trace amounts of the radionuclide are involved in the test.
- The patient must remain still while the scan is being performed.
- No fasting is required before the test.
- Obtain a signed informed consent.

Procedure

- The radiopharmaceutical is administered by intravenous injection in a peripheral vein.
- The patient is assisted to a supine position on the examination table.
- A scintillation camera is positioned over the right upper quadrant of the patient's abdomen. This camera takes a radioactivity reading from the body. This information is transformed into a two-dimensional picture of the area.
- Scans are obtained 30 minutes post-injection. Scans with the patient in the lateral and prone positions are also performed.
- Gloves are worn during the radionuclide injection.

Post-Test Nursing Care

- Check the injection site for redness or swelling.
- If a woman who is lactating *must* have a nuclear scan, she should not breast feed the infant until the radionuclide has been eliminated, possibly for 3 days.
- Although the amount of diagnostic radionuclide excreted in the urine is low, the urine should not be used for any laboratory tests for the time period indicated by the nuclear medicine department. Clients should be told to flush the toilet three times after voiding.
- Gloves are worn when dealing with the urine.
- Encourage fluid intake by the patient to enhance excretion of the radionuclide.
- Report abnormal findings to the primary care provider.

• • • • • • • • • • • • • • • • • • • •

Low-Density Lipoprotein
(LDL)

Cholesterol is synthesized in the liver from dietary fats. It is transported in the blood by the low density lipoproteins (LDLs, or "bad" cholesterol) and high density lipoproteins (HDLs, or "good" cholesterol). LDLs carry cholesterol from the liver to other parts of the body. Thus, high levels of LDL are associated with an increased risk for coronary heart disease. As a part of evaluating this risk, the low-density lipoprotein (LDL) level is measured as part of the lipid profile. In addition to actual measurement of the LDL, it can be calculated with the following formula:

$$LDL = \text{Total Cholesterol} - \left[HDL + \frac{(Triglycerides)}{2} \right]$$

Normal Values

Desirable:	< 130 mg/dL (<3.36 mmol/L, SI units)

Abnormal Values

Borderline high risk:	130–159 (3.36–4.11 mmol/L, SI units)
High risk:	>159 mg/dL (>4.11 mmol/L, SI units)

Possible Meanings of Abnormal Values

Increased	Decreased
Diabetes mellitus	Malabsorption
Hepatic disease	Malnutrition
High cholesterol diet	
Hyperlipidemia	
Hypothyroidism	
Multiple myeloma	

Increased	Decreased
Nephrotic syndrome	
Porphyria	
Pregnancy	

Contributing Factors to Abnormal Values

- Drugs that may *increase* LDL levels: androgens, catecholamines, diuretics, glucocorticoids, oral contraceptives.
- Drugs that may *decrease* LDL levels: cholestyramine, clofibrate, estrogens, neomycin sulfate, nicotinic acid, probucol, thyroxine.

Pre-Test Nursing Care

- Explain to the patient the purpose of the test and the need for a blood sample to be drawn.
- Fasting for 12 hours is required before the test. Water is permitted.

Procedure

- A 7-mL blood sample is drawn in a collection tube containing EDTA.
- Gloves are worn throughout the procedure.

Post-Test Nursing Care

- Apply pressure at venipuncture site. Apply dressing, periodically assessing for continued bleeding.
- Label the specimen and transport it to the laboratory.
- Report abnormal findings to the primary care provider.
- For individuals with elevated LDL levels, counseling is needed regarding dietary changes, weight loss, and exercise.

• • • • • • • • • • • • • •

Lung Biopsy

Lesions of the lung may be studied through such tests as chest x-ray, computed tomography (CT) scan, and bronchoscopy. However, determination of the nature of a lesion, that is, whether a mass is benign or malignant, can only be made by obtaining a biopsy of the tissue. In a lung biopsy, a sample of lung tissue is removed for histologic study. The tissue sample may be obtained by needle biopsy through the chest wall, by tissue sampling during fiberoptic bronchoscopy, or by open biopsy during a thoracotomy. This discussion will be limited to that of needle biopsy of the lung.

Normal Values

No abnormal cells or tissue present.

Possible Meanings of Abnormal Values

Adenocarcinoma
Granuloma
Oat cell carcinoma
Pulmonary infection
Sarcoidosis
Squamous cell carcinoma

CONTRAINDICATIONS

- Patients with bleeding disorders.
- Patients with hypoxia, pulmonary hypertension, or cardiac disease with cor pulmonale.
- Patients with hyperinflation of the lung.
- Patients unable to cooperate with the examination.

Pre-Test Nursing Care

- Explain to the patient the purpose of the test and the procedure to be done. Explain to the patient that a local anesthetic will be used, but that transient sharp pain may be experienced when the biopsy needle touches the lung. Remind the patient that no movement, such as coughing, can occur during the biopsy.
- Obtain baseline chest x-ray and coagulation tests (partial thromboplastin time, platelet count, prothrombin time).
- Fasting after midnight before the test is usually required.
- Obtain a signed informed consent.
- Obtain baseline vital signs.

Procedure

- The patient is assisted to a sitting position with the arms supported on a pillow on an overbed table.
- The skin is cleansed with an antiseptic and draped.
- A local anesthetic is administered.
- A small incision is made in the posterior chest wall at the selected intercostal space.
- The biopsy needle is introduced through the incision, chest wall, and pleura, and into the tissue or mass to be biopsied.
- The specimen is obtained and the needle removed.
- A portion of the tissue to be studied for histology is placed in a container with a formaldehyde solution. The remaining tissue sample is placed in a sterile container for microbiologic study.
- Pressure is exerted on the biopsy site, followed by application of a sterile dressing.
- Gloves are worn throughout the procedure.

Post-Test Nursing Care

Possible complications:
- **Bleeding**
- **Hemothorax**
- **Infection**
- **Pneumothorax**

- Assist the patient into a semi-Fowler's position.
- Monitor the patient's vital signs, breath sounds, and comfort level, and check the dressing for drainage every 15 to 30 minutes until stable.
- Observe for indications of hemothorax or pneumothorax: rapid, shallow respirations, dyspnea, air hunger, chest pain, cough, hemoptysis, and absence of breath sounds over area.
- Observe for signs of infection: elevated temperature, chest pain, yellow sputum, and abnormal breath sounds.
- Administer analgesics as needed.
- Provide emotional support as the patient awaits test results.
- Report abnormal findings to the primary care provider.

• • • • • • • • • • • • • • • •

Lung Scan
(Lung Perfusion Scan, Lung Ventilation Scan, Ventilation/Perfusion Scanning)

The *lung perfusion scan* is performed to detect pulmonary emboli, and to assess arterial perfusion of the lungs. The scan involves injection of a radiopharmaceutical, followed by scanning. The radiolabeled particles filter out of the capillary membrane and become trapped in the lung tissue, allowing the camera to detect areas of obstructed blood flow. The lung perfusion scan is performed prior to, but in association with, the lung ventilation scan. The *lung ventilation scan* is used to delineate areas of the lung ventilated during respiration. For this scan, the patient inhales a radioactive gas. The results of both scans are reviewed to help in diagnosis. In cases of pulmonary embolism, perfusion is decreased while ventilation is maintained; in pneumonia, perfusion may be normal, but ventilation is decreased.

Normal Values
Uniform uptake pattern during both perfusion and ventilation portions of the test.

Possible Meanings of Abnormal Values
Asthma
Atelectasis
Bronchitis
Emphysema
Pneumonia
Pulmonary embolism
Tumors
Tuberculosis

Contributing Factors to Abnormal Values

- Any movement by the patient may alter quality of films taken.
- Pulmonary parenchymal problems, such as pneumonia, may mimic a perfusion defect.

 ## CONTRAINDICATIONS

- Pregnant women (*Caution:* A woman in her childbearing years should undergo radiography only during her menses or 12–14 days after its onset to avoid any exposure to a fetus.).
- Patients who are lactating.
- Patients who are unable to cooperate because of age, mental status, pain, or other factors.

Pre-Test Nursing Care

- Explain to the patient the purpose of the test. Provide any written teaching materials available on the subject. Note that discomfort involved with this test is primarily owing to lying on a hard table for an extended period of time and the needle puncture. Reassure the patient that only trace amounts of the radionuclide are involved in the test.
- The patient must remain still while the scan is being performed.
- No fasting is required prior to the test, unless sedation is going to be used during the test. If so, fasting for 4 hours is required before the test.
- Obtain a signed informed consent.

Procedure

Perfusion Scan

- The radiopharmaceutical is administered by intravenous injection in a peripheral vein.
- The patient is assisted to a supine position on the examination table.
- A scintillation camera is positioned over the patient's chest. This camera takes a radioactivity reading from the body. This information is transformed into a two-dimensional picture of the area.
- Scans with the patient in the prone and several lateral positions are also performed.
- Gloves are worn during the radionuclide injection.

Ventilation Scan

- The patient breathes the radioactive gas (krypton 85 or xenon 133) through a face mask.
- Scanning of the chest to show gas distribution is completed.

Post-Test Nursing Care

- Check the injection site for redness or swelling.
- If a woman who is lactating *must* have a nuclear scan, she should not breast feed the infant until the radionuclide has been eliminated, possibly for 3 days.
- Although the amount of diagnostic radionuclide excreted in the urine is low, the urine should not be used for any laboratory tests for the time period indicated by the nuclear medicine department. Clients should be told to flush the toilet three times after voiding.
- Gloves are worn when dealing with the urine.
- Encourage fluid intake by the patient to enhance excretion of the radionuclide.
- Report abnormal findings to the primary care provider.

• • • • • • • • • • • • • • •

Lupus Erythematosus Test
(LE Cell Prep, LE Test)

Systemic lupus erythematosus (SLE) is an autoimmune disease characterized by inflammatory changes in the vascular and connective tissue. SLE is most common among females, ages 15–40, and involves multiple body systems. Clinical manifestations may include such signs and symptoms as arthralgias, a butterfly-shaped rash across the bridge of the nose and cheeks, pericarditis, pleuritis, and generalized lymphadenopathy.

One of the diagnostic findings in SLE is the presence of *LE cells*. These cells are autoantibodies; that is, they are antibodies against the contents of the SLE patient's body. The degree of LE cell formation tends to correlate with the severity of the SLE.

The LE cell prep is considered less sensitive and reliable than either the antinuclear antibody (ANA) or the anti-DNA antibody tests. In this test, a sample of the patient's blood is mixed with a specific antigen. If the patient's blood contains ANA, this antibody reacts with the antigen, causing cell lysis. Phagocytic cells engulf the cell debris, including a great deal of DNA from the cell nucleus, forming LE cells. These cells are then able to be seen when stained for microscopic examination.

Normal Values

No LE cells present.

Possible Meanings of Abnormal Values

Positive

Chronic active hepatitis
Rheumatoid arthritis
Scleroderma
Systemic lupus erythematosus

Contributing Factors to Abnormal Values

- Hemolysis of the blood sample may alter test results.
- Drugs that may cause *false-positive* LE cell results: acetazolamide, chlorothiazide, chlorpromazine, chlorprothixene, clofibrate, ethosuximide, gold salts, griseofulvin, hydralazine hydrochloride, isoniazid, lithium, mephenytoin, methyldopa, methysergide, oral contraceptives, para-aminosalicylic acid, penicillamine, phenylbutazone, phenytoin, primidone, procainamide hydrochloride, propylthiouracil, quinidine, reserpine, streptomycin, sulfasalazine, sulfonamides, tetracyclines, trimethadione.
- Drugs that may cause *false-negative* LE cell results: heparin, steroids.

Pre-Test Nursing Care

- Explain to the patient the purpose of the test and the need for a blood sample to be drawn.
- No fasting is required before the test.

Procedure

- A 7-mL blood sample is drawn in a collection tube containing no additives.
- Gloves are worn throughout the procedure.

Post-Test Nursing Care

Possible complication: Infection at venipuncture site owing to immunocompromised state.

- Apply pressure at venipuncture site. Apply dressing, periodically assessing for continued bleeding.
- Teach the patient to monitor the site and notify the health care provider if signs or symptoms of infection occur, such as drainage, redness, warmth, edema, pain at the site, or fever.
- Report abnormal findings to the primary care provider.

• • • • • • • • • • • • • • • •

Luteinizing Hormone
(LH)

Luteinizing hormone (LH), like follicle-stimulating hormone (FSH), is secreted by the anterior pituitary gland. FSH promotes maturation of the ovarian follicle, which is needed for production of estrogen. As estrogen levels rise, luteinizing hormone (LH) is produced. FSH and LH are both needed in order for ovulation to occur in women and for the transformation of the ovarian follicle into the corpus luteum, a process known as *luteinization*. The corpus luteum secretes progesterone. In males, LH and FSH stimulate the testes to release testosterone, which is needed for spermatogenesis to occur. This test is used to determine whether ovulation has occurred, and to evaluate amenorrhea and infertility. LH and FSH are usually measured at the same time.

Normal Values

Females:

Follicular phase:	5–30 U/mL (5–30 Arb. units, SI units)
Midcycle:	75–150 U/mL (75–150 Arb. units, SI units)
Luteal phase:	3–40 U/mL (3–40 Arb. units, SI units)
Postmenopausal:	30–200 U/mL (30–200 Arb. units, SI units)

Males:

6–23 U/mL (6–23 Arb. units, SI units)

Possible Meanings of Abnormal Values

Increased	Decreased
Acromegaly (early)	Anorexia nervosa
Amenorrhea	Hypogonadotropism
Congenital absence of ovaries	Hypopituitarism
Hyperpituitarism	Hypothalamic dysfunction

Increased	Decreased
Klinefelter's syndrome	Malnutrition
Menopause	
Menstruation	
Primary gonadal dysfunction	
Stein-Leventhal syndrome	
Turner's syndrome	

Contributing Factors to Abnormal Values

- Hemolysis of the blood sample or having a radioactive scan within 1 week of the test may alter test results.
- Drugs that may *increase* LH levels: anticonvulsants, clomiphene citrate, naloxone hydrochloride, spironolactone.
- Drugs that may *decrease* LH levels: digoxin, estrogens, oral contraceptives, phenothiazines, progesterone, testosterone.

Pre-Test Nursing Care

- Explain to the patient the purpose of the test and the need for a blood sample to be drawn.
- No fasting is required before the test.
- If possible, withhold drugs that may alter test results for 48 hours before the test.

Procedure

- A 7-mL blood sample is drawn in a collection tube containing a silicone gel.
- Gloves are worn throughout the procedure.

Post-Test Nursing Care

- Apply pressure at venipuncture site. Apply dressing, periodically assessing for continued bleeding.
- Label the specimen and transport it to the laboratory.
- For female patients: on the laboratory slip, include the date on which the patient began her last menstrual period.
- Resume medications as taken before the test.
- Report abnormal findings to the primary care provider.

• • • • • • • • • • • • • • •

Lyme Disease Antibody Test

Lyme disease is caused by the tick-transmitted spirochete *Borrelia burgdorferi*. The incubation period for the infection is 14 to 23 days. Lyme disease has three stages. The first stage involves a lesion and erythema around the bite, followed by regional lymphadenopathy, malaise, fever, headache, myalgia, arthralgia, and possibly conjunctivitis. The second stage, which occurs weeks to months later, may be associated with a rash and neurologic abnormalities, including meningitis, encephalitis, and Bell's palsy. The third stage, the chronic form of the disease, is characterized by arthritis, skin lesions, and additional neurologic problems.

Diagnosis of Lyme disease is made through determination of the presence of *Borrelia* antibodies. Antibody titers are usually low during the first several weeks of the illness, reach peak levels months later, and remain elevated for several years. Once the disease has been diagnosed, treatment can begin. Such treatment includes administration of tetracycline and penicillin.

Normal Values

Negative

Possible Meanings of Abnormal Values

Increased

Lyme disease

Contributing Factors to Abnormal Values

- False-positive results may occurs in persons with high rheumatoid factor (RF) levels.

Pre-Test Nursing Care

- Explain to the patient the purpose of the test and the need for a blood sample to be drawn.
- No fasting is required before the test.

Procedure

- A 7-mL blood sample is drawn in a collection tube containing no additives.
- Gloves are worn throughout the procedure.

Post-Test Nursing Care

- Apply pressure at venipuncture site. Apply dressing, periodically assessing for continued bleeding.
- Label the specimen and transport it to the laboratory.
- Report abnormal findings to the primary care provider.

• • • • • • • • • • • • • • • • •

Lymphangiography
(Lymphography)

Lymphangiography is the term used to indicate visualization of the lymphatic system. A contrast medium is injected into each foot. Visualization is then possible of the lymphatic system from the feet up to the thoracic duct. The test is used to detect and stage lymphomas and to assist in the differential diagnosis of lymphedema. The contrast medium remains in the body for 1 to 2 years, thus allowing subsequent films to be made in order to monitor disease progression and assess any response of the patient to therapy.

Normal Values

Normal lymphatic vessels and nodes.

Possible Meanings of Abnormal Values

Hodgkin's lymphoma
Lymphadenopathy
Metastatic involvement of the lymph nodes
Non-Hodgkin's lymphoma
Primary lymphedema
Secondary lymphedema

Contributing Factors to Abnormal Values

- Any movement by the patient may alter quality of films taken.

CONTRAINDICATIONS

- Patients who are allergic to iodine, shellfish, or contrast medium dye.
- Pregnant women (*Caution:* A woman in her childbearing years should undergo radiography only during her menses or 12–14 days after its onset to avoid any exposure to a fetus.).
- Patients who are unable to cooperate because of age, mental status, pain, or other factors.
- Patients with renal failure or those susceptible to dye-induced renal failure (dehydrated patients).
- Patients with compromised functioning of the cardiac, pulmonary, hepatic, or renal systems.

Pre-Test Nursing Care

- Explain to the patient the purpose of the test. Provide any written teaching materials available on the subject. Note that discomfort involved with this test is primarily owing to lying on a hard table for an extended period of time and the needle punctures. Explain that some discomfort may be felt in the popliteal or inguinal areas when the dye is first injected. Inform the patient that the dye will turn the urine and stool blue for 48 hours. The patient's skin and vision may have a blue tint for 48 hours.
- Check for allergies to iodine, shellfish, or contrast medium dye. Inform the radiologist of such possible allergy and obtain order for an antihistamine and corticosteroid to be administered before the test.
- Patients receiving metformin (Glucophage) for non–insulin-dependent diabetes mellitus should discontinue the drug 2 days before elective surgery or angiographic exams. This is because of the possible occurrence of lactic acidosis, a potentially fatal complication of biguanide therapy.
- No fasting is required before the test.
- Obtain a signed informed consent.

Procedure

- The patient is assisted to a supine position on the examination table.
- The skin over the dorsum of each foot is cleansed. Blue contrast dye is injected intradermally between each of the first three toes of each foot. In 15 to 30 minutes the lymphatic vessels will appear as small blue lines.
- In the dorsum of each foot, a local anesthetic is injected and a 1-in. incision is made.
- Because of the extreme smallness of the lymphatic vessels, a 30- gauge needle is inserted into the vessel. The contrast dye is then infused over a 60– to 90-minute period of time.

- When the contrast dye reaches the level of the third and fourth lumbar vertebrae, as visualized by fluoroscopy, the infusion is discontinued.
- The needles are removed, the incisions sutured, and sterile dressings are applied.
- Radiographic films are taken at this time and again in 24 hours.
- Gloves are worn throughout the procedure.

Post-Test Nursing Care

Possible complications:

- **Allergic reaction to dye**
- **Bleeding at puncture site**
- **Infection at the puncture site**
- **Lipid pneumonia from embolization of the contrast medium**
- **Renal failure**

  - Most allergic reactions to radiopaque dye occur within 30 minutes of administration of the contrast medium. Observe the patient closely for: respiratory distress, hypotension, edema, hives, rash, tachycardia, and/or laryngeal stridor. Emergency resuscitation equipment must be readily accessible.
  - Continue to observe the patient for allergic reaction for 24 hours.
  - Check the incisional sites for bleeding and signs of infection at frequent intervals. Sutures are removed in 7–10 days.
  - The patient should maintain bedrest with the feet elevated for 24 hours. Ice bags may be applied to the feet to help reduce swelling.
  - Observe for signs of pulmonary complications: shortness of breath, pleuritic pain, hypotension, low-grade fever, and cyanosis.
  - Renal function should be assessed before metformin is restarted.
  - Report abnormal findings to the primary care provider.

• • • • • • • • • • • • • • • • •

Magnesium

Magnesium (Mg^{2+}) is primarily an ion of the intracellular fluid. Only a very small amount of magnesium is found in the blood. The majority of magnesium is found in the bones, combined with calcium and phosphorus. Because of the close relationship among these electrolytes, changes in serum magnesium also affect serum levels of calcium and phosphorus. Like potassium, the excretion of magnesium by the kidneys is controlled by aldosterone. Magnesium is essential for proper neuromuscular functioning, blood clotting, and the activation of some enzymes.

Patients experiencing increased serum magnesium levels (*hypermagnesemia*) will have lethargy, flushing, hypotension, respiratory depression, bradycardia, and weak or absent deep tendon reflexes. Patients with *hypomagnesemia,* or decreased serum magnesium levels, will have muscle twitching and tremors, tetany, cardiac arrhythmias, and hyperactive deep tendon reflexes.

Normal Values

1.5–2.0 mEq/L (0.8–1.0 mmol/L, SI units)

Possible Meanings of Abnormal Values

Increased (Hypermagnesemia)	Decreased (Hypomagnesemia)
Addison's disease	Alcoholism
Adrenalectomy	Chronic malnutrition
Dehydration	Chronic pancreatitis
Hypothyroidism	Chronic renal disease
IV administration of	Diabetic acidosis
magnesium sulfate	Diarrhea
Renal failure	Draining GI fistulas
Uncontrolled diabetes	Hemodialysis
	Hepatic cirrhosis
	Hyperaldosteronism
	Hypercalcemia
	Hyperthyroidism
	Hypoalbuminemia
	Hypoparathyroidism
	Malabsorption
	Toxemia of pregnancy
	Ulcerative colitis

Contributing Factors to Abnormal Values

- Use of a tourniquet during acquisition of the blood sample may alter test results.
- Hemolysis of the blood sample may alter test results.
- Drugs that may *increase* serum magnesium levels: aminoglycosides, antacids, cathartics, Epsom salts, ethacrynic acid, lithium, loop diuretics, salicylates, thyroid medications.
- Drugs that may *decrease* serum magnesium levels: aminoglycosides, amphotericin, calcium gluconate, cisplatin, corticosteroids, cyclosporine, diuretics, insulin.

Pre-Test Nursing Care

- Explain to the patient the purpose of the test and the need for a blood sample to be drawn.
- No fasting is required before the test.
- Drugs containing magnesium salts, such as Epsom salts and Milk of Magnesia, should be withheld for 3 days before the test.

Procedure

- A 7-mL blood sample is drawn in a collection tube containing a silicone gel, avoiding use of a tourniquet, if possible.
- Gloves are worn throughout the procedure.

Post-Test Nursing Care

- Apply pressure at venipuncture site. Apply dressing, periodically assessing for continued bleeding.
- Label the specimen and transport it to the laboratory.
- Report abnormal findings to the primary care provider.

• • • • • • • • • • • • • •

Magnetic Resonance Imaging
(MRI)

Magnetic resonance imaging (MRI) is based upon the knowledge that a magnetic field causes atoms, especially the nuclei of hydrogen ions, to line up in a parallel configuration. Radio-frequency energy is then directed at the atoms, knocking them out of their alignment and causing them to spin. When the radio-frequency energy is discontinued, the atoms realign themselves within the magnetic field. During their realignment, the atoms emit radio-frequency energy as a tissue-specific signal based on the relative density of their nuclei and their realignment time. These signals are interpreted by the MRI computer, which then produces a very high-resolution image.

The MRI holds several advantages over computed tomography (CT). The image provided by the procedure is of excellent quality. The MRI uses no contrast medium and no radiation, thus it presents no hazards of allergic reaction or radiation exposure to the patient. Bone artifacts that can obscure the viewing in a CT scan do not occur with an MRI. Blood vessels appear dark on the MRI, so that they can be easily viewed. MRI is quickly replacing other diagnostic tests as the standard of care for various conditions. MRI can evaluate cerebral infarction within hours of the event. It is used for diagnosis of most abnormalities of the brain and spine, has almost entirely replaced arthrography for diagnosis of knee injuries, and has virtually eliminated the need for myelography. A disadvantage is that the MRI is more expensive to perform than the CT; however, its diagnostic value is well worth the additional cost.

The MRI machine is enclosed in a special room designed to protect it from interference by outside radio signals. The magnetic field in the room is always present and will cause watches to stop and will erase the magnetic strips found on the back of credit cards. The magnetic field also affects the functioning of computer-based equipment such as electronic infusion devices and ventilators. The magnet may move metal objects that may be present in the body; therefore, the test is contraindicated for any patient with a pacemaker, intracranial aneurysm clips, inner ear implants, metal fragments in the eyes, or gunshot wounds to the head. The patient is put on a moving pallet that is pushed into a large cylinder that houses the magnet. As the radio signals are switched on and off, the patient hears a variety of noises.

Normal Values

No evidence of pathology.

Possible Meanings of Abnormal Values

Abscesses
Acute tubular necrosis
Aortic aneurysm
Arteriovenous malformation
Atherosclerotic plaques
Avascular necrosis
Cerebral infarction
Cerebral lesions
Congenital heart disease
Degenerative vertebral disks

M

Dementia
Edema
Gaucher's disease
Glomerulonephritis
Hemorrhage
Hydronephrosis
Hyperparathyroidism
Joint disorders
Marfan's syndrome
Multiple sclerosis
Myocardial infarction
Osteomyelitis
Renal vein thrombosis
Seizures
Spinal cord injuries
Subarachnoid hemorrhage
Tumor detection and staging

Contributing Factors to Abnormal Values

- Excessive movement by the patient can blur images.

CONTRAINDICATIONS

- Patients who are morbidly obese.
- Patients who are pregnant, although there is no evidence of teratogenic or development abnormalities associated with MRI.
- Patients who are unable to cooperate during the procedure.
- Patients who are claustrophobic.
- Patients who require continuous life-support equipment that cannot be used inside the MRI room.
- Patients with implantable metal objects, such as pacemakers, intracranial aneurysm clips, infusion pumps, inner ear implants, or heart valves manufactured before 1964, or those with metal fragments in the eye(s) or gunshot wounds of the head. (*Note:* Most stainless steel orthopedic implants and prosthetic devices are not ferromagnetic and are not affected by MRI.)

Pre-Test Nursing Care

- Explain to the patient the purpose of the test and the procedure to be performed. Note that no radiation exposure is involved in this test. Explain that the patient will be moved into a large cylinder for the test and will need to remain completely still during the test. A variety of noises will be heard during the test.
- No fasting is required before the test.
- Obtain a signed informed consent.
- Pre-procedure medication with anti-anxiety drugs for those patients with claustrophobia may be needed.
- Remove all metal objects from the body before the test.
- Instruct the patient to void before the test.
- Sedation may be ordered for patients who are very young, uncooperative, or claustrophobic.

M

Procedure

- The patient is assisted to a supine position on the padded table and moved into the MRI cylinder.
- The patient and MRI staff may communicate via microphone during the procedure.

Post-Test Nursing Care

- If sedation was given prior to the exam, ensure the patient is fully awake prior to ambulation.
- Report abnormal findings to the primary care provider.

• • • • • • • • • • • • • • • • • •

Mammography

Mammography is a radiographic technique in which x-ray films are made of the breast. The mammogram is considered a routine screening procedure to detect the presence of tumors too small to be discovered by palpation. It is also used to further investigate questionable areas found on breast palpation. Suspicious areas found by mammography are then biopsied in order to confirm the presence of malignancy. The test has a high rate of false-positive results.

The American Cancer Society and the American College of Radiologists recommend a baseline mammogram be performed on all women between the ages of 35 and 40. Both groups agree that after age 50, women should have yearly mammograms. Women between the ages of 40 and 50 should check with their physician regarding suggested frequency of the exam. Women considered high risk owing to fibrocystic breast disease, family history of breast cancer, or personal history of any type of cancer, should begin screening at an earlier age and be tested on a more frequent basis.

Normal Values

Negative

M

Possible Meanings of Abnormal Values

Benign cyst
Breast abscess
Fibrocystic changes
Malignant tumor
Suppurative mastitis

Contributing Factors to Abnormal Values

- Very glandular breast tissue, previous breast surgery, and breast implants hinder accurate analysis of the mammogram.
- Powders and salves on the breast may appear as calcifications on the mammograms, thus causing false-positive results.

CONTRAINDICATIONS

- Pregnant women (*Caution:* A woman in her childbearing years should undergo radiography only during her menses or 12–14 days after its onset to avoid any exposure to a fetus.).

Pre-Test Nursing Care

- Explain to the patient the purpose of the test and the procedure to be performed. Note that some discomfort will be felt during compression of the breast.
- No fasting is required before the test.
- All jewelry and clothing are to be removed from above the waist. An x-ray gown that opens in the front is worn for the test.

Procedure

- The patient is either seated on a chair or standing in front of the mammogram machine.
- One breast is placed on a platform above the x-ray plate.
- The breast is compressed from above as the craniocaudal film is taken.
- The machine is then rotated, the breast is compressed from the side, and the lateral, or axillary, film is taken.
- The procedure is repeated for the other breast.

Post-Test Nursing Care

- The patient is asked to remain in the x-ray department until the films are developed and found to be readable.
- Instruct the patient in breast self-examination, as appropriate.
- Report abnormal findings to the primary care provider.

• • • • • • • • • • • • • • • •

Meckel Scan
(Meckel's Diverticulum Nuclear Scan)

M

The causes of abdominal pain or occult gastrointestinal bleeding are many, but one, Meckel's diverticulum, is a common congenital abnormality of the intestinal tract. Although located in the intestinal tract, approximately one-fourth of the diverticulum are lined with *gastric* mucosa. This type of mucosa secretes acid, which causes ulceration of intestinal tissue. This results in the abdominal pain and occult blood in stools that causes the patient to seek health care.

In the Meckel scan, technetium-99m pertechnetate is administered by intravenous injection. This particular radionuclide concentrates in gastric mucosal tissue, whether located in the stomach or in Meckel's diverticulum. Scanning then detects this concentration. The scan will not detect Meckel's diverticulum that do not contain gastric mucosa.

Normal Values

Negative (no increased uptake of radionuclide in right lower quadrant).

Possible Meanings of Abnormal Values

Meckel's diverticulum

Contributing Factors to Abnormal Values

- Any movement by the patient may alter quality of films taken.
- Retained barium from previous exams may interfere with the test.

CONTRAINDICATIONS

- Pregnant women (*Caution:* A woman in her childbearing years should undergo radiography only during her menses or 12–14 days after its onset to avoid any exposure to a fetus.).
- Patients who are lactating.
- Patients who are unable to cooperate because of age, mental status, pain, or other factors.

Pre-Test Nursing Care

- Explain to the patient the purpose of the test. Provide any written teaching materials available on the subject. Note that discomfort involved with this test is primarily owing to lying on a hard table for an extended period of time and the needle puncture. Reassure the patient that only trace amounts of the radionuclide are involved in the test.
- The patient must remain still while the scan is being performed.
- Fasting for 6 to 12 hours is required before the test.
- Obtain a signed informed consent.
- Administer a histamine H_2-receptor antagonist 1–2 days prior to the test, as ordered.

Procedure

- The patient should empty the bladder before the exam.
- The radiopharmaceutical is administered by intravenous injection in a peripheral vein.
- The patient is assisted to a supine position on the examination table.
- A scintillation camera is positioned over the right lower quadrant of the patient's abdomen. This camera takes a radioactivity reading from the body. This information is transformed into a two-dimensional picture of the area.
- Scans are obtained every 5 minutes for 1 hour.
- Gloves are worn during the radionuclide injection.

Post-Test Nursing Care

- Check the injection site for redness or swelling.
- If a woman who is lactating *must* have a nuclear scan, she should not breast feed the infant until the radionuclide has been eliminated, possibly for 3 days.
- Although the amount of diagnostic radionuclide excreted in the urine is low, the urine should not be used for any laboratory tests for the time period indicated by the nuclear medicine department. Patients should be told to flush the toilet three times after voiding.
- Gloves are worn when dealing with the urine.
- Encourage fluid intake by the patient to enhance excretion of the radionuclide.
- Report abnormal findings to the primary care provider.

Mediastinoscopy

Mediastinoscopy is the direct visualization of the contents of the mediastinum, including the heart and its vessels, the trachea, esophagus, thymus, and lymph nodes. This is accomplished via a mediastinoscope inserted at the suprasternal notch. Biopsy of the lymph nodes can be performed, allowing detection of lymphoma, sarcoidosis, and staging of lung cancer. Diagnosis of bronchogenic carcinoma can be made at an early stage using this procedure.

Normal Values

Normal mediastinal lymph nodes.

Possible Meanings of Abnormal Values

Coccidioidomycosis
Esophageal cancer
Histoplasmosis
Lung cancer
Lymphoma (including Hodgkin's disease)
Metastasis
Pneumocystis carinii
Sarcoidosis
Tuberculosis

CONTRAINDICATIONS

- Patients with scarring of the mediastinal area from previous mediastinoscopy.

Pre-Test Nursing Care

- Explain to the patient the purpose of the test and the procedure to be done. Note that the patient will receive a general anesthetic and may experience a sore throat after the procedure caused by the placement of an endotracheal tube. Note that temporary chest and incisional pain is also common.
- Fasting for 8 hours is required before the test.
- Obtain a signed written consent.
- Administer pre-procedure medication as ordered.

Procedure

- This sterile procedure is conducted in the operating room.
- The patient is given a general anesthetic, and an endotracheal tube is inserted.
- A small incision is made in the suprasternal notch.
- The mediastinoscope is inserted, and tissue samples are collected.
- Videotaping of the procedure may be done via a camera attached to the mediastinoscope.
- The mediastinoscope is removed, the incision is closed with sutures, and a sterile dressing is applied.

Post-Test Nursing Care

Possible complications:

- **Hemorrhage**
- **Laryngeal nerve damage**
- **Pneumothorax**
- **Puncture of the esophagus, trachea, or blood vessels**

- Monitor vital signs every 15 minutes for 1 hour, every 30 minutes for 2 hours, every hour for 4 hours, and then every 4 hours.
- Check the dressing for drainage, and the wound for hematoma formation.
- Assess the patient for fever, crepitus, dyspnea, cyanosis, diminished breath sounds, tachycardia, and hypotension.
- Send tissue specimen to the laboratory immediately.
- When fully awake, resume diet as taken before the procedure.
- Report abnormal findings to the primary care provider.

• • • • • • • • • • • • • • • •

Metyrapone Test
(Cortisol Test)

Metyrapone is an inhibitor of 11-betahydroxylase, an enzyme that converts 11-deoxycortisol to cortisol. With administration of metyrapone, less cortisol is produced, which normally stimulates the pituitary to produce adrenocorticotropic hormone (ACTH) through a negative feedback mechanism. Although cortisol itself is not able to be synthesized, the cortisol precursors such as 11-deoxycortisol, are present in the blood or the urine.

This test is used in the differential diagnosis of adrenal hyperplasia from a primary adrenal tumor. If adrenal hyperplasia is present, the amount of cortisol precursors is significantly increased. If, however, the problem is owing to an adrenal tumor, there is no response to metyrapone administration.

M

Normal Values

Blood

11-Deoxycortisol	>7 mcg/dL (>202 nmol/L, SI units)
Cortisol	<3 mcg/dL (<83 nmol/L, SI units)

24-Hour Urine

17-Ketosteroids:	>2 times base level
17-OHCS:	3–5 times base level

Possible Meanings of Abnormal Values

Increased	Decreased
Cushing's syndrome	Addison's disease
	Hypopituitarism

327

Contributing Factors to Abnormal Values
- Radioactive scans within 7 days prior to the test will alter test results.
- Drugs that may *decrease* plasma metyrapone levels: amitriptyline, chlordiazepoxide, estrogens, glucocorticoids, methysergide, oral contraceptives, phenobarbital, phenothiazines, progestins.

 ### CONTRAINDICATIONS
- Do *not* perform this test if primary adrenal insufficiency is likely. Metyrapone inhibits cortisol production.

Pre-Test Nursing Care
- Explain to the patient the purpose of the test and the need for two blood samples to be drawn. Also explain the need for multiple 24-hour urine collections.
- Stress the importance of saving *all* urine in the 24-hour period. Instruct the patient to avoid contaminating the urine with toilet paper or feces.
- Inform the patient of the presence of a preservative in the collection bottle.
- No fasting is required before the test.

Procedure

Blood
- A 7-mL blood sample is drawn in a collection tube containing EDTA. This is the baseline cortisol level.
- Administer metyrapone (30 mg/ky) orally with milk at 11 PM.
- Another 7-mL blood sample is drawn the next morning.
- Gloves are worn throughout the procedure.

24-Hour Urine
- A baseline 24-hour urine specimen is collected.
- Obtain the proper container containing the appropriate preservative from the laboratory.
- Begin the testing period in the morning following the patient's first voiding, which is discarded.
- Timing of the 24-hour period begins at the time the first voiding is discarded.
- *All* urine for the next 24 hours is collected in the container, which is to be kept refrigerated or on ice.
- If any urine is accidentally discarded during the 24-hour period, the test must be discontinued and a new test begun.
- The ending time of the 24-hour collection period should be posted in the patient's room.
- Administer adult patients metyrapone 500 to 750 mg orally every 4 hours for 6 doses (dosage for children is reduced; refer to reference laboratory) beginning at 11 PM.
- Begin additional 24-hour urine collection at 8 AM the next morning, following the same collection procedure as described.
- Gloves are to be worn when dealing with the specimen collection.

Post-Test Nursing Care

Possible complication: Addisonian crisis.

- Monitor for symptoms of Addisonian crisis: muscle weakness, mental and emotional changes, anorexia, nausea, vomiting, hypotension, hyperkalemia, severe abdominal, back, and leg pain, hyperpyrexia followed by hypothermia, vascular collapse. Treatment goals include: reverse shock, restore blood circulation, and replenish body with essential steroids.

Blood

- Apply pressure at venipuncture site. Apply dressing, periodically assessing for continued bleeding.
- Label specimen and transport it to the laboratory.

24-Hour Urine

- Label the container and transport it on ice to the laboratory as soon as possible following the end of each of the 24-hour collection periods.
- Report abnormal findings to the primary care provider.

• • • • • • • • • • • • • • • •

Mononucleosis Test

(Epstein-Barr Virus [EBV] Antibody Test, Heterophil Antibody Titer [HAT], Infectious Mononucleosis Testing, Monospot Test)

Infectious mononucleosis is caused by a herpesvirus, the Epstein-Barr virus (EBV). It is characterized by fatigue, sore throat, fever, pharyngitis, lymphadenopathy, splenomegaly, and the presence of lymphocytosis. It is a self-limiting condition, with treatment aimed at symptom control.

In addition to the increased production of lymphocytes and monocytes in the lymph nodes, infectious mononucleosis also stimulates the production of heterophil antibodies. This IgM type of antibody, which is not normally present in human beings, causes agglutination of sheep or horse red blood cells. The antibodies usually form within 5 to 7 days of the onset of the illness.

A positive *heterophil antibody titer (HAT)* assists in the diagnosis of infectious mononucleosis. A more rapid test is the *Monospot test*. In this test, two types of antigens are used, the heterophil antigen and the Forssman antigen, which can be present in normal people and agglutinates with sheep red blood cells. On one slide, the patient serum is mixed with guinea pig kidney antigen, which contains Forssman antigen. On another slide, the patient's serum is mixed with beef red blood cells, which contain infectious mononucleosis antigen. Horse red blood cells, which contain both types of antigens, are then added to each slide. The test is considered positive for infectious mononucleosis if agglutination of the beef red blood cells occurs. Positive results to this testing may occur with other conditions as well.

Normal Values

Negative

Possible Meanings of Abnormal Values

Positive

Burkitt's lymphoma
Chronic fatigue (EBV) syndrome
Cytomegalovirus
Epstein-Barr virus
Hodgkin's disease
Infectious mononucleosis
Izumi fever
Lymphocytic leukemia
Malaria
Nasopharyngeal cancer
Pancreatic cancer
Rheumatoid arthritis
Rubella
Sarcoidosis
Systemic lupus erythematosus
Viral hepatitis

Contributing Factors to Abnormal Values

- Hemolysis of the blood sample may alter test results.

Pre-Test Nursing Care

- Explain to the patient the purpose of the test and the need for a blood sample to be drawn.
- No fasting is required before the test.
- (*Note:* A white blood count with differential should be done concurrently to identify the lymphocytosis and the presence of atypical lymphocytes usually found in infectious mononucleosis.)

Procedure

- A 7-mL blood sample is drawn in a collection tube containing no additives.
- Gloves are worn throughout the procedure.

Post-Test Nursing Care

- Apply pressure at venipuncture site. Apply dressing, periodically assessing for continued bleeding.
- Label the specimen and transport it to the laboratory.
- Report abnormal findings to the primary care provider.

• • • • • • • • • • • • • • • •

Myelography

Myelography is the radiographic study of the subarachnoid space of the spinal column. This is accomplished through injection of a water-soluble contrast dye into the spinal subarachnoid space via a lumbar puncture. Air may be injected in place of dye, but this is rarely done. The filling of the space with the dye can be viewed via fluoroscopy. Disorders that can be visualized through use of myelography include tumors, changes in bone structure, and herniations or protrusions of intervertebral disks. The procedure, although still used, is becoming less popular since the advent of magnetic resonance imaging (MRI).

Normal Values

Normal spinal canal with no obstruction or structural abnormalities.

Possible Meanings of Abnormal Values

Arachnoiditis
Arthritic bone spurs
Astrocytomas
Congenital abnormalities
Herniated intervertebral disks
Meningiomas
Metastatic tumors
Neurofibromas
Primary tumors
Spinal nerve root injury

CONTRAINDICATIONS

- Patients who are allergic to iodine, shellfish, or contrast medium dye.
- Pregnant women (*Caution:* A woman in her childbearing years should undergo radiography only during her menses or 12–14 days after its onset to avoid any exposure to a fetus.).
- Patients with increased intracranial pressure.
- Patients with infection at the puncture site.
- Patients with multiple sclerosis.
- Patients who are unable to cooperate because of age, mental status, pain, or other factors.

Pre-Test Nursing Care

- Explain to the patient the purpose of the test. Provide any written teaching materials available on the subject. Note that discomfort during the test is owing to insertion of the needle, and that during injection of the dye, transient sensations, including warmth, flushing, a salty taste, and nausea, may be experienced. Explain that movement will not be allowed during the test.
- Check for allergies to iodine, shellfish, or contrast medium dye. Inform the radiologist of such possible allergy and obtain order for an antihistamine and corticosteroid to be administered before the test. A hypoallergenic nonionic contrast medium may be used for the test in allergic patients.

M

- Patients receiving metformin (Glucophage) for non–insulin-dependent diabetes mellitus should discontinue the drug 2 days before elective surgery or angiographic examinations. This is owing to the possible occurrence of lactic acidosis, a potentially fatal complication of biguanide therapy.
- Fasting for 8 hours is required before the test. The patient should be well hydrated before beginning the fasting period.
- Instruct the patient to void before the procedure.
- If a water-soluble contrast medium such as metrizamide (Amipaque) is to be used during the procedure, drugs that decrease the seizure threshold should be withheld for 48 hours before the test. This drugs include phenothiazines, tricyclic antidepressants, central nervous system (CNS) stimulants, and amphetamines.

Procedure

- The patient is assisted to a side-lying position on the radiography table, with the knees drawn up to the abdomen and the chin on the chest.
- A lumbar puncture is performed. Fifteen milliliters of cerebrospinal fluid are removed and an equal amount of contrast dye is injected.
- With the needle in place, the patient is turned to the prone position and the table is tilted to assist with the flow of the dye. The chin is hyperextended to prevent the dye from entering the cranium.
- Radiographic films are taken.
- At the end of the procedure, the needle is removed and a sterile dressing is applied to the site.
- Gloves are worn during the venipuncture.

Post-Test Nursing Care

Possible complications:
- **Allergic reaction to dye**
- **Headache**
- **Herniation of the brain**
- **Meningitis**
- **Seizures**

- Most allergic reactions to radiopaque dye occur within 30 minutes of administration of the contrast medium. Observe the patient closely for respiratory distress, hypotension, edema, hives, rash, tachycardia, and/or laryngeal stridor. Emergency resuscitation equipment must be readily accessible.
- Observe for allergic reaction to the dye for at least 6 hours post-procedure.
- The patient is to remain on bedrest for 8 hours with the head of the bed elevated no more than 45 degrees. Specific positioning instructions should be ordered by the physician.
- Observe the patient for indications of meningeal irritation, as characterized by headache, irritability, neck stiffness, fever, and photophobia. If present, keep the room quiet and dark, and provide analgesic medication.
- Monitor vital signs at least every 30 minutes for 4 hours, then every 4 hours for 24 hours.
- Check the dressing for drainage with each vital sign assessment.
- Assess the patient's ability to void.
- Encourage fluid intake to enhance excretion of the dye.

- The patient may resume pre-procedure diet and activities the day following the test. A clear liquid diet is usually preferred following the test.
- Renal function should be assessed before metformin is restarted.
- Report abnormal findings to the primary care provider.

• • • • • • • • • • • • • • • • •

Myoglobin

Myoglobin is a heme-containing, oxygen-binding protein present in the cytoplasm of cardiac and skeletal muscle cells. It serves as a reservoir of oxygen to meet very short-term needs. When muscle cell injury occurs through disease, as in myocardial infarction, or through trauma, myoglobin is released into the blood. This usually occurs within 2 to 6 hours following muscle tissue damage. Myoglobin is excreted by the kidneys (myoglobinuria) and is detected in the urine up to 1 week following muscle tissue injury.

Normal Values

0–85 ng/mL (0–85 nmol/L, SI units)

Possible Meanings of Abnormal Values

Increased

Glycogen and lipid storage diseases
Hyperthermia
Muscle enzyme deficiencies
Muscle injury
Muscular dystrophy
Myocardial infarction
Polymyositis
Renal failure
Rhabdomyolysis
Severe burns
Surgical procedure
Trauma
Viral infection

Contributing Factors to Abnormal Values

- Hemolysis of the blood sample and recent radioactive scans will alter test results.
- Intramuscular (IM) injections may *increase* myoglobin levels.

Pre-Test Nursing Care

- Explain to the patient the purpose of the test and the need for a blood sample to be drawn.
- No fasting is required before the test.

M

Procedure

- A 7-mL blood sample is drawn in a collection tube containing no additives.
- Gloves are worn throughout the procedure.

Post-Test Nursing Care

- Apply pressure at venipuncture site. Apply dressing, periodically assessing for continued bleeding.
- Label the specimen and transport it to the laboratory.
- Report abnormal findings to the primary care provider.

• • • • • • • • • • • • • • •

Nonstress Test
(NST, Fetal Activity Study)

The nonstress test (NST) is a noninvasive technique used to evaluate the status of the fetus. Unlike the contraction stress test, the NST does not include stimulation with oxytocin. The fetal activity monitored in this test may be spontaneous or induced by uterine contraction or external manipulation. Normally, the fetal heart rate (FHR) should accelerate in response to fetal movement. The fetus is reported as being "reactive" when two or more FHR accelerations are detected within a 20-minute period. Each of the accelerations must be at least 15 beats per minute and last for at least 15 seconds. The NST is highly reliable for determining fetal viability. Only with a "nonreactive" result is a contraction stress test (CST) indicated.

Normal Values

"Reactive" fetus

Possible Meanings of Abnormal Values

Nonreactive fetus

Pre-Test Nursing Care

- Explain to the patient the purpose of the test and the procedure to be done. Note that there is no discomfort associated with the NST.
- No fasting is required before the test. Instruct the patient to eat before the test to ensure a high maternal serum glucose level, which enhances fetal activity.

Procedure

- The patient is instructed to void.
- The patient is assisted into a Sims' position.
- An external fetal monitor is applied to the patient's abdomen, which will provide a graph of FHR and uterine contractions.
- The patient is instructed to push a button on the fetal monitor whenever she feels fetal movement. This is then indicated on the graph, allowing correlation to be made with the FHR at that time.

- If there is no fetal movement for 20 minutes, the fetus is externally stimulated by rubbing or compressing the patient's abdomen or by producing a loud noise near the abdomen.

Post-Test Nursing Care
- Report abnormal findings to the primary care provider.
- If the test finds the fetus to be nonreactive, the patient is scheduled for a CST.

• • • • • • • • • • • • • • • • • •

5′-Nucleotidase
(5′N)

Testing for 5′-nucleotidase is used in conjunction with alkaline phosphatase (ALP) to differentiate between hepatobiliary diseases and bone diseases. 5′-Nucleotidase is an enzyme found in the plasma membranes of liver cells and cells of the bile duct. Its limited location makes this test relatively specific in nature. When both 5′-nucleotidase and ALP are elevated, the presence of liver metastases is probable.

Normal Values

1–11 U/L (0.02-0.18 microkat/L, SI units)

Possible Meanings of Abnormal Values

Increased

Biliary obstruction
Cholestasis
Cirrhosis
Hepatitis
Late pregnancy
Liver disease
Liver metastases

Contributing Factors to Abnormal Values
- Drugs that may *increase* 5′-nucleotidase levels: codeine, hepatotoxic drugs, meperidine hydrochloride, morphine, phenothiazines.

Pre-Test Nursing Care
- Explain to the patient the purpose of the test and the need for a blood sample to be drawn.
- No fasting is required before the test.

N

Procedure

- A 5-mL blood sample is drawn in a collection tube containing no additives.
- Gloves are worn throughout the procedure.

Post-Test Nursing Care

Possible complication: With liver dysfunction, patient may have prolonged clotting time.

- Apply pressure 3 to 5 minutes at venipuncture site. Apply dressing, periodically assessing for continued bleeding.
- Teach the patient to monitor the site. If the site begins to bleed, the patient should apply direct pressure and, if unable to control the bleeding, return to the laboratory or notify the nurse.
- Label the specimen and transport it to the laboratory.
- Report abnormal findings to the primary care provider.

• • • • • • • • • • • • • • • • •

Oculoplethysmography
(OPG)

One of the major contributors to sufficient cerebral circulation is adequate blood flow through the internal carotid artery. For patients who have had carotid endarterectomy performed and for patients who are experiencing dizziness, ataxia, syncope, carotid bruits, or transient ischemic attacks, ensuring the adequacy of the blood through the internal carotid artery is very important. One way to do so is to measure the blood flow in the ophthalmic artery, the first major branch of the internal carotid.

Oculoplethysmography (OPG) is a noninvasive test used to indirectly measure ocular artery pressure. In this test, eyecups are applied to the cornea of each eye, whose blood flow comes from the ophthalmic artery. Photoelectric cells are attached to the patient's earlobes, whose blood supply comes from the external carotid artery. The pulse arrival times in the eyes are compared with those of the ears. If the blood flow is adequate within the internal carotid artery, the pulse arrival times should be the same to both the eyes and the ears. If *internal* carotid stenosis is present, blood flow to the ophthalmic artery, and thus to the eye, will be slowed.

Normal Values

All pulses (in both the eyes and the ears) should occur simultaneously.

Possible Meanings of Abnormal Values

Decreased

Carotid occlusive disease

CONTRAINDICATIONS

- Patients who have had eye surgery within 6 months.
- Patients with conjunctivitis, uncontrolled glaucoma, cataracts, or enucleation.

- Patients who have had retinal detachment or lens implantation.
- Patients with a hypersensitivity to local anesthetics.

Pre-Test Nursing Care

- Explain to the patient the purpose of the test and procedure to be followed.
- No fasting is required before the test.
- Obtain a signed informed consent.
- Have the patient remove contact lenses, if applicable.
- Patients who normally receive eye drops may continue to do so before the test.

Procedure

- The patient is assisted to a supine position.
- Anesthetic eyedrops are administered.
- Small photoelectric cells are applied to the earlobes.
- Eyecups are applied to the corneas and held in place with light suction.
- Recordings are made of pulsations in each of the eyes and ears and compared with each other.

Post-Test Nursing Care

Possible complications:

- **Conjunctival hemorrhage**
- **Corneal abrasion**
- **Transient photophobia**

- After the eyecups are removed, the eyes may appear bloodshot and have mild burning for several hours. Instruct the patient not to rub the eyes or insert contact lenses for at least 2 hours after the test. Artificial tears may be used, if needed, for eye irritation. Sunglasses should be worn if photophobia occurs.
- Instruct the patient to report severe burning or pain in the eyes.
- Report abnormal findings to the primary care provider.

• • • • • • • • • • • • • • • •

Osmolality, Blood
(Serum Osmolality)

The osmolality of the blood measures the number of osmotically active particles in the serum. The test is useful in assessing fluid and electrolyte imbalances and in determining fluid requirements. It provides valuable information regarding a patient's hydration status, the concentration of the urine, and the status of ADH (antidiuretic hormone) secretion, and is used in toxicology workups. The serum osmolality is calculated with the following formula:

$$2 \text{ (Sodium level)} + \frac{BUN}{2.8} + \frac{Blood\ glucose}{18} = Serum\ osmolality$$

Normal Values

280–296 mOsm/Kg of H_2O (280–296 mmol/Kg, SI units)

Abnormal Values

Respiratory arrest may occur with values > 360 mOsm/Kg.

Possible Meanings of Abnormal Values

Increased	Decreased
Acidosis	Addison's disease
Advanced liver disease	Congestive heart failure
Alcoholism	Edema
Azotemia	Hepatic cirrhosis
Burns	Hepatic failure with ascites
Convulsions	Lung cancer
Dehydration	Overhydration
Diabetes insipidus	Postoperative
Diabetes mellitus	Syndrome of inappropriate
Edema	ADH secretion (SIADH)
High protein diet	
Hyperaldosteronism	
Hyperbilirubinemia	
Hypercalcemia	
Hyperglycemia	
Hypernatremia	
Hypokalemia	
Ketoacidosis	
Methanol poisoning	
Shock	
Trauma	
Uremia	

Contributing Factors to Abnormal Values

- Test results may be altered because of hemolysis of the blood sample.
- Drugs that may alter test results: mineralocorticoids, osmotic diuretics.

Pre-Test Nursing Care

- Explain to the patient the purpose of the test and the need for a blood sample to be drawn.
- No fasting is required before the test.

Procedure

- A 7-mL blood sample is drawn in a collection tube containing a silicone gel.
- Gloves are worn throughout the procedure.

Post-Test Nursing Care

- Apply pressure at venipuncture site. Apply dressing, periodically assessing for continued bleeding.
- Label the specimen and transport it to the laboratory.
- Report abnormal findings to the primary care provider.

• • • • • • • • • • • • • • • •

Osmolality, Urine
(Urine Osmolality)

The urine osmolality measures the number of osmotically active particles in the urine, or the concentration of the urine. This, in turn, reflects the ability of the kidneys to concentrate urine. The test is useful in assessing fluid and electrolyte imbalances and in determining fluid requirements. Following an overnight fast, the urine osmolality should be at least three times the osmolality of the blood.

Normal Values

500–800 mOsm/Kg water (500–800 mmol/Kg, SI units)

Possible Meanings of Abnormal Values

Increased	Decreased
Addison's disease	Aldosteronism
Azotemia	Diabetes insipidus
Congestive heart failure	Edema
Dehydration	Fever
Diabetes mellitus	Glomerulonephritis
Diarrhea	High protein diet
Edema	Hypercalcemia
Glycosuria	Hypokalemia
Hepatic cirrhosis	Hyponatremia
Hyperglycemia	Multiple myeloma
Ketoacidosis	Overhydration
Postoperative	Sickle cell anemia
Sodium overload	Urinary tract obstruction
Syndrome of inappropriate ADH secretion (SIADH)	
Uremia	

Contributing Factors to Abnormal Values

- Abnormal results may occur with intake of antibiotics, dextran, diuretics, glucose, mannitol, and radiographic contrast agents.

Pre-Test Nursing Care

- Explain to the patient the purpose of the test and the need for a urine specimen.
- No fasting is required for random testing.
- Overnight fasting is required before the test, if ordered as a fasting urine specimen.

Procedure

- 10 mL of urine is collected in a plastic specimen container.
- Gloves are worn throughout the procedure.

Post-Test Nursing Care

- Label the specimen and transport it to the laboratory immediately.
- Report abnormal findings to the primary care provider.

• • • • • • • • • • • • • • • •

Oximetry
(Ear Oximetry, Pulse Oximetry, Oxygen Saturation, SaO₂)

Oximetry is a noninvasive procedure used to monitor the oxygen saturation of arterial blood. Because of the simplicity and convenience of the procedure, oximetry is used in a variety of settings where monitoring of oxygenation status is needed. Examples of oximetry use include during surgical procedures, during mechanical ventilation, and during diagnostic testing such as stress testing.

Oximetry measures the percentage of oxygen being carried by the hemoglobin. To perform this measurement, a light-emitting sensor is attached to a site such as a finger. The sensor emits beams of light through the skin tissue. A light-detecting sensor then records the amount of light absorbed by the oxygenated hemoglobin. This absorption rate is converted to the percentage of oxygen saturation present in the blood, which is shown on the monitor.

Normal Values

96%–100%

Possible Meanings of Abnormal Values

Increased	Decreased
Adequate oxygen therapy	Carbon monoxide poisoning
	Hypoxia

Contributing Factors to Abnormal Vales

- False alarms may occur because of movement of the site to which the sensor is attached, equipment problems, or inadequate blood flow to the site.
- Inaccurate readings may occur if the patient is anemic or has received contrast media, or if there are bright lights in the room.

Pre-Test Nursing Care

- Explain to the patient the purpose of the test, noting that no discomfort is associated with this procedure.
- Inform the patient of the presence of alarms. Explain that the alarm will sound should the sensor become displaced. Also inform the patient of steps that will be taken should the oxygen saturation be found to be low.
- No fasting is required before the test.

Procedure

- The site must have good circulation. Examples of possible sites include fingers, earlobes, and toes.
- Ensure that the skin is clean and dry. Rub the area to increase its blood flow.
- Apply the sensor to the chosen site.

Post-Test Nursing Care

- Report abnormal findings to the primary care provider.

• • • • • • • • • • • • • • • •

Pancreatic Enzymes

See:
Amylase, Serum
Amylase, Urine
Lipase

• • • • • • • • • • • • • • • •

Papanicolaou Smear
(Exfoliative Cytologic Study, Pap Smear, Pap Test)

The Papanicolaou (Pap) smear can be performed on many body secretions, including gastric secretions, prostatic secretions, sputum, and urine. However, the term usually refers to a test for detection of cervical cancer. A vaginal examination is performed and cells are obtained from the cervix. These cells are then classified according to a grading system ranging from normal cells to the presence of cancer. Following are two systems used for grading of Pap smear results:

P

Older system

Grade I: Normal-appearing cells
Grade II: Atypical, but no evidence of malignancy
Grade III: Suggestion of malignancy, but not conclusive
Grade IV: Strongly suggestive of malignancy
Grade V: Conclusive for malignancy

Newer system

Normal
Inflammatory
Mild-cervical intraepithelial neoplasia
Severe-cervical intraepithelial neoplasia
Cancer

It is recommended that women between ages 20 and 40 who are not considered high risk have a Pap test every 3 years, after three initial smears performed 1 year apart are normal. Annual Pap tests are recommended for women after age 40, for women considered as high-risk, and for any woman who has had a positive Pap test. Any abnormal Pap smear result should be closely monitored, with biopsy performed as needed.

Normal Values

No abnormal cells

Possible Meanings of Abnormal Values

Cervical cancer
Fungal infections
Inflammatory processes
Parasitic infestations
Venereal disease

Contributing Factors to Abnormal Values

- Pap test results may be altered by allowing the cells of the specimen to dry, using lubricating jelly on the vaginal speculum, douching, tub bathing, menstrual flow, and infections.
- Drugs that may alter test results include digitalis and tetracycline.

CONTRAINDICATIONS

- Patients currently having menses.

Pre-Test Nursing Care

- Explain to the patient the purpose of the test and the need for a vaginal examination to be done. Note that minimal discomfort is felt during the insertion of the vaginal speculum.
- No fasting is required before the test.
- Instruct the patient not to douche or tub bathe for 24 hours before the examination.
- Instruct the patient to void before the examination.

Procedure

- The patient is assisted into the lithotomy position with her legs supported in the stirrups.
- A vaginal speculum lubricated only with saline or warm water is inserted into the vagina.
- Secretions are collected from the cervix and the endocervical canal.
- Slides are prepared from the secretions.
- Gloves are worn throughout the procedure.

Post-Test Nursing Care

- Assist the patient to an upright position.
- Explain to the patient that a very small amount of bleeding from the cervix may occur after the procedure.
- Report abnormal findings to the primary care provider.

• • • • • • • • • • • • • • • •

Paracentesis
(Abdominal Paracentesis, Abdominal Tap, Peritoneal Fluid Analysis, Peritoneal Tap)

Paracentesis refers to the removal of fluid from the peritoneal cavity. This cavity is the space between the visceral peritoneum, which covers the abdominal organs, and the parietal peritoneum, which lines the abdominal cavity. In some conditions, such as cardiac disease, infection, neoplasia, sodium retention, and cirrhosis of the liver, serous fluid accumulates in the peritoneal cavity, an assessment finding known as *ascites*.

Paracentesis may be done for a diagnostic purpose to determine the cause of the ascites, or for therapeutic purposes to remove up to 1000 mL of the ascites at any one time. The test is also performed in cases of abdominal trauma to check for bleeding into the peritoneal cavity. The fluid analysis includes red and white blood cell counts, cytologic studies, bacterial and fungal cultures, and determination of alkaline phosphatase, ammonia, amylase, glucose, lactic dehydrogenase, and protein levels.

Normal Values

Gross appearance:	clear to pale yellow in color, odorless
Amount:	<50 mL
Bacteria:	None
Cell counts:	Red blood cells: Negative
	White blood cells: <300/µL
Cytology:	No malignant cells present
Fungi:	None
Alkaline phosphatase:	
Male >age 18:	90–239 U/L
Female <age 45:	76–196 U/L
Female >age 45:	87–250 U/L
Ammonia:	<50 mg/dL
Amylase:	138–404 U/L

P

Glucose:	70–100 mg/dL
Lactic dehydrogenase:	Equal to serum level
Protein:	0.3–4.1 g/dL

Possible Meanings of Abnormal Values

Color

Milk colored:	Chyle present from blocked thoracic lymphatic ducts owing to: carcinoma, lymphoma, tuberculosis.
Cloudy fluid:	Inflammation owing to: appendicitis, pancreatitis, peritonitis.
Bloody fluid:	Owing to hemorrhagic pancreatitis, traumatic tap, tumor.
Green fluid:	Bile-stained owing to acute pancreatitis, perforated intestines, ruptured gallbladder.

Alkaline Phosphatase

Increased

Intestinal strangulation
Ruptured intestine

Ammonia

Increased

Intestinal strangulation
Ruptured appendix
Ruptured intestine
Ruptured ulcer

Amylase

Increased

Acute pancreatitis
Intestinal necrosis
Intestinal strangulation
Pancreatic pseudocyst
Pancreatic trauma

Bacteria

Increased

Appendicitis
Pancreatitis
Tuberculosis
Ovarian disease

Fungi

Increased

Candidiasis
Coccidioidomycosis
Histoplasmosis

Glucose

Decreased

Peritoneal carcinomatosis
Tuberculous peritonitis

Lactic Dehydrogenase

Increased

Malignancy
Pancreatic ascites
Tuberculous ascites

Protein

Increased

Cancer
Peritonitis
Tuberculosis

Red Blood Cells

Increased

Intra-abdominal trauma
Neoplasm
Tuberculosis

White Blood Cells

Increased

Bacterial peritonitis
Chylous ascites
Cirrhosis
Tuberculous peritonitis

Contributing Factors to Abnormal Values

- Injury to underlying organs may contaminate the sample with bile, blood, urine, or feces.
- Contamination of the specimen will alter white blood cell count.

 CONTRAINDICATIONS
- Patients with bleeding disorders.

Pre-Test Nursing Care

- Explain to the patient the purpose of the test and the procedure to be done. Explain that a local anesthetic will be used, but that a pressure-like pain will occur as the needle pierces the peritoneum.
- No fasting is required before the test.
- Obtain a signed informed consent.

- The patient needs to empty the bladder before the procedure to avoid accidental puncture of the bladder.
- Obtain baseline assessment information, including vital signs, weight, and abdominal girth.

Procedure

- Assist the patient to a sitting position with the feet on the floor and the back well supported. If the patient cannot tolerate this position, a high Fowler's position may be used.
- Monitor vital signs every 15 minutes during the procedure.
- Sterile technique is used throughout the procedure.
- The usual site to be used for the puncture is located midway between the umbilicus and the symphysis pubis. Alternate sites are the flank, the iliac fossa, the border of the rectus, or, when assessing for abdominal bleeding, at each quadrant of the abdomen.
- The area is shaved, cleansed, and draped.
- A local anesthetic is administered.
- A small incision is made at the site if a trocar and cannula are to be inserted. Otherwise, a needle is inserted through the peritoneum.
- A sample of the fluid is obtained.
- If additional fluid is to be drained, connect a tubing between the cannula and the collection receptacle.
- A maximum of 1000 mL is allowed to drain slowly from the site. Rapid drainage, and thus hypovolemia, can be avoided by either raising the collection receptacle to slow the draining or by clamping the tubing.
- When the procedure is complete, the trocar or needle is removed. A pressure dressing is applied.

Post-Test Nursing Care

Possible complications:

- **Hemorrhage**
- **Hepatic coma**
- **Perforation of abdominal organs**
- **Peritonitis**
- **Shock and hypovolemia**

- Monitor vital signs until stable.
- Check the dressing frequently for drainage. Assess for hemorrhage, for increasing pain, and for abdominal tenderness.
- If a large amount of fluid is drained from the peritoneal cavity, a fluid shift may occur from the vascular space to the peritoncal cavity. Assess for elevated pulse and respirations, decreased blood pressure, mental status changes, and dizziness. Intravenous fluids or albumin will probably be ordered.
- Observe for hepatic coma in patients with severe hepatic disease, as evidenced by mental status changes, drowsiness, and stupor.
- Weigh the patient and measure the abdominal girth for comparison with pre-test values, as indications of fluid loss.
- Monitor urinary output for 24 hours. Observe for hematuria.
- Label the specimen and transport it to the laboratory immediately.
- Report abnormal findings to the primary care provider.

• • • • • • • • • • • • • • •

Parathyroid Hormone
(PTH, Parathormone)

Parathyroid hormone (PTH) is produced by the parathyroid glands, four glands located within the fascial capsule of the thyroid gland. Through the work of PTH, calcium and phosphorus levels in the body are maintained. This balance is accomplished through promotion of intestinal absorption of calcium, through mobilization of calcium and phosphorus from the bone, and through renal tubular reabsorption of calcium and excretion of phosphorus. The results of this test, along with determination of calcium levels, assist in the differential diagnosis of parathyroid disorders.

Normal Values

10–60 pg/mL (10–60 ng/L, SI units)

Possible Meanings of Abnormal Values

Increased	Decreased
Calcium malabsorption	Autoimmune disease
Chronic renal failure	Graves' disease
Ectopic PTH production	Hypercalcemia
Hypocalcemia	Hypoparathyroidism
Lactation	Milk-alkali syndrome
Pregnancy	Parathyroidectomy
Primary hyperparathyroidism	Sarcoidosis
Renal hypercalciuria	Vitamin A and D toxicity
Rickets	
Secondary hyperparathyroidism	
Squamous cell carcinoma	
Vitamin D deficiency	

Contributing Factors to Abnormal Values

- Falsely low values may occur following ingestion of milk.
- Drugs that may *decrease* PTH levels: thiazide diuretics.

Pre-Test Nursing Care

- Explain to the patient the purpose of the test and the need for a blood sample to be drawn.
- Fasting for 8 to 10 hours is required before the test.

Procedure

- A 7-mL *morning* blood sample is drawn in a collection tube containing no additives.
- Gloves are worn throughout the procedure.

Post-Test Nursing Care

- Apply pressure at venipuncture site. Apply dressing, periodically assessing for continued bleeding.
- Label the specimen, place it on ice and transport it to the laboratory immediately.
- Report abnormal findings to the primary care provider.

• • • • • • • • • • • • • • • • • •

Partial Thromboplastin Time
(PTT, Activated Partial Thromboplastin Time [APTT])

The process of hemostasis involves numerous steps and the proper functioning of a variety of coagulating factors and other substances. The *partial thromboplastin time (PTT)* is used to evaluate how well the coagulation process is functioning. This test is useful for detecting bleeding disorders caused by either deficient or defective coagulation factors that compose the intrinsic system. These factors include I, II, V, VIII, IX, X, XI, and XII. (For review of the entire coagulation process, see Coagulation Studies.)

The PTT is also used to monitor heparin therapy. Heparin inactivates prothrombin and prevents the formation of thromboplastin. Thus, in conditions in which prevention of thrombus formation is essential, heparin is given, usually in the form of a continuous intravenous infusion. It is important that the patient's response to this anticoagulant therapy be appropriate; that is, enough for prevention of clot formation, but not so much as to cause spontaneous bleeding. This delicate balance can be monitored through use of the PTT.

The PTT involves measuring the amount of time it take for a clot to form in a plasma sample to which calcium and partial thromboplastin have been added. If additional chemicals are added to standardize and accelerate the test, the result is reported as an *activated partial thromboplastin time (APTT)*. A normal range for PTT is 60 to 90 seconds, whereas for APTT the normal range is 24 to 37 seconds. Laboratories report the actual PTT or APTT values along with the control value for reference. The therapeutic level for a patient receiving heparin is 1.5 to 2.5 times the control value. If the value falls below the therapeutic level for a patient on heparin, an increase in anticoagulation, and thus, dosage is needed. If the APTT is greater than 100 seconds, the patient is at high risk for spontaneous bleeding. In the case of heparin overdose with resultant hemorrhage, the antidote is protamine sulfate, with each 1 mg reversing 100 units of heparin.

Normal Values

APTT: 24–37 seconds
PTT: 60–90 seconds
Therapeutic level for anticoagulant therapy: 1.5–2.5 times the control value.

Possible Meanings of Abnormal Values

Increased	Decreased
Abruptio placentae	Acute hemorrhage
Afibrinogenemia	Advanced cancer

Increased	Decreased
Autologous blood transfusion	Hypercoagulability
Bleeding disorders	Very early DIC
Cardiac surgery	
Cirrhosis	
Disseminated intravascular coagulation	
Dysfibrinogenemia	
Hemodialysis	
Hemophilia A (factor VIII deficiency)	
Hemophilia B (factor IX deficiency)	
Hypoprothrombinemia	
Liver disease	
Vitamin K deficiency	
von Willebrand's disease	

Contributing Factors to Abnormal Values

- Hemolysis of the blood sample may alter test results.
- Drugs that may *increase* PTT: antihistamines, ascorbic acid, chlorpromazine, dicumarol, dipyridamole, heparin, salicylates.
- Drugs that may *decrease* PTT: antihistamines, digitalis, nicotine, oral contraceptives, tetracyclines.

Pre-Test Nursing Care

- Explain to the patient the purpose of the test and the need for a blood sample to be drawn.
- If the patient is receiving a continuous heparin infusion, inform the patient that a blood sample will be drawn daily for monitoring response to the medication.
- No fasting is required before the test.
- If the patient is receiving heparin intermittently, draw the PTT 30 to 60 minutes before the next dose. If receiving heparin by continuous infusion, the PTT can be drawn at any time.
- Do *not* draw the sample from the arm in which heparin is infusing.
- If the blood sample is to be drawn from an arterial line with a heparin-flush pressure bag, withdraw at least 10 mL of blood before drawing the sample for the PTT.

Procedure

- A 7-mL blood sample is drawn in a collection tube containing sodium citrate and citric acid.
- Gloves are worn throughout the procedure.

Post-Test Nursing Care

Possible complications:

- **Hematoma at site owing to prolonged bleeding time**
- **Spontaneous bleeding with PTT > 100 seconds**

  - Assess patient for spontaneous bleeding: epistaxis, bleeding gums, low back pain from possible retroperitoneal bleeding, joint pain, bruising, petechiae, hematuria, or melena.
  - Apply pressure 3–5 minutes at venipuncture site. Apply dressing, periodically assessing for continued bleeding.

P

- Teach the patient to monitor the site. If the site begins to bleed, the patient should apply direct pressure and, if unable to control the bleeding, return to the laboratory or notify the nurse.
- Report abnormal findings to the primary care provider.

• • • • • • • • • • • • • • • • •

Pelvic Ultrasonography
(Gynecologic Sonogram, Obstetric Sonogram, Pelvic Echogram)

Ultrasonography is a noninvasive method of diagnostic testing in which ultrasound waves are sent into the body with a small transducer pressed against the skin. The transducer not only sends the sound waves into the body but also receives any returning sound waves, which are deflected back as they bounce off various structures. The transducer converts the returning sound waves into electric signals that are then transformed by a computer into a visual display on a monitor.

In this particular form of ultrasonography, the female reproductive tract is evaluated, along with an assessment of, if present, the fetus and fetal sac. Pelvic ultrasonography is used for evaluation of suspected pelvic disease and monitoring of fetal growth. It is helpful in the diagnosis of fetal death, placenta previa, and abruptio placentae. It also provides guidance for amniocentesis, fetoscopy, or intrauterine procedures.

Normal Values
Normal fetal and placental size and position.
No pelvic organ abnormalities.

Possible Meanings of Abnormal Values
Abnormal fetal structure
Abruptio placentae
Abscesses
Ectopic pregnancy
Fetal death
Fetal malpresentation (breech, transverse)
Fibroids
Foreign body (e.g., intrauterine device)
Hydatidiform mole
Inappropriate fetal size
Multiple pregnancy
Pelvic tumor
Placenta previa

Contributing Factors to Abnormal Values
- The transducer must be in good contact with the skin as it is being moved. A lubricant, such as mineral oil, glycerin, or a water-based jelly, is used to ensure good contact with the skin.
- Retained barium from previous exams or bowel gas may alter test results.

Pre-Test Nursing Care

- Explain to the patient the purpose of the test. Provide any written teaching materials available on the subject. Note that there is no discomfort involved with this test.
- No fasting is required before the test.
- A full bladder is needed during the examination. Instruct the patient to drink 1 liter of water 1 hour before the procedure and remind her not to void until the test is completed.

Procedure

- The patient is assisted to a supine position on the ultrasonography table.
- A coupling agent, such as a water-based gel, is applied to the abdominal and pelvic area.
- A transducer is placed on the skin and moved as needed to provide good visualization of the pelvic structures and the fetus.
- The sound waves are transformed into a visual display on the monitor. Printed copies of this display are made.

Post-Test Nursing Care

- Cleanse the patient's skin of remaining coupling agent.
- Allow the patient to void immediately after the test is completed.
- Report abnormal findings to the primary care provider.

• • • • • • • • • • • • • • • • •

Percutaneous Transhepatic Cholangiography

Percutaneous transhepatic cholangiography is the fluoroscopic examination of the biliary ducts using an iodine-based contrast dye that is injected directly into a biliary radicle. This test is performed in jaundiced patients since, in these patients, the cells of the liver are unable to transport the dye if administered orally or by intravenous infusion. With this procedure, the cystic, hepatic, and common bile ducts can be visualized and their diameter and filling evaluated. This allows differential diagnosis of obstructive jaundice and nonobstructive jaundice. If the ducts are found to be of normal size and intrahepatic cholestasis is indicated, further testing, such as a biopsy of the liver, is needed to distinguish among other problems such as cirrhosis or hepatitis.

Because this is an invasive procedure, there is the chance of complications such as bleeding and peritonitis occurring. However, for patients who are jaundiced, this procedure and endoscopic retrograde cholangiopancreatography (ERCP) are the only methods available for visualization of the biliary tree. Thus, benefits and risks to the patient must be weighed. Currently, ERCP is more commonly performed owing to its lower complication rate.

P

Normal Values

Normal diameter and filling of the cystic, hepatic, and common bile ducts.

Possible Meanings of Abnormal Values

Biliary sclerosis
Biliary tract carcinoma

Carcinoma of the papilla of Vater
Carcinoma of the pancreas
Cholelithiasis
Sclerosing cholangitis
Strictures of the ducts

Contributing Factors to Abnormal Values

- Under- or overexposure of the film may alter film quality.
- When patients are unable to hold still, because of pain or mental status, the quality of the film may be affected.
- Retained barium from other examinations will affect test results.

 ## CONTRAINDICATIONS

- Pregnant women (*Caution:* A woman in her childbearing years should undergo radiography only during her menses or 12–14 days after its onset to avoid any exposure to a fetus.).
- Patients with hypersensitivity to iodine, seafood, or contrast media.
- Patients with cholangitis, since injection of the dye will increase biliary pressure and cause bacteremia.
- Patients with massive ascites.
- Patients with uncontrolled coagulopathy (platelet count < 50,000/mm^3, prolonged bleeding time).
- Patients who are unable to cooperate because of age, mental status, pain, or other factors.

Pre-Test Nursing Care

- *Note:* If a barium swallow or an upper gastrointestinal and small-bowel series test is ordered, these should be completed *after* the cholangiography is performed. Otherwise the barium sulfate ingested during the other examinations may obscure the films made of the ducts.
- Explain to the patient the purpose of the test and the benefits and risks associated with the test. Provide any written teaching materials available on the subject. Explain that the patient will experience discomfort when the injection site is anesthetized and as the dye is injected.
- Obtain a signed informed consent from the patient.
- The patient is given a low-fat or fat-free diet for 1 day before the test.
- Inform the radiologist of any potential allergy to the contrast dye and obtain order for anti-histamine and corticosteroid to be given prior to the procedure.
- Patients receiving metformin (Glucophage) for non–insulin-dependent diabetes mellitus should discontinue the drug 2 days before elective surgery or angiographic examinations. This is because of the possible occurrence of lactic acidosis, a potentially fatal complication of biguanide therapy.
- Obtain baseline laboratory tests to assess for coagulopathy (clotting time, platelet count, and prothrombin time).
- The patient is to be NPO after midnight before the test.
- Additional aspects of the preparation *may* include:
  - type and crossmatch of blood in case of bleeding during the procedure.
  - administration of intravenous antibiotics 24 to 48 hours before the procedure.
  - administration of a sedative prior to the procedure.
- Instruct the patient to remove all objects containing metal, such as jewelry or undergarments, as these will show on the film.

P

Procedure

- The patient is secured in a supine position on the examination table.
- The skin of the right upper quadrant is cleansed, draped, and anesthetized with Xylocaine.
- The patient is instructed to inhale and exhale several times and then to hold the breath after a full expiration. A long, flexible needle is inserted into the liver and advanced under fluoroscopy until bile is aspirated from the duct. Placement of the needle is checked by injecting a small amount of the dye. If visualization by fluoroscopy verifies correct placement, the remaining dye is injected. As the flow of the dye is observed, films are periodically taken.
- When the films are found to be satisfactory for diagnostic purposes, the needle is removed, and a sterile dressing is applied.

Post-Test Nursing Care

Possible complications:

- **Adverse reaction or allergy to dye**
- **Peritonitis caused by bile extravasation from the liver after needle removal**
- **Hemorrhage**
- **Tension pneumothorax**

- Most allergic reactions to radiopaque dye occur within 30 minutes of administration of the contrast medium. Observe the patient closely for: respiratory distress, hypotension, edema, hives, rash, tachycardia, or laryngeal stridor. Emergency resuscitation equipment must be readily accessible.
- Assess the patient's vital signs until stable. Observe for signs of respiratory distress, hemorrhage, and peritonitis (chills, fever, abdominal pain, distention, and tenderness).
- Check the puncture site for bleeding, swelling, and tenderness often.
- Assist the patient to a right side-lying position, which is to be maintained for 6 hours.
- Resume the patient's diet and medications as taken before the test. Encourage fluid intake.
- Provide emotional support as the patient awaits the test results.
- Renal function should be assessed before metformin is restarted.
- Report abnormal findings to the primary care provider.

• • • • • • • • • • • • • • • • • •

Pericardiocentesis
(Pericardial Fluid Analysis)

Pericardiocentesis refers to the removal of fluid from the pericardial cavity. This cavity is the space between the visceral pericardium, which is the serous inner layer of the pericardium, and the parietal pericardium, which is the outer fibrous layer of the pericardium. In some conditions, such as inflammatory diseases of the heart, myocardial rupture, and penetrating trauma to the heart, a large amount of fluid may accumulate in the pericardial cavity, an assessment finding known as *pericardial effusion.*

Pericardiocentesis may be done for a diagnostic purpose to determine the cause of the fluid production, or for emergency therapeutic purposes. In the case of penetrating trauma, the rapidly forming effusion causes increased intrapericardial pressure, which reduces cardiac output, a situation known as *cardiac tamponade.* In this type of emergency, the pericardiocentesis must be done immediately, without waiting for signed informed consent.

Normal Values

Gross appearance:	Clear, straw-colored
Amount:	10–50 mL
Bacteria:	None
Cell counts:	No red blood cells
	No white blood cells
Cytology:	No abnormal cells present
Glucose:	Equal to serum level

Possible Meanings of Abnormal Values

Acute myocardial infarction
Bacterial pericarditis
Cardiac trauma
Congestive heart failure
Fungal pericarditis
Myocardial rupture
Neoplasm
Rheumatoid disease
Rupture of ventricular aneurysm
Systemic lupus erythematosus
Traumatic tap
Tuberculous pericarditis

Contributing Factors to Abnormal Values

- Antimicrobial therapy, if started prior to the test, may decrease the bacterial count.
- Contamination of the specimen through break in sterile technique will alter white blood cell count.

CONTRAINDICATIONS

- Patients with bleeding disorders.
- Patients who are unable to cooperate during the procedure.

Pre-Test Nursing Care

- Explain to the patient the purpose of the test and the procedure to be done. Explain that a local anesthetic will be used, but that a pressure-like pain will occur as the needle pierces the pericardial sac. Explain that no movement, including deep breathing or coughing, can occur during the test.
- No fasting is required before the test.
- Obtain a signed informed consent. (*Note:* If emergency situation, inform the patient's family of the immediate need for the procedure.)
- Pre-procedure echocardiography should be performed before the test to locate the fluid and to avoid accidental puncture of the heart.
- Obtain baseline vital signs.

- Resuscitation and suctioning equipment must be readily available.
- Pulse oximetry may be ordered for use throughout the procedure.

Procedure

- Assist the patient to the supine position with the head of the bed elevated 60 degrees.
- Initiate a maintenance intravenous line, and administer premedication as ordered.
- Monitor vital signs every 15 minutes during the procedure.
- Sterile technique is used throughout the procedure.
- The skin from the left costal margin to the xiphoid process is cleansed and draped.
- A local anesthetic is administered.
- A 16- to 18-gauge cardiac needle attached to a 50-mL syringe and a three-way stopcock is inserted through the chest wall between the left costal margin and the xiphoid process (in the subxyphoid space) into the pericardial sac. An ECG lead is attached to the needle with a clip. The ECG must be monitored throughout the procedure for the following changes:
  - *Elevation of the PR segment* indicates the needle is touching the atrial surface.
  - An *ST-segment elevation* indicates the needle is touching the epicardial surface and needs to be pulled back slightly.
  - An *abnormally shaped QRS complex* may indicate myocardial perforation.
  - *Premature ventricular contractions* usually indicate the needle is touching the ventricular wall.
- When the pocket of fluid is reached, a Kelly clamp is applied to the needle at the skin surface to prevent it from entering further. A 50-mL sample of the fluid is then obtained.
- When the procedure is complete, the needle is removed. Pressure is immediately applied and maintained for 3–5 minutes. A dressing is then applied.

Post-Test Nursing Care

Possible complications:

- **Cardiac tamponade syndrome from laceration of coronary artery or rapid reaccumulation of fluid**
- **Myocardial laceration**
- **Pleural effusion**
- **Puncture of lung, liver, or stomach**
- **Vasovagal arrest**
- **Ventricular fibrillation**

- Monitor vital signs every 15 minutes for 1 hour, every 30 minutes for 2 hours, every hour for 4 hours, and then every 4 hours.
- Check the dressing frequently for drainage.
- Continue to observe the patient for any respiratory or cardiac distress: muffled and distant heart sounds, distended neck veins, paradoxical pulse, and shock.
- Label the specimen and transport it to the laboratory immediately.
- Report abnormal findings to the primary care provider.

• • • • • • • • • • • • • • • • •

P

Phenylketonuria Test
(PKU Test, Guthrie Test, Phenylalanine)

Phenylalanine hydroxylase is an enzyme that converts phenylalanine to tyrosine. A deficiency of this enzyme leads to a buildup of phenylalanine that results in severe mental retardation. This condition, known as *phenylketonuria (PKU)*, is an autosomal recessive inborn error of metabolism. Screening of all newborns for PKU is required in all states. Testing is done either on the serum (Guthrie test) or on the urine. Testing is not valid until the newborn has ingested an ample amount of the amino acid phenylalanine, which is found in human and cow's milk. Two or three days of intake is usually sufficient for the Guthrie test. Urine PKU testing is usually done after the infant is 4 to 6 weeks old.

Normal Values

Blood:	Negative
Urine:	No green discoloration

Possible Meanings of Abnormal Values

Increased

Delayed enzyme system development
Galactosemia
Hepatic disease
Phenylketonuria

Contributing Factors to Abnormal Values
- Testing for PKU too early may lead to *false-negative* results.
- Drugs that may alter test results: antibiotics, aspirin, salicylates.

Pre-Test Nursing Care
- Explain the purpose of the test to the mother and the need for a blood sample to be drawn.
- No fasting is required before the test.

Procedure

Guthrie (Serum) Test
After the newborn has been taking in ample amounts of milk for 2 to 3 days, the test may be performed.
- Cleanse the newborn's heel with alcohol and allow to air dry.
- Puncture the heel with a lancet, allowing several drops of blood to collect on the filter paper for the Guthrie test.

Urine Test
Urine testing for PKU may be performed after 4 to 6 weeks of age.
- This is accomplished by either dropping 10% ferric chloride solution on a diaper containing fresh urine, or by pressing a Phenistix test stick against the urine on the diaper.

P

- With either method, a green discoloration is indicative of PKU.
- Gloves are worn throughout the preceding procedures.

Post-Test Nursing Care
- Apply pressure on the newborn's heel for 5–10 minutes and then leave the site open to the air for healing.
- Report abnormal findings to the primary care provider.

• • • • • • • • • • • • • • • • • •

Phonocardiography
(PCG)

As blood flows through the heart and the great vessels, low-frequency sound waves are produced. The phonocardiograph (PCG) graphically picks up these sounds through a microphone placed on the patient's chest. The PCG documents the occurrence, timing, and length of sounds of the heart cycle. The test is very useful in locating and timing abnormal heart sounds that have been detected on auscultation, including those owing to valvular dysfunction. The PCG is recorded simultaneously with carotid pulse, electrocardiogram (ECG), and respiration.

Normal Values
Normal heart sounds.

Possible Meanings of Abnormal Values
Bundle branch block
Coronary artery disease
Hypertension
Hypertrophic cardiomyopathy
Left ventricular failure
Mitral valve prolapse
Myocarditis
Pericardial effusion
Pulmonary embolism
Right ventricular overload
Valve regurgitation
Valvular stenosis

Contributing Factors to Abnormal Values
- Incorrect microphone placement, background noise, patient movement, and patient obesity affect the accuracy of the test results.

Pre-Test Nursing Care
- Explain to the patient the purpose of the test. Note that the test will cause no discomfort.
- No fasting is required before the test.

P

Procedure

- The patient is assisted into a supine position.
- ECG leads are placed on all four extremities.
- Monitors for the pulse (using a cuff around the neck) and respiration recordings are prepared.
- Recordings of the heart sounds are made under the following conditions:
  - The microphones are placed over the apex and pulmonary area. The patient is requested to inhale and then exhale. The recording is made while the expiration is held.
  - The microphone is moved from the pulmonary area to the aortic area. The patient is requested to inhale and then exhale. The recording is made while the expiration is held.
  - The cuff is removed from the neck and the microphone is placed at the fourth intercostal space at the border of the left sternum. The patient is requested to inhale and then exhale. The recording is made while the expiration is held.
  - The heart sounds may also be recorded with the patient in different positions, while varying the respiratory patterns, or while performing exercises.

Post-Test Nursing Care

- The electrodes are moved and the skin is cleansed of any electrode paste.
- Report abnormal findings to the primary care provider.

• • • • • • • • • • • • • • • •

Phosphorus
(P, Phosphate, PO₄)

Phosphorus is the main anion in the intracellular fluid. It has several functions, including a role in glucose and lipid metabolism, storage and transfer of energy within the body, generation of bony tissue, and maintenance of acid-base balance. Like calcium, phosphorus is controlled by the parathyroid hormone (PTH). It holds an inverse relationship with calcium; an excess in the serum of one results in the kidneys excreting the other. An elevated serum phosphorus level is known as *hyperphosphatemia;* decreased level, *hypophosphatemia.*

Normal Values

2.6–4.5 mg/dL (0.84–1.45 mmol/L, SI units)

Elderly: Decreased

Possible Meanings of Abnormal Values

Increased (Hyperphosphatemia)	Decreased (Hypophosphatemia)
Acromegaly	Antacid abuse
Addison's disease	Carbohydrate loading
Bone tumors	Chronic alcoholism
Excessive intake of alkali	Diabetic acidosis/coma

Increased (Hyperphosphatemia)	Decreased (Hypophosphatemia)
Healing fracture	Diuresis
Hypocalcemia	Hypercalcemia
Hypoparathyroidism	Hyperinsulinism
Massive blood transfusions	Hyperparathyroidism
Nephritis	Malabsorption
Prepuberty	Malnutrition
Renal failure	Osteomalacia
Sarcoidosis	Rickets
Uremia	Salicylate intoxication
Vitamin D intoxication	Vitamin D deficiency

Contributing Factors to Abnormal Values

- Use of a tourniquet during acquisition of the blood sample may alter test results.
- Hemolysis of the blood sample may alter test results.
- Owing to increased carbohydrate metabolism causing decreased phosphorus levels, glucose solutions should not be infused before the test.
- Drugs that may *increase* serum phosphorus levels: heparin, methicillin sodium, phenytoin, phosphate enemas, or infusions.
- Drugs that may *decrease* serum phosphorus levels: anabolic steroids, androgens, antacids, diuretics, epinephrine, glucagon, glucose, insulin, mannitol, salicylates.

Pre-Test Nursing Care

- Explain to the patient the purpose of the test and the need for a blood sample to be drawn.
- No fasting is required before the test.

Procedure

- A 7-mL blood sample is drawn in a collection tube containing a silicone gel, avoiding use of a tourniquet, if possible.
- Gloves are worn throughout the procedure.

Post-Test Nursing Care

- Apply pressure at venipuncture site. Apply dressing, periodically assessing for continued bleeding.
- Label the specimen and transport it to the laboratory.
- Report abnormal findings to the primary care provider.

• • • • • • • • • • • • • • • •

P

Plasminogen

When injury to a blood vessel or tissue occurs, the process of hemostasis is initiated and results in the formation of a fibrin clot. Plasminogen is a beta-globulin protein normally found in fibrin clots in an inactive form. Once healing has occurred and the fibrin clots are no longer needed, enzymes within the endothelial cells trigger the conversion of plasminogen to plasmin. The production of plasmin, which is a fibrinolytic enzyme, results in lysis of the fibrin clot.

Plasmin cannot be directly measured since it is not present in the circulation in its active form. Thus, measurement of its inactive form, plasminogen, is used to evaluate this fibrinolytic system. The test is performed by adding a plasminogen activator, streptokinase, to the patient's blood sample. This causes plasminogen to convert to active plasmin, which in turn causes a chemical substance in the solution to change color. This colored substance, which can be measured, is proportional to the functional plasminogen level.

Normal Values

3.8–8.4 CTA (Council on Thrombolytic Agents) U/mL

Possible Meanings of Abnormal Values

Increased	Decreased
Anxiety	Cirrhosis
Deep vein thrombosis	Coagulation
Infection	Disseminated intravascular
Inflammation	Eclampsia
Malignancy	Hyaline membrane disease
Myocardial infarction	Liver disease
Pregnancy	Nephrosis
Stress	Pre-eclampsia
Surgery	Tumors

Contributing Factors to Abnormal Values

- Hemolysis of the blood sample may alter test results.
- Falsely decreased values may occur if the tourniquet remains in place a prolonged time before the venipuncture.
- Drugs that may *increase* plasminogen levels: oral contraceptives.
- Drugs that may *decrease* plasminogen levels: L-asparaginase, streptokinase, urokinase.

Pre-Test Nursing Care

- Explain to the patient the purpose of the test and the need for a blood sample to be drawn.
- No fasting is required before the test.

P

Procedure

- A 7-mL blood sample is drawn in a collection tube contain sodium citrate and citric acid.
- Gloves are worn throughout the procedure.

Post-Test Nursing Care

Possible complication: Hematoma at site owing to prolonged bleeding time.

- Apply pressure 3–5 minutes at venipuncture site. Apply dressing, periodically assessing for continued bleeding.
- Teach the patient to monitor the site. If the site begins to bleed, the patient should apply direct pressure and, if unable to control the bleeding, return to the laboratory or notify the nurse.
- Label the specimen and transport it to the laboratory.
- Report abnormal findings to the primary care provider.

• • • • • • • • • • • • • • • •

Platelet Activity Tests

See:
Bleeding Time
Capillary Fragility Test
Platelet Aggregation Test
Platelet Count
Platelet, Mean Volume

• • • • • • • • • • • • • • •

Platelet Aggregation Test

The *platelet aggregation test* evaluates the ability of the platelets to adhere to each other. When there is an injury to the wall of a blood vessel, any bleeding through the vessel wall is brought under control through the formation of a platelet plug. Several substances and processes are required for this plug to form. There must be an adequate number of platelets in the circulation. There must also be platelet agonists, such as thrombin, which assist the platelets to aggregate or clump, and proteins such as fibrinogen that are able to bind to the surface of the platelets.

In this test, the patient's platelets are mixed with platelet agonists such as adenosine diphosphate (ADP), arachidonic acid, collagen, epinephrine, ristocetin, and thrombin. After clumping of the platelets has occurred, a measurement is made of the amount of light passing through the solution. The transmission of light through the plasma solution should be increased after platelet aggregation.

Normal Values

Depends on reagent used. Check with reference laboratory.

Possible Meanings of Abnormal Values

Increased	Decreased
Atheromatosis	Afibrinogenemia
Diabetes mellitus	Bernard-Soulier syndrome
Hypercoagulability	Beta-thalassemia major
Hyperlipemia	Cirrhosis
Polycythemia vera	Glanzmann's thrombasthenia
	Idiopathic thrombocytopenic purpura
	Macroglobulinemia
	Myeloid metaplasia
	Plasma cell dyscrasias
	Preleukemia
	Scurvy
	Systemic lupus erythematosus
	Thrombocythemia
	Uremia
	von Willebrand's disease
	Wiskott-Aldrich syndrome

Contributing Factors to Abnormal Values

- Hemolysis of the blood sample, lipemia, hyemoglobinemia, or bilirubinemia may alter the test results.
- Drugs that may *decrease* platelet aggregation: antibiotics, antihistamines, anti-inflammatory drugs, aspirin, carbenicillin, cephalothin, chlordiazepoxide, chloroquine hydrochloride, clofibrate, cocaine, corticosteroids, cyproheptadine hydrochloride, dextropropoxyphene, diazepam, diphenhydramine hydrochloride, dipyridamole, furosemide, gentamicin, guaifenesin, heparin, ibuprofen, imipramine hydrochloride, indomethacin, marijuana, mefenamic acid, naproxen, nitrofurantoin, nortriptyline hydrochloride, penicillin G, phenothiazines, phenylbutazone, promethazine hydrochloride, propranolol hydrochloride, pyrimidine compounds, sodium warfarin, sulfinpyrazone, theophylline, tricyclic antidepressants, vitamin E.

Pre-Test Nursing Care

- Explain to the patient the purpose of the test and the need for a blood sample to be drawn.
- No fasting is required before the test.

Procedure

- A 7-mL blood sample is drawn in a collection containing sodium citrate and citric acid.
- Gloves are worn throughout the procedure.

Post-Test Nursing Care

Possible complication: Hematoma at site owing to prolonged bleeding time.

- Apply pressure 3–5 minutes at venipuncture site. Apply dressing, periodically assessing for continued bleeding.
- Teach the patient to monitor the site. If the site begins to bleed, the patient should apply direct pressure and, if unable to control the bleeding, return to the lab or notify the nurse.
- Label the specimen and transport it to the laboratory.
- Report abnormal findings to the physician or nurse practitioner.

• • • • • • • • • • • • • • • •

Platelet Antibody Test
(Antiplatelet Antibody Detection, Platelet Antibody Detection Test)

Platelet autoantibodies are IgG immunoglobulins which develop in individuals when they become sensitized to platelet antigens of transfused blood. When platelet autoantibodies are present, both donor and recipient platelets are destroyed. These autoantibodies are present in all cases of idiopathic thrombocytopenic purpura (ITP). Drug-induced immunologic thrombocytopenia may be caused by such drugs as chlordiazepoxide, diphenylhydantoin, gold, heparin, quinidine, quinine sulfate, and sulfa drugs.

Normal Values
Negative

Possible Meanings of Abnormal Values

Increased

Drug-induced immunologic thrombocytopenia
Idiopathic thrombocytopenic purpura
Neonatal thrombocytopenia
Paroxysmal hemoglobinuria
Postransfusion purpura

Contributing Factors to Abnormal Values
- Hemolysis of the blood sample will alter test results.
- Blood transfusions may result in the development of isoantibodies.

Pre-Test Nursing Care
- Explain to the patient the purpose of the test and the need for a blood sample to be drawn.
- If possible, the blood sample should be drawn before any blood transfusion.
- No fasting is required before the test.

Procedure
- A 10- to 30-mL blood sample is drawn in two collection tubes containing sodium citrate and citric acid.
- Gloves are worn throughout the procedure.

Post-Test Nursing Care

Possible complication: Prolonged bleeding owing to thrombocytopenia.

- Apply pressure 3–5 minutes at venipuncture site. Apply dressing, periodically assessing for continued bleeding.
- Teach the patient to monitor the site. If the site begins to bleed, the patient should apply direct pressure and, if unable to control the bleeding, return to the laboratory or notify the nurse.
- Label the specimen and transport it to the laboratory.
- Report abnormal findings to the primary care provider.

• • • • • • • • • • • • • • • •

Platelet Count
(Thrombocyte Count)

Platelets, or thrombocytes, are fragments of megakaryocytes which are formed in the bone marrow. They circulate in the bloodstream for a lifespan of 8–12 days, at which time they are removed from the circulation by the spleen. Platelets are essential to hemostasis and blood clotting. When a blood vessel wall is injured, the platelets adhere to its wall and aggregrate, forming a platelet plug. They also release phospholipids that are required by the intrinsic coagulation pathway.

Patients with platelet counts between 50,000 and 150,000/mm^3 usually show few, if any, signs of bleeding. Spontaneous bleeding of a minor nature and prolonged bleeding following surgery or trauma are seen in patients with platelet counts ranging between 20,000 and 50,000/mm^3. The most serious risk lies with patients whose platelet counts are fewer than 20,000/mm^3. In these patients, spontaneous bleeding of a more serious nature occurs.

The platelet count may be done by machine or by microscopic examination. Obtaining the platelet count is helpful in the diagnosis of *thrombocytopenia* (decreased platelet count) and *thrombocytosis* (increased number of platelets), provides information about platelet production, and allows monitoring of the effect of antineoplastic drug therapy and radiation therapy on platelet production.

Normal Values

150,000–350,000/mm^3 (150–350 × 10^9/L, SI units)

Possible Meanings of Abnormal Values

Increased	Decreased
Acute infection	Acute leukemia
Asphyxiation	Acquired Immunodeficiency Syndrome (AIDS)
Chronic leukemia	Allergic conditions
Chronic pancreatitis	Aplastic anemia

Increased	Decreased
Cirrhosis	Autotransfusion
Collagen disease	Clostridial infection
Heart disease	Disseminated intravascular
Inflammation	coagulation
Iron-deficiency anemia	Exposure to DDT
Malignant tumors	Extracorporeal bypass
Multiple myeloma	Hemolytic anemia
Myeloproliferative disease	Hypersplenism
Polycythemia vera	Idiopathic thrombocytopenic
Posthemorrhagic anemia	purpura
Postpartum	Lymphoproliferative diseases
Post-splenectomy	Menstruation
Pregnancy	Multiple myeloma
Rheumatoid arthritis	Pernicious anemia
Sickle cell anemia	Radiation
Trauma	Splenomegaly
Tuberculosis	Systemic lupus erythematosus
	Viral infections

Contributing Factors to Abnormal Values

- Conditions in which platelet count is *increased:* high altitudes, persistent cold temperatures, strenuous exercise, excitement.
- Condition in which platelet count is *decreased:* prior to menstruation.
- Drugs that may *increase* the platelet count: epinephrine, oral contraceptives.
- Drugs that may *decrease* the platelet count: acetazolamide, acetohexamide, aminosalicylic acid, amphotericin B, ampicillin, antineoplastics, arsenicals, aspirin, aurothiglucose, barbiturates, brompheniramine maleate, carbamazepine, chloramphenicol, chlorpropamide, chloroquine hydrochloride, chlorothiazide, colchicine, diazoxide, digitoxin, furosemide, gold, hydroxychloroquine sulfate, indomethacin, isoniazid, mefenamic acid, meprobamate, methazolamide, methimazole, methyldopa, oral hypoglycemics, oxytetracycline, penicillamine, penicillins, phenylbutzone, phenytoin, pyrimethamine, quinidine, quinine sulfate, rifampin, salicylates, streptomycin, sulfonamides, thiazides, tobutamide, tricyclic antidepressants, vaccines.

Pre-Test Nursing Care

- Explain to the patient the purpose of the test and the need for a blood sample to be drawn.
- No fasting is required before the test.

Procedure

- A 5-mL blood sample is drawn in a collection tube containing EDTA.
- Gloves are worn throughout the procedure.

P

Post-Test Nursing Care

Possible complications:
- **Hematoma at site owing to prolonged bleeding time**
- **Spontaneous bleeding with platelet count <20,000/mm.[3]**

- Assess patient for spontaneous bleeding: epistaxis, bleeding gums, low back pain from possible retroperitoneal bleeding, joint pain, bruising, petechiae, hematuria, or melena.
- Apply pressure 3–5 minutes at venipuncture site. Apply dressing, periodically assessing for continued bleeding.
- Teach the patient to monitor the site. If the site begins to bleed, the patient should apply direct pressure and, if unable to control the bleeding, return to the laboratory or notify the nurse.
- Label the specimen and transport it to the laboratory.
- Report abnormal findings to the primary care provider.

• • • • • • • • • • • • • • •

Platelet, Mean Volume
(Mean Platelet Volume, [MPV])

Platelets, or thrombocytes, are fragments of megakaryocytes that are formed in the bone marrow. They are essential to hemostasis and blood clotting. When a blood vessel wall is injured, the platelets adhere to its wall and aggregrate, or clump, forming a platelet plug. It is advantageous to this process for the platelets to be large. When bone marrow function declines, the megakaryocytes are small, resulting in small platelets. If a condition other than bone marrow dysfunction is the cause of a low platelet count, the bone marrow tries to compensate by releasing larger platelets. Thus, measurement of the mean platelet volume assists in the diagnosis of thrombocytopenic disorders, those conditions in which there is a decreased platelet count.

Normal Values

25 micrometers in diameter (8–10 fL, SI units)

Possible Meanings of Abnormal Values

Increased	Decreased
Bernard-Soulier syndrome	Aplastic anemia
Diabetes mellitus	Hypersplenism
Disseminated intravascular coagulation	Megaloblastic anemia
	Wiskott-Aldrich syndrome
Hyperthyroidism	
Leukemia	
May-Hegglin anomaly	
Myeloproliferative disorders	

Increased	Decreased
Rheumatic heart disease	
Systemic lupus erythematosus	
Valvular heart disease	

Pre-Test Nursing Care

- Explain to the patient the purpose of the test and the need for a blood sample to be drawn.
- No fasting is required before the test.

Procedure

- A 7-mL blood sample is drawn in a collection tube containing EDTA.
- Gloves are worn throughout the procedure.

Post-Test Nursing Care

Possible complication: Hematoma at site owing to prolonged bleeding time.

- Apply pressure 3–5 minutes at venipuncture site. Apply dressing, periodically assessing for continued bleeding.
- Teach the patient to monitor the site. If the site begins to bleed, the patient should apply direct pressure and, if unable to control the bleeding, return to the laboratory or notify the nurse.
- Label the specimen and transport it to the laboratory.
- Report abnormal findings to the physician or nurse practitioner.

• • • • • • • • • • • • • • • • • •

Plethysmography, Arterial
(Pneumoplethysmography)

Arterial plethysmography is a manometric test that evaluates the arterial blood flow in the lower extremities. This test involves the placement of pressure cuffs at various levels on the legs. Arterial waveforms are then recorded. A normal waveform is characterized by a sharp rise to a peak, a dicrotic notch, and then a downslope to the baseline. In the case of arterial occlusive disease, the waveforms are abnormal, with a lower height, a rounding of the peaks, and a loss of the dicrotic notch.

Normal Values

Normal arterial waveforms.

Possible Meanings of Abnormal Values

Arterial embolism
Arterial insufficiency
Arterial trauma
Arteriosclerosis

Diabetic ischemia
Raynaud's disease

Contributing Factors to Abnormal Values

- Since nicotine constricts the blood vessels, smoking within 2 hours before the examination will affect the test results.
- The temperature of the testing area may alter the peripheral circulation, thus affecting the test results.
- Arterial occlusion proximal to the extremity can prevent blood flow to the limb and affect the test results.

 ## CONTRAINDICATIONS

- The test should not be performed on an extremity that is cold and pale or cyanotic, since blood flow is obviously compromised to the limb.

Pre-Test Nursing Care

- Explain to the patient the purpose of the test and the procedure to be done.
- Inform the patient that the procedure is painless, but that no movement of the extremities can occur during the test.
- No fasting is required before the test.
- All clothing must be removed from the extremities.
- Obtain signed informed consent if required by the institution.

Procedure

- The patient is assisted into a semi-Fowler's position.
- Pressure cuffs are applied to the upper thigh, above the knee, below the knee, and above the ankle of each leg.
- The first cuff is inflated to 75 mm Hg for 2 seconds and then lowered to 65 mm Hg. The waveforms are recorded.
- The procedure is repeated for each cuff on each leg.

Post-Test Nursing Care

- The cuffs are removed and the patient is allowed to dress.
- Ensure that each set of waveforms are labeled with the correct cuff site.
- Report abnormal findings to the primary care provider.

• • • • • • • • • • • • • • • •

P

Plethysmography, Venous
(Impedance Plethysmography)

V*enous plethysmography* is a manometric test that evaluates changes in venous capacity and out-flow of the lower extremities. The test involves the placement of pressure cuffs at the level of the thigh and the calf. Each cuff is inflated to temporarily stop venous flow. Each one is then de-flated to allow venous flow to resume. Venous waveforms are recorded throughout the procedure. Normal waveforms are characterized by a steady upslope after the cuff is inflated as the vein fills to capacity. After the cuff is deflated, there is a sharp downslope documenting rapid venous out-flow. When there is an obstruction in the vein, as in deep vein thrombosis, the downslope of the line after cuff deflation is less steep, indicating minimal venous blood flow owing to the obstruc-tion.

Normal Values

Normal venous waveforms.

Possible Meanings of Abnormal Values

Deep vein thrombosis
Partial venous obstruction
Superficial thrombophlebitis
Total venous obstruction

Contributing Factors to Abnormal Values

- Since nicotine constricts the blood vessels, smoking within 2 hours before the exam will af-fect the test results.
- The temperature of the testing area may alter the peripheral circulation, thus affecting the test results.

Pre-Test Nursing Care

- Explain to the patient the purpose of the test and the procedure to be done.
- Inform the patient that the procedure is painless, but that no movement of the extremities can occur during the test.
- No fasting is required before the test.
- All clothing must be removed from the extremities.
- Obtain signed informed consent if required by the institution.

Procedure

- The patient is assisted into a supine position.
- Pressure cuffs are applied to the thigh and the calf of the affected leg.
- The calf cuff is inflated to 15 mm Hg and the thigh cuff is inflated to 55 mm Hg. The mini-mal pressure at the calf level allows monitoring of venous inflow. The thigh pressure ob-structs the venous outflow and causes engorgement of the veins.
- The waveform is recorded as the veins fill to capacity.

P

- Once the waveform indicates full venous capacity has been reached, the pressure cuff on the thigh is deflated.
- The procedure is repeated for 3–5 waveforms.
- The procedure is repeated on the unaffected leg, which is used for comparison.

Post-Test Nursing Care

- The cuffs are removed and the patient is allowed to dress.
- Ensure that each set of waveforms are labeled with the correct cuff site.
- Report abnormal findings to the primary care provider.

Pleural Biopsy

Pleural biopsy is generally performed after the pleural fluid removed during a thoracentesis suggests infection, neoplasia, or tuberculosis. Determination of the nature of the problem can only be made by obtaining a biopsy of the tissue. In a pleural biopsy, a sample of pleural tissue is removed for histologic study. The tissue sample may be obtained by needle biopsy through the chest wall, as part of a thoracentesis, or by open biopsy during a thoracotomy. This discussion will be limited to that of needle biopsy of the pleura.

Normal Values

No abnormal cells or tissue present.

Possible Meanings of Abnormal Values

Collagen vascular disease
Fungal disease
Malignancy
Parasitic disease
Tuberculosis
Viral disease

CONTRAINDICATIONS

- Patients with bleeding disorders.
- Patients unable to cooperate with the examination.

P

Pre-Test Nursing Care

- Explain to the patient the purpose of the test and the procedure to be done. Explain to the patient that a local anesthetic will be used.
- Obtain baseline chest x-ray and coagulation tests (partial thromboplastin time, platelet count, prothrombin time).
- No fasting is required before the test.
- Obtain a signed informed consent.
- Obtain baseline vital signs.

Procedure

- The patient is assisted to a sitting position with the arms supported on a pillow on an overbed table.
- The skin is cleansed with an antiseptic and draped.
- A local anesthetic is administered.
- The needle is inserted through the posterior chest wall at the selected intercostal space, and into the biopsy site. A Vim-Silverman needle or Cope's needle is usually used for obtaining the biopsy.
- The specimen is obtained and the needle removed.
- The tissue is placed in a container with a formaldehyde solution.
- Pressure is exerted on the biopsy site, followed by application of a sterile dressing.
- Gloves are worn throughout the procedure.

Post-Test Nursing Care

Possible complications:

- **Bleeding**
- **Hemothorax**
- **Infection**
- **Pneumothorax**

- Assist the patient into a semi-Fowler's position.
- Monitor the patient's vital signs, breath sounds, and comfort level, and check the dressing for drainage every 15–30 minutes until stable.
- Observe for indications of hemothorax or pneumothorax: rapid, shallow respirations, dyspnea, air hunger, chest pain, cough, hemoptysis, and absence of breath sounds over area.
- Observe for signs of infection: elevated temperature, chest pain, yellow sputum, and abnormal breath sounds.
- Administer analgesics as needed.
- Provide emotional support as the patient awaits test results.
- Report abnormal findings to the primary care provider.

• • • • • • • • • • • • • • • • •

Porphyrins
(Coproporphyrin, Porphobilinogen [PBG], Uroporphyrin, Urinary Porphyrins)

P

Several substances known as "porphyrins", including coproporphyrin, porphobilinogen [PBG], and uroporphyrin, are involved in the synthesis of heme of hemoglobin (see Aminolevulinic Acid for diagram of synthesis pathway). Aminolevulinic acid (ALA) is the precursor for the formation of porphobilinogen. With a disturbance of the heme synthesis pathway, as in the case of porphyria, large amounts of porphyrins are excreted. Since porphyrins are considered urine pigments, their presence causes the urine to be amber to burgundy in color.

Normal Values

Qualitative random sample

Coproporphyrins:	3–20 µg/dL
Porphobilinogen:	Negative
Uroporphyrins:	Negative

Quantitative 24-hour test

Coproporphyrins:	50–160 µg/24 hours or 0.075-0.24 µmol/24 hours (SI units)
Porphobilinogen:	0.1.5 mg/24 hours or 0–4.4 µmol/24 hours (SI units)
Uroporphyrins:	up to 50 µg/24 hours or up to 0.06 µmol/ 24 hours (SI units)

Possible Meanings of Abnormal Values

Increased

Cirrhosis of the liver
Infectious mononucleosis
Lead poisoning
Porphyrias
Viral hepatitis

Contributing Factors to Abnormal Values

- Pregnancy and menstruation may alter test results.
- Drugs that *increase* the porphyrin levels are: antibiotics (penicillin, tetracyclines), antiseptics (phenazopyridine hydrochloride), barbiturates, hypnotics, phenothiazines, procaine, sulfonamides.

Pre-Test Nursing Care

- Explain 24-hour urine collection procedure to the patient.
- Stress the importance of saving *all* urine in the 24-hour period. Instruct the patient to avoid contaminating the urine with toilet paper or feces.
- Inform the patient of the presence of a preservative in the collection bottle.

Procedure

For Qualitative (Screening) Tests

- Collect a random sample of at least 30 cc of urine during or immediately after an acute attack of porphyria, which is characterized by acute abdominal pain and neurologic changes.

For Quantitative (24-hour) Tests

- Obtain the proper container containing the appropriate preservative from the laboratory.
- Begin the testing period in the morning following the patient's first voiding, which is discarded.
- Timing of the 24-hour period begins at the time the first voiding is discarded.
- *All* urine for the next 24 hours is collected in the container, which is to be kept refrigerated or on ice, and protected from light. This is accomplished with either a dark container or a container covered with aluminum foil.

P

- If any urine is accidentally discarded during the 24-hour period, the test must be discontinued and a new test begun.
- The ending time of the 24-hour collection period should be posted in the patient's room.
- Gloves are worn when dealing with specimen collection.

Post-Test Nursing Care

- Label the container and send it on ice to the laboratory as soon as possible following the end of the 24-hour collection period.
- Report abnormal findings to the primary care provider.

• • • • • • • • • • • • • • • • •

Positron Emission Tomography
(PET, Single Photon Emission Computed Tomography, SPECT)

Positron emission tomography (PET) is a noninvasive radiographic method for studying blood flow and metabolic changes occurring in specific organs or regions of body tissues. PET scanning is especially useful in the measurement of brain activity, myocardial functioning, and the evaluation of malignant tumors.

For PET studies, the patient receives an injection of a biochemical substance tagged with a radionuclide. As the radionuclide disintegrates, positively charged particles, called *positrons* are emitted. As the positrons are combined with the negatively charged electrons normally found in the tissue cells, they emit gamma rays that can be detected with a scanning device. The PET scanner then translates the emissions into color-coded images.

PET has several advantages. Although computed tomography (CT) and magnetic resonance imaging (MRI) are used to diagnose internal problems, their focus is on the structural problems. PET and *SPECT (single photon emission computed tomography)*, however, measure functional problems. There is minimal radiation dosage received by the patient from the radionuclide, and the radiation of the PET scan itself is less than 25% of that required for a CT scan. A disadvantage of PET is that it is more costly than MRI testing and the number of institutions with PET scanning capabilities is limited at this time.

Normal Values

Normal patterns of tissue metabolism.

Possible Meanings of Abnormal Values

Alzheimer's disease
Brain tumor
Cerebrovascular accident
Coronary artery disease
Dementia
Epilepsy
Huntington's chorea
Migraine headache

P

Myocardial infarction
Parkinson's disease
Pneumonia
Pulmonary edema
Schizophrenia

Contributing Factors to Abnormal Values

- Movement may blur the PET images.
- Drugs that may influence test results: sedatives, tranquilizers.

 ## CONTRAINDICATIONS

- Pregnant women (*Caution:* A woman in her childbearing years should undergo radiography only during her menses or 12–14 days after its onset to avoid any exposure to a fetus.).
- Patients who are lactating.
- Patients who are unable to cooperate because of age, mental status, pain, or other factors.

Pre-Test Nursing Care

- Explain to the patient the purpose of the test and the procedure to be followed. Explain to the patient that movement is not allowed during the test. To assist with relaxation and to block any noises that occur during the testing, encourage the patient to listen to an audiotape during the procedure.
- No fasting is required before the test.
- Obtain a signed informed consent.
- Pre-procedure sedation may be ordered.
- Intake of caffeine or fluid should be discouraged for 2 hours before the test.

Procedure

- The patient is assisted to a supine position on the scanning table.
- An intravenous (IV) line is initiated.
- The patient is moved within the PET scanner.
- The radionuclide is administered either by the IV or by inhalation.

Post-Test Nursing Care

- Assist the patient to slowly rise from the lying position to avoid postural hypotension.
- Discontinue the IV site and check the site for bleeding.
- If a woman who is lactating *must* have this procedure, she should not breast feed the infant until the radionuclide has been eliminated, possibly for 3 days.
- Although the amount of diagnostic radionuclide excreted in the urine is low, the urine should not be used for any laboratory tests for the time period indicated by the nuclear medicine department. Clients should be told to flush the toilet three times after voiding.
- Gloves are worn whenever dealing with the urine.
- Encourage fluid intake to enhance elimination of the radionuclide from the body.
- Report abnormal findings to the primary care provider.

• • • • • • • • • • • • • • • •

Potassium, Blood

Potassium (K^+) is the major cation in the intracellular fluid. It is also present in small amounts in the extracellular fluid. There is an inverse relationship between potassium and sodium. Potassium is responsible for maintenance of acid-base balance, regulation of cellular osmotic pressure, and electrical conduction in muscle cells, especially cardiac and skeletal muscles.

Patients with elevated serum potassium levels (*hyperkalemia*) have weakness, malaise, nausea, diarrhea, muscle irritability, oliguria, and bradycardia. *Hypokalemic* patients, those patients whose serum potassium level is below normal, experience mental confusion, anorexia, muscle weakness, paresthesia, hypotension, rapid weak pulse, and decreased reflexes.

It is important to note that hypokalemia enhances the effect of digitalis preparations, making the patient prone to digitalis toxicity. Many patients receive both digitalis and a diuretic that causes loss of potassium. The resultant hypokalemia can lead to potentially fatal cardiac arrhythmias. Patients with hyperkalemia *or* hypokalemia may experience cardiac arrhythmias.

Serum potassium levels are most often used in evaluating patients with cardiac dysrhythmias, renal dysfunction, mental confusion, and GI distress. Should intravenous replacement therapy of potassium be deemed necessary, the solution should be administered via an electronic infusion device.

Normal Values

3.5–5.0 mEq/L (3.5–5.0 mmol/L, SI units)

Possible Meanings of Abnormal Values

Increased (Hyperkalemia)	Decreased (Hypokalemia)
Acute renal failure	Chronic fever
Addison's disease	Chronic stress
Adrenal cortical insufficiency	Cushing's syndrome
Diabetic acidosis	Cystic fibrosis
Excessive potassium intake	Diarrhea
Nephritis	Extensive burns
Sickle cell anemia	Liver disease
Systemic lupus erythematosus	Malabsorption
	Neoplasms
	Primary aldosteronism
	Pyloric obstruction
	Renal tubular acidosis
	Salicylate intoxication
	Saline intravenous infusions
	Starvation
	Vomiting

P

Contributing Factors to Abnormal Values

- Use of a tourniquet during acquisition of the blood sample may alter test results. Use of a tourniquet and pumping of the patient's hand can increase the value by up to 20%.
- Hemolysis of the blood sample may alter test results.
- Drugs that may *increase* serum potassium levels: aminocaproic acid, antibiotics, antineoplastics, captopril, cyclophosphamide, digoxin, ephedrine, epinephrine, estrogens, heparin, histamine, ibuprofen, indomethacin, isoniazid, lithium, mannitol, methicillin sodium, nonsteroidal anti-inflammatory drugs, potassium bicarbonate, potassium chloride, potassium citrate, potassium gluconate, propranolol hydrochloride, spironolactone, tetracyclines, timolol maleate, triamterene.
- Drugs that may *decrease* serum potassium levels: acetazolamide, albuterol, aminosalicylic acid, ammonium chloride, amphotericin, aspirin, bisacodyl, bronchodilators, carbenicillin, chlorthalidone, cisplatin, corticosteroids, corticotropin, EDTA, estrogens, ethacrynic acid, furosemide, gentamicin, glucose, insulin, laxatives, licorice, mercurial diuretics, penicillin G, phenothiazines, piperacillin, salicylates, sodium bicarbonate, sodium chloride, thiazides, thiopental, ticarcillin, trimethaphan camsylate.

Pre-Test Nursing Care

- Explain to the patient the purpose of the test and the need for a blood sample to be drawn.
- No fasting is required before the test.

Procedure

- A 7-mL blood sample is drawn in a collection tube containing a silicone gel, avoiding the use of a tourniquet, if possible.
- Gloves are worn throughout the procedure.

Post-Test Nursing Care

- Apply pressure at venipuncture site. Apply dressing, periodically assessing for continued bleeding.
- Label the specimen and transport it to the laboratory.
- Report abnormal findings to the primary care provider.
- Patients with low potassium levels should be informed of dietary sources of potassium: apricots, bananas, meats, potatoes, prunes, and tomatoes.

• • • • • • • • • • • • • • • • •

Potassium, Urine

Potassium is the major cation in the intracellular fluid. It is also present in small amounts in the extracellular fluid. There is an inverse relationship between potassium and sodium. Potassium is responsible for maintenance of acid-base balance, regulation of cellular osmotic pressure, and electrical conduction in muscle cells, especially cardiac and skeletal muscles. Measurement of the amount of potassium excreted in the urine in a 24-hour period provides data regarding the electrolyte balance of the body. This knowledge aids in the diagnosis of adrenal and renal disorders.

Normal Values

25–123 mEq/24 hours (25–134 mmol/day, SI units)

Possible Meanings of Abnormal Values

Increased	Decreased
Alkalosis	Acute renal failure
Chronic renal failure	Adrenal cortical insufficiency
Cushing's disease	Diarrhea
Dehydration	Excessive aldosterone activity
Diabetic ketoacidosis	Hyperkalemia
Excessive potassium intake	Malabsorption
Fever	Nephrotic syndrome
Hypokalemia	Syndrome of inappropriate ADH
Primary aldosteronism	secretion (SIADH)
Renal tubular acidosis	
Salicylate intoxication	
Starvation	

Contributing Factors to Abnormal Values

- Drugs that may *increase* urinary potassium levels: acetazolamide, ammonium chloride, glucocorticoids, loop diuretics, mercurial diuretics, potassium, salicylates, thiazide diuretics.
- Drugs that may *decrease* urinary potassium levels: laxatives, licorice (contains a mineralocorticoid compound).

Pre-Test Nursing Care

- Explain 24-hour urine collection procedure to the patient.
- Stress the importance of saving *all* urine in the 24-hour period. Instruct the patient to avoid contaminating the urine with toilet paper or feces.

Procedure

- Obtain the proper container containing no preservative from the laboratory.
- Begin the testing period in the morning following the patient's first voiding, which is discarded.
- Timing of the 24-hour period begins at the time the first voiding is discarded.
- *All* urine for the next 24 hours is collected in the container, which is to be kept refrigerated or on ice.
- If any urine is accidentally discarded during the 24-hour period, the test must be discontinued and a new test begun.
- The ending time of the 24-hour collection period should be posted in the patient's room.
- Gloves are to be worn when dealing with the specimen collection.

P

Post-Test Nursing Care

- Label the container and transport it on ice to the laboratory as soon as possible following the end of the 24-hour collection period.
- Report abnormal findings to the primary care provider.

• • • • • • • • • • • • • • • •

Pregnancy Test
(Human Chorionic Gonadotropin [HCG])

Human chorionic gonadotropin (HCG) is a hormone secreted exclusively by the placenta; thus its measurement is useful in determining pregnancy. HCG is produced, and thus can be detected in the blood, 8 to 10 days after conception. This time period correlates with the implantation of the fertilized ovum into the uterine wall. The HCG level increases until it peaks at 8 to 12 weeks gestation. It then decreases slowly during the remainder of the pregnancy. The hormone is no longer detectable approximately 2 weeks after delivery.

The test is performed by mixing the patient's serum with anti-HCG. If HCG is present in the patient's serum, it combines with and inactivates the anti-HCG antibodies. When indicator cells coated with HCG are then added, the cells do not clump since the anti-HCG antibodies have been inactivated. This indicates a positive pregnancy test. If clumping does occur, this means that anti-HCG antibodies have not been inactivated by HCG. Thus, the test is negative.

Pregnancy testing can also be performed on urine specimens. Home pregnancy testing is available. These tests confirm pregnancy by detecting the presence of HCG in the urine.

Normal Values

Negative

Possible Meanings of Abnormal Values

Increased	Decreased
Breast cancer	Abortion
Bronchogenic carcinoma	Ectopic pregnancy
Choriocarcinoma	Threatened abortion
Embryonal carcinoma	
Hydatidiform mole	
Liver cancer	
Malignant melanoma	
Multiple myeloma	
Pancreatic cancer	
Pregnancy	
Tumors	

P

Contributing Factors to Abnormal Values

- Drugs that may cause *false-positive* results: anticonvulsants, antiparkinsonian agents, hypnotics, and tranquilizers.
- *False-negative* results may occur if the test is performed too early in the pregnancy.

Pre-Test Nursing Care

- Explain to the patient the purpose of the test and the need for a blood sample to be drawn.
- No fasting is required before the test.

Procedure

- A 5 mL blood sample is drawn in a collection tube containing a silicone gel.
- Gloves are worn throughout the procedure.

Post-Test Nursing Care

- Apply pressure at venipuncture site. Apply dressing, periodically assessing for continued bleeding.
- Label the specimen and transport it to the laboratory.
- Report abnormal findings to the primary care provider.

• • • • • • • • • • • • • • • •

Pregnanediol

Progesterone is a steroid sex hormone secreted by the corpus luteum, by the placenta during pregnancy, and by the adrenal cortex. The primary metabolite of progesterone is *pregnanediol*. This test is used to evaluate placental and ovarian function. Excretion of pregnanediol is typically high in pregnancy and low in luteal deficiency or placental insufficiency.

Normal Values

Female: 0.2–6.0 mg/day (0.6–18.7 µmol/day, SI units)
Third trimester of pregnancy:
               27–47 mg/day (84–147 µmol/day SI units)
Male: 0.2–1.2 mg/day (0.6–3.7 µmol/day, SI units)

Possible Meanings of Abnormal Values

Increased	Decreased
Adrenal hyperplasia	Amenorrhea
Biliary tract obstruction	Anovulation
Hyperadrenocorticism	Breast neoplasm
Metastatic ovarian cancer	Fetal death
Ovarian cyst	Hydatidiform mole
Ovulation	Ovarian neoplasm
Pregnancy	Placental insufficiency

P

Increased	Decreased
	Pre-eclampsia
	Threatened abortion
	Toxemia of pregnancy

Contributing Factors to Abnormal Values

- Drugs that may *increase* pregnanediol levels: corticotropin, methenamine mandelate.
- Drugs that may *decrease* pregnanediol levels: oral contraceptives, progesterones.

Pre-Test Nursing Care

- Explain 24-hour urine collection procedure to the patient.
- Stress the importance of saving *all* urine in the 24-hour period. Instruct the patient to avoid contaminating the urine with toilet paper or feces.
- Inform the patient of the presence of a preservative in the collection bottle.

Procedure

- Obtain the proper container containing the appropriate preservative from the laboratory.
- Begin the testing period in the morning following the patient's first voiding, which is discarded.
- Timing of the 24-hour period begins at the time the first voiding is discarded.
- *All* urine for the next 24 hours is collected in the container, which is to be kept refrigerated or on ice.
- If any urine is accidentally discarded during the 24-hour period, the test must be discontinued and a new test begun.
- The ending time of the 24-hour collection period should be posted in the patient's room.
- Gloves are to be worn whenever dealing with the specimen collection.

Post-Test Nursing Care

- Label the container and transport it on ice to the laboratory as soon as possible following the end of the 24-hour collection period.
- For female patients: on the laboratory slip, include the date on which the patient began her last menstrual period or, if pregnant, the approximate week of gestation.
- Report abnormal findings to the primary care provider.

• • • • • • • • • • • • • • • • • •

P

Pregnanetriol

Pregnanetriol is involved in the synthesis of adrenal corticoids. It is a metabolite of 17-hydroxyprogesterone and is normally excreted in the urine in very small amounts. In adrenogenital syndrome, cortisol synthesis is blocked at the point at which 17-hydroxyprogesterone converts to cortisol. This results in a buildup of 17-hydroxyprogesterone and increased amounts of its metabolite, pregnanetriol, are excreted in the urine.

The reduced plasma cortisol levels stimulate the secretion of ACTH, which normally leads to increased cortisol levels. However, since cortisol synthesis is impaired, pregnanetriol levels continue to rise instead. High levels of 17-hydroxyprogesterone and ACTH lead to virilization in females and sexual precocity in young males.

Normal Values

Adult:	0.5–2.0 mg/day (1.5–6.0 µmol/day, SI units)
2–16 years:	0.3–1.1 mg/day (0.9–3.3 µmol/day, SI units)
<2 years:	0-0.2 mg/day (0-0.6 µmol/day, SI units)

Possible Meanings of Abnormal Values

Increased

Adrenocortical tumor
Adrenogenital syndrome
Congenital adrenocortical hyperplasia
Hirsutism
21-Hydroxylase deficiency
Overian tumor
Stein-Leventhal syndrome
Virilization

Contributing Factors to Abnormal Values

- Exercise may alter test results.

Pre-Test Nursing Care

- Explain 24-hour urine collection procedure to the patient.
- Stress the importance of saving *all* urine in the 24-hour period. Instruct the patient to avoid contaminating the urine with toilet paper or feces.
- Inform the patient of the presence of a preservative in the collection bottle.
- Encourage the patient to avoid excessive physical activity during the testing period.

Procedure

- Obtain the proper container containing the appropriate preservative from the laboratory.
- Begin the testing period in the morning following the patient's first voiding, which is discarded.
- Timing of the 24-hour period begins at the time the first voiding is discarded.
- *All* urine for the next 24 hours is collected in the container, which is to be kept refrigerated or on ice.
- If any urine is accidentally discarded during the 24-hour period, the test must be discontinued and a new test begun.
- The ending time of the 24-hour collection period should be posted in the patient's room.
- Gloves are to be worn when dealing with the specimen collection.

P

Post-Test Nursing Care

- Label the container and transport it on ice to the laboratory as soon as possible following the end of the 24-hour collection period.
- Report abnormal findings to the primary care provider.

• • • • • • • • • • • • • • • •

Proctosigmoidoscopy
(Anoscopy, Proctoscopy, Sigmoidoscopy)

Proctosigmoidoscopy is the direct visualization of the distal sigmoid colon, the rectum, and the anus through the use of a flexible fiberoptic endoscope. This endoscope is a multilumen instrument that allows viewing of the organ linings, insufflation of air, aspiration of fluid, removal of foreign objects, obtaining of tissue biopsies, and passage of a laser beam for obliteration of abnormal tissue or control of bleeding. This procedure is performed when the patient has experienced lower abdominal pain, a change in bowel habits, or passage of blood, mucus, or pus in the stool.

Normal Values

Normal sigmoid colon, rectum, and anus.

Possible Meanings of Abnormal Values

Anal fissures
Anal fistula
Anorectal abscesses
Benign lesions
Crohn's disease
Hemorrhoids
Hypertrophic anal papilla
Irritable bowel syndrome
Polyps
Pseudomembranous colitis
Tumors
Ulcerative colitis

Contributing Factors to Abnormal Values

- Retention of barium following previous tests, active gastrointestinal bleeding, or inadequate colon preparation hinders successful completion of this test.

STOP CONTRAINDICATIONS

- Patients with acute diverticulitis.
- Patients with suspected perforation of the colon.
- Patients who are medically unstable.
- Patients unable to cooperate with the examination.

Pre-Test Nursing Care

- Explain to the patient the purpose of the test. Provide any written teaching materials available on the subject. Inform the patient that pressure may be experienced during movement of the endoscope and during insufflation with air or carbon dioxide.
- Obtain a signed informed consent.
- The colon is prepared for the examination as follows:
  - clear liquid diet for 2 days before the test.
  - an enema the morning of the test.
- No fasting is required before the test.
- Resuscitation and suctioning equipment should be readily available.

Procedure

- The patient is assisted into the left lateral decubitus or knee-chest position on the endoscopy table.
- The physician inserts a well-lubricated index finger into the anus and rectum to palpate for tenderness. The finger is withdrawn and checked for the presence of blood, mucus, or stool.
- The sigmoidoscope is inserted into the anus and advanced into the distal sigmoid colon.
- During the procedure, insufflation of the bowel with air is used for better visualization.
- The sigmoid colon, rectum, and anus are visualized.
- Encourage the patient to take slow, deep breaths to induce relaxation and to minimize the urge to defecate.
- Biopsy forceps may be used to remove a tissue specimen, or a cytology brush may be used to obtain cells from the surface of a lesion. Removal of foreign bodies or polyps is accomplished, if needed.
- Videotaping of the procedure is often done via a camera attached to the endoscope.
- Gloves are worn throughout the procedure.

Post-Test Nursing Care

Possible complications:

- **Bleeding**
- **Perforation of the bowel**

- Monitor vital signs every 15 minutes until stable.
- Observe the patient for indications of bowel perforation: rectal bleeding, abdominal pain and distention, and fever.
- Inform the patient that passage of a large amount of flatus is normal after this procedure.
- Report abnormal findings to the primary care provider.

• • • • • • • • • • • • • • • •

P

Progesterone

Progesterone is a steroid sex hormone secreted via three sources:

1. by the corpus luteum, which causes thickening of the endometrium in preparation for implantation of a fertilized egg;
2. by the placenta during pregnancy, which causes continued thickening of the endometrium for provision of nutrients for the developing fetus and decreased myometrial excitability and uterine contractions, and also prepares the breasts for lactation; and
3. by the adrenal cortex in men.

Measurement of progesterone levels is useful in studies of the corpus luteum and placental function.

Normal Values

Female:
Follicular phase:	0–1.5 ng/mL (0–4.7 nmol/L, SI units)
Luteal phase:	2–30 ng/mL (6.3–94.5 nmol/L, SI units)
Postmenopausal:	0–1.5 ng/mL (0–4.7 nmol/L, SI units)
Pregnancy:	Peaks in third trimester as high as 200 ng/mL (630 nmol/L, SI units)

Male: 0–1.0 ng/mL (0–3.2 nmol/L, SI units)

Possible Meanings of Abnormal Values

Increased	Decreased
Adrenal hyperplasia	Adrenogenital syndrome
Adrenal neoplasms	Amenorrhea
Chorionepithelioma of ovary	Anovular menstruation
Corpus luteum cyst	Fetal death
Molar pregnancy	Menstrual disorders
Ovarian neoplasms	Ovarian failure
Precocious puberty	Placental insufficiency
Pregnancy	Pre-eclampsia
Retained placental tissue	Stein-Leventhal syndrome
	Threatened abortion
	Toxemia of pregnancy
	Turner's syndrome

Contributing Factors to Abnormal Values

- Hemolysis of the blood sample or having a radioactive scan within 1 week of the test may alter test results.
- Drugs that may *increase* progesterone levels: adrenocortical hormones, estrogens, progesterones.

Pre-Test Nursing Care

- Explain to the patient the purpose of the test and the need for a blood sample to be drawn.
- No fasting is required before the test.

Procedure

- A 7-mL blood sample is drawn in a collection tube containing a silicone gel.
- Gloves are worn throughout the procedure.

Post-Test Nursing Care

- Apply pressure at venipuncture site. Apply dressing, periodically assessing for continued bleeding.
- Label the specimen and transport it to the laboratory.
- On the laboratory slip, include the date on which the patient began her last menstrual period or, if pregnant, the trimester of the pregnancy.
- Report abnormal findings to the primary care provider.

• • • • • • • • • • • • • • • • •

Prolactin Level
(PRL, Human Prolactin [HPRL], Lactogen, Lactogenic Hormone)

Like growth hormone, prolactin (PRL) is secreted by the anterior pituitary gland. This hormone is responsible for growth of breast tissue and the promotion and maintenance of lactation. Determination of prolactin levels is used to diagnose pituitary and hypothalamic dysfunction and to evaluate amenorrhea and galactorrhea.

Normal Values

Female:	0–15 ng/mL (0–15 µg/L, SI units)
Male:	0–10 ng/mL (0–10 µg/L, SI units)
Pregnancy:	
First trimester:	<80 ng/mL (<80 µg/L, SI units)
Second trimester:	<160 ng/mL (<160 µg/L, SI units)
Third trimester:	<400 ng/mL (<400 µg/L, SI units)

Possible Meanings of Abnormal Values

Increased	Decreased
Acromegaly	Gynecomastia
Addison's disease	Hirsutism
Amenorrhea	Osteoporosis
Anorexia nervosa	Pituitary infarction
Breast stimulation	Pituitary necrosis
Chronic renal failure	
Ectopic tumors	

P

Increased	Decreased
Endometriosis	
Exercise	
Galactorrhea	
Hyperpituitarism	
Hypothalamic disorders	
Hypothyroidism	
Hysterectomy	
Lactation	
Pituitary tumors	
Plycystic ovaries	
Pregnancy	
Sleep	
Stress	

Contributing Factors to Abnormal Values

- Prolactin levels are increased following exercise.
- Diagnostic tests using radioactive materials, recent surgery, or hemolysis of the blood sample may alter test results.
- Drugs that may *increase* prolactin levels: amitriptyline, amoxapine, amphetamines, antihistamines, chlorprothixene, desipramine, doxepin hydrochloride, droperidol, estrogens, halperidol, histamine antagonists, imipramine hydrochloride, isoniazid, maprotiline hydrochloride, meprobamate, methyldopa, metoclopramide, monoamine oxidase inhibitors, nortriptyline hydrochloride, opiates, oral contraceptives, phenothiazines, procainamide hydrochloride, protriptyline, reserpine, thiothixene, thyrotropin, triavil, trimipramine maleate, verapamil hydrochloride.
- Drugs that may *decrease* prolactin levels: apomorphine hydrochloride, clonidine hydrochloride, bromocriptine mesylate, dopamine hydrochloride, ergot alkaloid derivatives, levodopa.

Pre-Test Nursing Care

- Explain to the patient the purpose of the test and the need for a blood sample to be drawn.
- No fasting is required before the test.
- The patient should rest 30 minutes before the test.
- The sample should be drawn in the morning.

Procedure

- A 7-mL blood sample is drawn in a collection tube containing a silicone gel.
- Gloves are worn throughout the procedure.

Post-Test Nursing Care

- Apply pressure at venipuncture site. Apply dressing, periodically assessing for continued bleeding.
- Label the specimen and transport it to the laboratory.
- Report abnormal findings to the primary care provider.

• • • • • • • • • • • • • • • •

Prostate Sonogram
(Prostate Ultrasound, Transrectal Sonogram)

Ultrasonography is a noninvasive method of diagnostic testing in which ultrasound waves are sent into the body with a small transducer pressed against the skin. The transducer not only sends the sound waves into the body but also receives any returning sound waves, which are deflected back as they bounce off various structures. The transducer converts the returning sound waves into electric signals that are then transformed by a computer into a visual display on a monitor.

The prostate sonogram is used in the early diagnosis of cancer the prostate gland. It is used as an adjunct to digital examination of the prostate and to tests such as the prostate-specific antigen (PSA) test. The sonogram demonstrates the size and shape of the prostate gland and is thus helpful in monitoring patient response to therapy for prostate disease. It also provides guidance for prostate biopsy.

Normal Values

Normal size, shape, and consistency of the prostate gland.

Possible Meanings of Abnormal Values

Benign prostatic hypertrophy
Perirectal abscess
Perirectal tumor
Prostate abscess
Prostate cancer
Prostatitis
Rectal tumor
Seminal vesicle tumor

Contributing Factors to Abnormal Values

- The transducer must be in good contact with the skin as it is being moved. A lubricant, such as mineral oil, glycerin, or a water-based jelly, is used to ensure good contact with the skin.
- Retained barium from previous tests or stool within the rectum will hinder accurate test results.

Pre-Test Nursing Care

- Explain to the patient the purpose of the test. Provide any written teaching materials available on the subject. Note that rectal pressure will be felt during the test.
- No fasting is required before the test.
- Some institutions may require a signed informed consent form to be completed.
- For transrectal sonography, a small enema is administered 1 hour before the test.

Procedure

- The patient is assisted to a supine position on the ultrasonography table.
- A transabdominal sonogram and a suprapubic examination of the prostate is performed.

P

- The patient is then assisted to a knee-elbow or lateral decubitus position.
- The transducer is covered with a transparent cover, lubricated, and inserted into the rectum.
- The transducer is angled toward the prostate to provide good visualization of the gland.
- The sound waves are transformed into a visual display on the monitor. Printed copies of this display are made.
- Gloves are worn throughout the procedure.

Post-Test Nursing Care

- Cleanse the patient's skin of any lubricant.
- Report abnormal findings to the primary care provider.

• • • • • • • • • • • • • • • •

Prostate-Specific Antigen
(PSA)

Prostate-specific antigen (PSA) is a glycoprotein found only in the prostate epithelium. PSA is considered a reliable tumor marker for prostate cancer. Measurement of the PSA level is performed to screen patients for the presence of prostate cancer, to monitor the progression of the disease, and to monitor the response of the patient to treatment for prostate cancer.

Two commercial assays are available to use in determining the PSA level: the Pro-Check and Tandem-R. With both tests, a value of greater than 10 ng/mL is highly suggestive of prostate cancer. Values greater than 100 ng/mL indicate probable metastatic cancer of the prostate. However, most important to note and that which requires further investigation, is an upward trend in the PSA level. Even if the value is within the normal range, an increase of at least 0.75 ng/mL per year is considered abnormal.

Normal Values

Pro-Check:	0–2.5 ng/mL (0–2.5 mcg/L, SI units)
Tandem-R:	0–4 ng/mL (0–4 mcg/L, SI units)

Possible Meanings of Abnormal Values

Increased

Benign prostatic hypertropy
Cirrhosis
Impotence
Prostate cancer
Prostatitis
Urinary retention

Contributing Factors to Abnormal Values

- Falsely elevated PSA values occur following palpation of the prostate or any manipulation such as through cystoscopy, transrectal ultrasound, or prostatic biopsy.
- Drug that may *decrease* PSA level: finasteride.

P

Pre-Test Nursing Care

- Explain to the patient the purpose of the test and the need for a blood sample to be drawn.
- No fasting is required before the test.
- The blood sample is collected before palpation of the prostate during rectal examination.

Procedure

- A 5-mL blood sample is drawn in a collection tube containing a silicone gel.
- Gloves are worn throughout the procedure.

Post-Test Nursing Care

- Apply pressure at venipuncture site. Apply dressing, periodically assessing for continued bleeding.
- Label the specimen and transport it to the laboratory.
- Report abnormal findings to the primary care provider.

• • • • • • • • • • • • • • • • •

Protein, Blood
(Total Protein, TP, Albumin, Alpha Globulins, Beta Globulins, Gamma Globulins)

The measurement of total protein in the blood includes values for both of the two main protein groups: albumin and globulins. *Albumin,* which is synthesized in the liver, has two very important functions. First, it is essential in maintaining oncotic pressure, for without albumin, fluid would be able to leak out of the instial spaces. Second, many substances such as bilirubin, fatty acids, drugs, and hormones are bound to albumin while they are circulating in the bloodstream, allowing them to be transported throughout the body.

There are three primary types of *globulins.* The *alpha globulins* are synthesized in the liver, and include both alpha$_1$ globulins, such as alpha$_1$-antitrypsin, alpha-fetoprotein, and thyroxine-binding globulin, and alpha$_2$ globulins, such as haptoglobin and ceruloplasmin. The *beta globulins,* also synthesized in the liver, include such substances as transferrin and the complement proteins. *Gamma globulins,* which are also called *immunoglobulins,* are produced by B-lymphocytes in response to stimulation by antigens. The gamma globulins include the IgA, IgD, IgE, IgG, and IgM antibodies, and are discussed in detail in the section Immunoelectrophoresis.

The exact amount of albumin and each of the globulin types are determined with a procedure called *protein electrophoresis.* If any of the gamma globulins are abnormal, an additional test, *immunoelectrophoresis,* is performed. Both of these tests are discussed under their individual test names.

Normal Values

Total protein:	6.0–8.0 g/dL (60–80 g/L, SI units)
Albumin:	3.1–4.3 g/dL (31–43 g/L, SI units)
Globulin:	2.6–4.1 g/dL (26–41 g/L, SI units)

Possible Meanings of Abnormal Values

Total Protein

Increased	Decreased
Addison's disease	Acute cholecystitis
Crohn's disease	Agammaglobulinemia
Dehydration	Diarrhea
Diarrhea	Excessive intravenous (IV) glucose
Hypergammaglobulinemia	Exfoliative dermatitis
Multiple meyloma	Fever
Renal disease	Hodgkin's disease
Sarcoidosis	Hyperthyroidism
Vomiting	Inflammatory processes
	Leukemia
	Malabsorption
	Malignancies
	Malnutrition
	Nephrotic syndrome
	Peptic ulcer disease
	Severe burns
	Severe liver disease
	Syndrome of inappropriate ADH secretion (SIADH)
	Ulcerative colitis

Albumin

Increased	Decreased
Dehydration	Acquired Immunodeficiency Syndrome (AIDS)
IV albumin infusions	Ascites
	Cirrhosis
	Diarrhea
	Eclampsia
	Edema
	Excessive IV glucose
	Exfoliative dermatitis
	Hyperthyroidism
	Infection
	Neoplasms
	Nephrosis
	Nephrotic syndrome
	Pre-eclampsia
	Severe burns
	Severe malnutrition
	Syndrome of inappropriate ADH secretion
	Trauma

P

Globulin

Increased	Decreased
Immunologic tumors	Immunologic deficiencies
	Malnutrition

Contributing Factors to Abnormal Values

- Testing with radiographic contrast dye within 48 hours will falsely increase total protein levels.
- Drugs that may *increase* total protein levels: bromosulfophthalein, clofibrate, corticosteroids, corticotropin, dextran, heparin, insulin, levothyroxine sodium, radiographic contrast dye, somatropin, somatrem, thyrotropin, tolbutamide.
- Drugs that may *decrease* total protein levels: ammonium ion, dextran glucose infusions, oral contraceptives, pyrazinamide, salicylates.

Pre-Test Nursing Care

- Explain to the patient the purpose of the test and the need for a blood sample to be drawn.
- No fasting is required before the test.
- No diet high in fat should be ingested for 8 hours before the test.

Procedure

- A 5-mL blood sample is drawn in a collection tube containing a silicone gel.
- Gloves are worn throughout the procedure.

Post-Test Nursing Care

- Apply pressure at venipuncture site. Apply dressing, periodically assessing for continued bleeding.
- Label the specimen and transport it to the laboratory.
- Report abnormal findings to the primary care provider.
- Should the total protein be found to be low, counsel the patient on dietary sources of protein, including such foods as eggs, cheese, fish, and meat.

• • • • • • • • • • • • • • • • •

Protein C
(PC)

After the process of hemostasis is completed, any excess amounts of clotting factors that remain are inactivated by fibrin inhibitors, such as antiplasmin, anti-thrombin III, and protein C. This prevents clotting from occurring indiscriminately. Protein C is a protein produced in the liver and circulating in the plasma. Vitamin K is essential for its production. Protein C acts as an anticoagulant by inactivating coagulation factors V and VIII. Protein S serves as a cofactor to enhance this anticoagulant effect. Testing for protein C is done when evaluating patients with severe thrombosis. When the level of protein C is found to be deficient, the patient is at increased risk of vascular thrombosis.

Normal Values

70%–140% (0.70–1.40, SI units)

Possible Meanings of Abnormal Values

Decreased

Cirrhosis
Disseminated intravascular coagulation
Vitamin K deficiency

Contributing Factors to Abnormal Values
- Hemolysis of the blood sample may alter test results.
- Drugs that may *decrease* protein C levels: anticoagulant drugs.

Pre-Test Nursing Care
- Explain to the patient the purpose of the test and the need for a blood sample to be drawn.
- No fasting is required before the test.

Procedure
- A 5-mL blood sample is drawn in a collection tube containing sodium citrate and citric acid.
- Gloves are worn throughout the procedure.

Post-Test Nursing Care
- Apply pressure at venipuncture site. Apply dressing, periodically assessing for continued bleeding.
- Label the specimen and transport it to the laboratory.
- Results are usually not available for 2–4 weeks.
- Report abnormal findings to the primary care provider.

• • • • • • • • • • • • • •

Protein Electrophoresis
(Serum Protein Electrophoresis [SPEP])

Total protein is composed of albumin and globulins. *Albumin,* which is synthesized in the liver, is essential in maintaining oncotic pressure and for transporting throughout the body substances, such as bilirubin, fatty acids, drugs, and hormones, which are bound to albumin while they are circulating in the bloodstream.

There are three primary types of *globulins*. The *alpha globulins* and *beta globulins*, which are synthesized in the liver, include alpha$_1$ globulins, such as alpha$_1$-antitrypsin, alpha-fetoprotein, and thyroxine-binding globulin, alpha$_2$ globulins, such as haptoglobin and ceruloplasmin and beta globulins, such as transferrin and the complement proteins. *Gamma globulins*, which are also called *immunoglobulins*, are produced by B-lymphocytes in response to stimulation by antigens, and include the IgA, IgD, IgE, IgG, and IgM antibodies. These are discussed in detail in the section Immunoelectrophoresis.

Protein electrophoresis is a commonly used method of measuring albumin and each of the globulin types. An electrical current is passed through the blood serum, causing the various proteins to separate according to their electrical charge, molecular size, and shape. Albumin moves farthest away from the current, followed by the alpha globulins, beta globulins, and, finally, the gamma globulins. The pattern that forms is compared with patterns characteristic of specific disease entities. Each of the components measured by protein electrophoresis may be reported as percentages or actual amounts.

Normal Values

Total protein		6.0–8.0 g/dL	(60–80 g/L, SI units)
Albumin	58%–74%	3.3–5.5 g/dL	(33–55 g/L, SI units)
Alpha$_1$ globulin	2%–3.5%	0.1-0.4 g/dL	(1–4 g/L, SI units)
Alpha$_2$ globulin	5.4%–10.6%	0.5–1.0 g/dL	(5–10 g/L, SI units)
Beta globulin	7%–14%	0.7–1.2 g/dL	(7–12 g/L, SI units)
Gamma globulin	8%–18%	0.8–1.6 g/dL	(8–16 g/L, SI units)

Possible Meanings of Abnormal Values

Total Protein

Increased	Decreased
Macroglobulinemia	Acute cholecystitis
Multiple myeloma	Analbuminemia
Sarcoidosis	Glomerulonephritis
	Hodgkin's disease
	Hypertension
	Hypogammaglobulinemia
	Leukemia
	Nephrosis
	Peptic ulcer disease
	Ulcerative colitis

Albumin

Increased	Decreased
Acute pancreatitis	Acute cholecystitis
	Analbuminemia
	Diabetes mellitus
	Gastrointestinal protein loss
	Glomerular protein loss
	Hepatic disease

P

Increased	Decreased
	Hodgkin's disease
	Hyperthyroidism
	Leukemia
	Malnutrition
	Peptic ulcer disease
	Rheumatoid arthritis
	Sarcoidosis
	Stress
	Systemic lupus erythematosus
	Ulcerative colitis

Alpha Globulin

Increased	Decreased
Acute infection	Cirrhosis
Acute inflammation	Hemolytic anemia
Carcinoma	Hepatic disease
Chronic glomerulonephritis	Hepatic metastases
Cirrhosis	Malabsorption
Diabetes mellitus	Pulmonary emphysema
Dysproteinemia	Scleroderma
Glomerular protein loss	Starvation
Hepatic damage	Steatorrhea
Hodgkin's disease	Viral hepatitis
Hypoalbuminemia	
Myocardial infarction	
Osteomyelitis	
Peptic ulcer disease	
Pregnancy	
Rheumatoid arthritis	
Sarcoidosis	
Stress	
Systemic lupus erythematosus	
Ulcerative colitis	

Beta Globulin

Increased	Decreased
Acute inflammation	Autoimmune disease
Analbuminemia	Hepatic disease
Diabetes mellitus	Leukemia
Dysproteinemia	Lymphoma
Glomerular protein loss	Malabsorption
Hypercholesterolemia	Malnutrition
Iron-deficiency anemia	Metastatic cancer
Nephrotic syndrome	Nephrosis
Obstructive jaundice	Scleroderma

P

Increased	Decreased
Pregnancy	Starvation
Rheumatoid arthritis	Systemic lupus erythematosus
Sarcoidosis	Ulcerative colitis
Viral hepatitis	

Gamma Globulin

Increased	Decreased
Advanced cancer	Agammaglobulinemia
Chronic hepatitis	Glomerular protein loss
Cystic fibrosis	Hypogammaglobulinemia
Hepatic disease	Leukemia
Hodgkin's disease	Lymphoma
Hypersensitivity reaction	Malabsorption
Leukemia	Nephrosis
Multiple myeloma	Nephrotic syndrome
Rheumatoid arthritis	Starvation
Sarcoidosis	Ulcerative colitis
Severe infection	
Systemic lupus erythematosus	
Viral infections	

Contributing Factors to Abnormal Values

- Drugs that may alter test results include aspirin, corticosteroids, estrogens, and penicillins.

Pre-Test Nursing Care

- Explain to the patient the purpose of the test and the need for a blood sample to be drawn.
- No fasting is required before the test.

Procedure

- A 7-mL blood sample is drawn in a collection tube containing a silicone gel.
- Gloves are worn throughout the procedure.

Post-Test Nursing Care

- Apply pressure at venipuncture site. Apply dressing, periodically assessing for continued bleeding.
- Label the specimen and transport it to the laboratory.
- Report abnormal findings to the primary care provider.

P

• • • • • • • • • • • • • • • •

Protein S

After the process of hemostasis is completed, any excess amounts of clotting factors that remain are inactivated by fibrin inhibitors, such as antiplasmin, anti-thrombin III, and protein C. This prevents clotting from occurring indiscriminately. Protein S is a protein produced in the liver and circulating in the plasma. Vitamin K is essential for its production. Protein S serves as a cofactor to enhance the anticoagulant effect of protein C, which inactivates coagulation factors V and VIII. Testing for protein S is done when evaluating patients for hypercoagulability states such as severe thrombosis. When the level of protein S is found to be deficient, the patient is at increased risk of vascular thrombosis.

Normal Values

70%–140% (0.70–1.40, SI units)

Possible Meanings of Abnormal Values

Decreased

Familial protein S deficiency

Interfering Factors

- Hemolysis of the blood sample may alter test results.

Pre-Test Nursing Care

- Explain to the patient the purpose of the test and the need for a blood sample to be drawn.
- No fasting is required before the test.

Procedure

- A 5-mL blood sample is drawn in a collection tube containing sodium citrate and citric acid.
- Gloves are worn throughout the procedure.

Post-Test Nursing Care

- Apply pressure at venipuncture site. Apply dressing, periodically assessing for continued bleeding.
- Label the specimen and transport it to the laboratory.
- Report abnormal findings to the primary care provider.

P

Prothrombin Time
(PT, PT Ratio/INR, Pro Time)

The process of hemostasis involves numerous steps and the proper functioning of a variety of coagulating factors and other substances. The *prothrombin time (PT)* is used to evaluate how well the coagulation process is functioning. This test is useful for detecting bleeding disorders caused by either deficient or defective coagulation factors that compose the extrinsic system. These factors include fibrinogen I, prothrombin II, V, VII, and X. If the patient's blood is deficient in one of these factors, the patient's PT in seconds will be higher than the control PT in seconds (or less than the control if using percentages). (For review of the entire coagulation process, see Coagulation Studies.)

The PT is also used to monitor the effectiveness of anticoagulant therapy with coumarin type drugs, such as warfarin sodium (Coumadin) and dicumarol (Bishydroxycoumarin). These drugs interfere with the production of vitamin K-dependent clotting factors, such as prothrombin.

The PT involves measuring the amount of time it take for a clot to form in a plasma sample to which calcium and tissue thromboplastin have been added. A normal range for PT is 8.8 to 11.6 seconds, but varies according to the norms established by individual laboratories. Laboratories report the actual PT value along with the control value for reference. The goal of oral anticoagulant therapy is to maintain the PT at 1.5 to 2 times the control value (in seconds). Thus, a therapeutic goal, if receiving Coumadin, would be a PT of 24 seconds, or 25% of normal activity.

If the value falls below the therapeutic level for a patient on an oral anticoagulant, an increase in anticoagulation, and thus, dosage is needed. If the PT is greater than 30 seconds, the patient is at high risk for spontaneous bleeding. In the case of coumarin overdose with resultant hemorrhage, the antidote is vitamin K, which reverses the action of a coumarin drug in 12 to 24 hours.

To provide standardization of PT reporting among different laboratories, the World Health Organization recommends the use of the *International Normalized Ratio (INR)* to express the intensity of therapy. Most laboratories now report both the PT and the INR.

Maintaining an INR of 2.0 to 3.0 is recommended for prophylaxis/treatment of venous thrombosis and thromboembolic complications associated with atrial fibrillation, for pulmonary embolism, for prophylaxis of systemic embolism after myocardial infarction, and for bioprosthetic cardiac valves. A higher INR, of 2.5 to 3.5, is recommended for cardiac valve replacement that involves mechanical valves. The frequency of testing to reach and maintain the recommended INR level is based on the individual patient's clinical status.

Normal Values

8.8–11.6 seconds; 60%–140% (varies according to laboratory)
Therapeutic level for anticoagulant therapy: 1.5–2 times the control value.

Possible Meanings of Abnormal Values

Increased (in seconds)	Decreased (in seconds)
Acute leukemia	Arterial occlusion
Afibrinogenemia	Deep vein thrombosis
Biliary obstruction	Hypercoagulability
Cirrhosis	Malignancy

Increased (in seconds)	Decreased (in seconds)
Colitis	Multiple myeloma
Congestive heart failure	Myocardial infarction
Chronic pancreatitis	Peripheral vascular disease
Disseminated intravascular coagulation	Pulmonary embolism
	Spinal cord injury
Factor deficiency (I/II/V/VII/X)	Transplant rejection
Hemorrhagic disease of the newborn	
Hepatitis	
Hypervitaminosis	
Liver disease	
Malabsorption	
Obstetric complications	
Obstructive jaundice	
Pancreatic cancer	
Polycythemia vera	
Reye's syndrome	
Salicylate toxicity	
Toxic shock syndrome	
Vitamin K deficiency	
Vomiting	

Contributing Factors to Abnormal Values

- Hemolysis of the blood sample may alter test results.
- Diarrhea, vomiting, and alcohol ingestion may *increase* PT results.
- Intake of a high-fat diet may *decrease* PT results.
- Drugs that may *increase* PT results include: acetaminophen, allopurinal, aminosalicyclic acid, anabolic steroids, anisindione, aspirin, cathartics, chloral hydrate, chloramphenicol, chlordiazepoxide, chlorpromazine, chlorthalidone, cholestyramine, cimetidine, clofibrate, corticotropin, diazoxide, dicumarol, disulfiram, diuretics, ethacrynic acid, ethyl alcohol, glucagon, guanethidine sulfate, heparin, indomethacin, kanamycin, levothyroxine sodium, mefenamic acid, mercaptopurine, methimazole, methyldopa, methylphenidate, mithramycin, MAOI, nalidixic acid, neomycin sulfate, nortriptyline hydrochloride, phenylbutazone, phenytoin, propylthiouracil, quinidine, quinine sulfate, reserpine, streptomycin, sulfinpyrazone, sulfonamides, tetracyclines, thyrotropin, tolbutamide, vitamin A, warfarin sodium.
- Drugs that may *decrease* PT results include: anabolic steroids, antacids, antihistamincs, ascorbic acid, aspirin, barbiturates, caffeine, chloral hydrate, cholestyramine, colchicine, cortisteroids, digitalis, diuretics, ethchlorvynol, glutethimide, griseofulvin, heptabarbital, menadiol sodium diphosphate, menadione, meprobamate, oral contraceptives, phenobarbital, phytonadione, pyrazinamide, rifampin, sodium benzoate, tetracyclines, theophylline, xanthines.

Pre-Test Nursing Care

- Explain to the patient the purpose of the test and the need for a blood sample to be drawn.
- Inform the patient that the PT test will probably be done on a daily basis until it is stabilized, followed by once every 4–6 weeks for long-term control.
- Obtain the blood sample before administration of any oral anticoagulant.

- No fasting is required before the test.

Procedure

- A 7-mL blood sample is drawn in a collection tube containing sodium citrate and citric acid.
- Gloves are worn throughout the procedure.

Post-Test Nursing Care

Possible complications:

- **Hematoma at site owing to prolonged bleeding time**
- **Spontaneous bleeding with PT >30 seconds**

- Assess patient for spontaneous bleeding: epistaxis, bleeding gums, low back pain from possible retroperitoneal bleeding, joint pain, bruising, petechiae, hematuria, or melena.
- Apply pressure 3–5 minutes at venipuncture site. Apply dressing, periodically assessing for continued bleeding.
- Teach the patient to monitor the site. If the site begins to bleed, the patient should apply direct pressure and, if unable to control the bleeding, return to the laboratory or notify the nurse.
- Label the specimen and transport it to the laboratory immediately.
- Report abnormal findings to the primary care provider.

• • • • • • • • • • • • • • • • • •

Pulmonary Angiography
(Pulmonary Arteriography)

Angiography is a general term used to indicate visualization of any blood vessels, whether they be arteries or veins. The more precise term for visualization of the arteries is *arteriography*. Arteriograms are extremely valuable for observing the blood flow to a part of the body and to detect lesions that may be amenable to surgical treatment. The purposes of pulmonary angiography are to detect pulmonary embolism, to assess for pulmonary vascular perfusion defects, and to evaluate the pulmonary circulatory system in patients with congenital heart disease.

Normal Values

Normal pulmonary vasculature.

Possible Meanings of Abnormal Values

Aneurysm
Pulmonary emboli
Pulmonary vascular filling defects
Pulmonary vascular stenosis
Tumors

Contributing Factors to Abnormal Values

- Any movement by the patient may alter quality of films taken.

CONTRAINDICATIONS

- Patients who are allergic to iodine, shellfish, or contrast medium dye.
- Patients with bleeding disorders.
- Pregnant women (*Caution:* A woman in her childbearing years should undergo radiography only during her menses or 12–14 days after its onset to avoid any exposure to a fetus.).
- Patients who are unable to cooperate because of age, mental status, pain, or other factors.
- Patients with renal failure or those susceptible to dye-induced renal failure (dehydrated patients).

Pre-Test Nursing Care

- Explain to the patient the purpose of the test. Provide any written teaching materials available on the subject. Note that discomfort involved with this test is primarily owing to lying on a hard table for an extended period of time and the needle puncture. Explain that for approximately 5 minutes after the injection, the patient may experience the urge to cough, a flush feeling, nausea, or a salty taste.
- Check for allergies to iodine, shellfish, or contrast medium dye. Inform the radiologist of such possible allergy and obtain order for an antihistamine and corticosteroid to be administered prior to the test.
- Patients receiving metformin (Glucophage) for non–insulin-dependent diabetes mellitus should discontinue the drug 2 days before elective surgery or angiographic exams. This is owing to the possible occurrence of lactic acidosis, a potentially fatal complication of biguanide therapy.
- Baseline laboratory data (CBC, PT, PTT) is obtained.
- Note any medications, such as anticoagulants or aspirin, which may prolong bleeding.
- Fasting for at least 8 hours is required before the test.
- Obtain a signed informed consent.
- Administer any pretest sedation after consent form is signed.
- Assess and document patient's peripheral pulses bilaterally before the test. Mark the location of the pulses with a marking pen.

Procedure

- The patient is assisted to a supine position on the examination table.
- A maintenance intravenous (IV) line is initiated.
- Cardiac monitoring is initiated.
- Resuscitation and suctioning equipment should be readily available.
- The femoral or antecubital site is cleansed and then anesthetized.
- An incision is made and a catheter is introduced into the vein, and advanced through the right atrium and ventricle and into the pulmonary artery. Positioning is monitored via fluoroscopy. Pressures are measured and blood samples are drawn from several portions of the pulmonary circulation.
- Once the catheter is in the correct position, contrast dye is injected through the catheter.
- Radiographic films are taken as the contrast dye circulates through the pulmonary artery and capillaries of the lung.
- After films of satisfactory quality are obtained, the catheter is removed and pressure held on the puncture site for at least 15 minutes.
- Gloves are worn throughout the procedure.

P

Post-Test Nursing Care
Possible complications:
- **Allergic reaction to dye**
- **Bleeding at puncture site**
- **Cardiac arrhythmias**
- **Infection at the puncture site**
- **Renal failure**

- Most allergic reactions to radiopaque dye occur within 30 minutes of administration of the contrast medium. Observe the patient closely for respiratory distress, hypotension, edema, hives, rash, tachycardia, or laryngeal stridor. Emergency resuscitation equipment must be readily accessible.
- A pressure dressing is applied to the puncture site. Check the dressing for bleeding and the area around the puncture site for swelling at frequent intervals.
- The patient is to remain on bedrest for 6–12 hours with the affected extremity immobilized.
- Maintain pressure on the puncture site with a sandbag.
- Monitor vital signs every 15 minutes for 1 hour, then every 30 minutes for 2 hours, then every hour for 4 hours, and then every 4 hours.
- Monitor urinary output.
- Assess the color, movement, temperature, and sensation (CMTS) and the pulse(s) of the affected extremity with each vital sign check. Compare with the other extremity.
- Encourage fluid intake to promote dye excretion.
- Renal function should be assessed before metformin is restarted.
- Report abnormal findings to the primary care provider.

• • • • • • • • • • • • • • • •

Pulmonary Function Tests
(PFT, Spirometry)

Pulmonary function testing (PFT) includes a series of measurements of pulmonary volume and capacity. These measurements are made by a spirometer, which is a breathing system that allows gas to be breathed in and out. An electrical recording is made of the gas amounts. Spirometry is used to determine the effectiveness of the movement of the lungs and chest wall. Test results provide information regarding the degree of obstruction to air flow or the restriction of the amount of air that can be inhaled.

Some of the test findings are obtained through actual testing, whereas others are determined through calculation. The information obtained through PFT includes information regarding airway flow rates and regarding lung volumes and capacities.

Airway flow rate information is obtained primarily through two measurements. *Forced vital capacity (FVC)* is the amount of air that can be forcefully exhaled from a maximally inflated lung. *Forced expiratory volume in 1 second (FEV$_1$)* is the volume of air expelled during the first second of the FVC.

Lung volumes and capacities are also measured or calculated during pulmonary function testing. The relationships among the various volumes and capacities are shown in Figure 6.

Lung Volumes			Lung Capacities	
Vital Capacity (VC) (IRV+VT+ERV)	Inspiratory Reserve Volume (IRV)		Inspiratory Capacity (IC) (IRV + VT)	Total Lung Capacity (TLC) (IRV+VT+ERV+RV) OR (VC + RV)
	Tidal Volume (VT)			
	Expiratory Reserve Volume (ERV)		Functional Residual Capacity (FRC) (ERV + RV)	
Residual Volume (RV)				

Figure 6 Pulmonary function testing.

Four volume measurements are essential parts of the PFT. The *tidal volume (VT)* is the normal volume of air inspired and expired with each regular respiration. The *expiratory reserve volume (ERV)* is the maximal volume of air that can be exhaled after a normal expiration. *Residual volume (RV)* is the volume of air remaining in the lungs following forced expiration. The *inspiratory reserve volume (IRV)* is the maximal volume of air that can be inspired from the end of a normal inspiration.

By combining two or more of these lung *volume* values, four lung *capacity* values can be calculated. The *inspiratory capacity (IC)*, which is the maximal amount of air that can be inspired after a normal expiration, is calculated by adding IRV and VT. *Functional residual capacity (FRC)*, the amount of air left in the lungs after a normal expiration, is calculated by adding ERV and RV. The *vital capacity (VC)*, which is the maximum amount of air that can be expired after a normal inspiration, is determined by added the IRV, VT, and ERV. And, finally, the total *lung capacity (TLC)*, the volume to which the lungs can be expanded with the greatest inspiratory effort, is calculated by adding the IRV, VT, ERV, and RV. Another way to determine TLC is to add the VC and RV values.

Normal Values

Note: Values vary with age, height, and sex.

Tidal volume:	500 cc
Expiratory reserve volume:	1500 cc
Residual volume:	1500 cc
Inspiratory reserve volume:	2000 cc

Possible Meanings of Abnormal Values

Allergy
Asbestosis
Asthma

Bronchiectasis
Chest trauma
Chronic bronchitis
Emphysema
Myasthenia gravis
Pulmonary fibrosis
Pulmonary tumors
Respiratory infections
Sarcoidosis

Contributing Factors to Abnormal Values

- Test results may be altered in the following situations or conditions: lack of patient cooperation during the testing, hypoxia, metabolic disturbances, pregnancy, gastric distention.

CONTRAINDICATIONS

- Patients with acute coronary insufficiency, angina, or recent myocardial infarction.
- Patients who are unable to cooperate because of pain, age, or mental status.

Pre-Test Nursing Care

- Explain to the patient the purpose of the test and the procedure to be done.
- No fasting is required before the test.
- Instruct the patient to use no bronchodilators for 6 hours before the test, if ordered by the physician.
- Instruct the patient not to smoke for 6 hours before the test.
- Measure the patient's height and weight.

Procedure

- The patient is in a sitting or standing position.
- The patient is fitted with a mouthpiece that is connected to the spirometer.
- A noseclip is used so that only mouth breathing is possible.
- The patient is instructed to:
  - to breathe normally for 10 breaths (VT).
  - to inhale deeply and then to exhale completely (VC).
    - This part of the test is usually repeated two additional times.
  - to breathe normally for several breaths and then to exhale completely (ERV).
  - to breathe normally for several breaths and then to inhale as deep as possible (IC).
  - to breathe normally into a spirometer containing a known concentration of an insoluble gas such as nitrogen. The point at which the concentration of gas in the spirometer is equal to that in the lungs is measured (FRC).

Post-Test Nursing Care

- Assess patient for dizziness or weakness following the testing. Allow the patient to rest as needed.
- Report abnormal findings to the primary care provider.

• • • • • • • • • • • • • • • •

P

Pyruvate Kinase
(PK)

Pyruvate kinase (PK) is a red blood cell glycolytic enzyme. Deficiency of this enzyme is an inherited, autosomal recessive trait. PK deficiency is the second most frequent cause, after glucose-6-phosphate dehydrogenase (G 6 PD) deficiency, of congenital nonspherocytic hemolytic anemia. Thus, this test is performed to determine the cause of hemolytic anemia.

Normal Values

Routine (ultraviolet assay): 2.0–8.8 U/g of hemoglobin

Possible Meanings of Abnormal Values

Decreased

Metabolic liver disease
Myelodysplastic syndromes
Pyruvate kinase deficiency

Contributing Factors to Abnormal Values

- Hemolysis of the blood sample may alter test results.
- Recent blood transfusions may alter test results.

Pre-Test Nursing Care

- Explain to the patient the purpose of the test and the need for a blood sample to be drawn.
- No fasting is required before the test.

Procedure

- A 7-mL blood sample is drawn in a collection tube containing EDTA.
- Gloves are worn throughout the procedure.

Post-Test Nursing Care

- Apply pressure at venipuncture site. Apply dressing, periodically assessing for continued bleeding.
- Label the specimen and transport it to the laboratory immediately.
- Report abnormal findings to the primary care provider.

P

Rabies Antibody Test
(Rabies Neutralizing Antibody Test)

This test is used to determine whether a person has been infected with the rabies virus. Rabies is an acute viral infection of the central nervous system that affects animals such as bats, cats, dogs, skunks, and squirrels. The virus is present in the saliva of the infected animal, making transmission to humans possible through animal bites. The infection is fatal if symptoms appear before treatment is begun. Treatment involves the administration of rabies immunoglobulin (RIG) as soon as possible following exposure to neutralize the virus in the wound. Human diploid cell rabies vaccine is given intramuscularly at the same time as the RIG is given, and again at 3, 7, 14, and 28 days after the initial dose.

This test is also used to measure the rabies neutralizing antibody titer to determine whether an individual who has received the human diploid cell rabies vaccine has developed adequate protection against the disease. This is especially important for individuals such as veterinarians, who work closely with animals. A rabies titer of at least 1:16 is considered protective.

Normal Values
Negative

Possible Meanings of Abnormal Values
Positive

Rabies

Pre-Test Nursing Care
- Explain to the patient the purpose of the test and the need for a blood sample to be drawn.
- No fasting is required before the test.

Procedure
- A 7-mL blood sample is drawn in a collection tube containing a silicone gel.
- Gloves are worn throughout the procedure.

Post-Test Nursing Care
- Apply pressure at venipuncture site. Apply dressing, periodically assessing for continued bleeding.
- Label the specimen and transport it to the laboratory.
- The animal's brain is examined along with the patient's blood sample.
- Report abnormal findings to the primary care provider.

R

Radioactive Iodine Uptake
(RAIU)

The radioactive iodine uptake (RAIU) test evaluates thyroid function by measuring the amount of radioactive iodine (^{123}I or ^{131}I) that accumulates in the thyroid gland 6 and 24 hours after oral ingestion of the substance. The test is used in the diagnosis of hyperthyroidism and hypothyroidism.

Normal Values

After 6 hours:	3%–16% absorbed by thyroid gland
After 24 hours:	8%–29% absorbed by thyroid gland

Possible Meanings of Abnormal Values

Increased	Decreased
Early Hashimoto's thyroidism	Hypothyroidism
Hyperthyroidism	Iodine overload
Hypoalbuminemia	Subacute thyroiditis
Iodine-deficient goiter	

Contributing Factors to Abnormal Values

- Any movement by the patient may alter quality of films taken.
- Patients taking exogenous iodine have decreased uptake, whereas iodine-deficient patients have increased uptake.
- Drugs that may *increase* uptake: barbiturates, estrogen, lithium, phenothiazines, and thyroid-stimulating hormone.
- Drugs that may *decrease* uptake: antihistamines, antithyroid drugs, corticosteroids, corticotropin, Lugol's solution, nitrates, potassium iodine, thyroid drugs, tolbutamide.

STOP CONTRAINDICATIONS

- Pregnant women (*Caution:* A woman in her childbearing years should undergo radiography only during her menses or 12 to 14 days after its onset to avoid any exposure to a fetus.)
- Patients who are lactating
- Patients who are allergic to iodine, shellfish, or contrast medium
- Patients who are unable to cooperate because of age, mental status, pain, or other factors

Pre-Test Nursing Care

- Explain to the patient the purpose of the test. Provide any written teaching materials available on the subject. Note that discomfort involved with this test is primarily owing to lying on a hard table for an extended period of time and the needle puncture. Reassure the patient that only trace amounts of the radionuclide are involved in the test.
- The patient must remain still while the scan is being performed.
- Fasting for 8 hours is required before the test by some laboratories.
- Obtain a signed informed consent.

R

Procedure

- Oral or intravenous radioactive iodine is administered.
- The patient is assisted to a supine position on the examination table.
- A scintillation camera is positioned over the patient's thyroid. This camera takes a radioactivity reading from the body. This information is transformed into a two-dimensional picture of the skeleton.
- Scanning is done at 6 hours and again at 24 hours.
- Gloves are worn during the radionuclide injection.

Post-Test Nursing Care

- Check the injection site for redness or swelling.
- If a woman who is lactating *must* have a nuclear scan, she should not breast feed the infant until the radionuclide has been eliminated, possibly for 3 days.
- Although the amount of diagnostic radionuclide excreted in the urine is low, the urine should not be used for any laboratory tests for the time period indicated by the nuclear medicine department. Clients should be told to flush the toilet three times after voiding.
- Gloves are worn when dealing with the urine.
- No other radionuclide tests should be scheduled for 24–48 hours.
- Encourage fluid intake by the patient to enhance excretion of the radionuclide.
- Report abnormal findings to the primary care provider.

• • • • • • • • • • • • • • • • •

Red Blood Cell Count
(erythrocyte count, RBC count)

The red blood cell (RBC) count is a measure of the number of red blood cells (erythrocytes) per cubic millimeter (mm^3) of blood. Red blood cells, which have a lifespan of 80–120 days, are produced by the bone marrow. These cells are important for the oxygen they carry on their hemoglobin molecules.

RBC production is stimulated by erythropoietin, a hormone secreted by the kidney. The amount of erythropoietin secreted increases whenever tissue hypoxia occurs. Such hypoxia occurs in individuals living at high altitudes. The result is the production of an increased number of red blood cells; this is known as *polycythemia*. If the number of red blood cells is decreased at least 10% below normal, the condition is known as *anemia*. There are several different types of anemia, with additional testing needed to differentiate among the various types.

Normal Values

4.15–4.90 × 10^6/mm^3 (4.15–4.90 × 10^{12}/L, SI units)

Pregnancy: Slightly decreased

R

Possible Meanings of Abnormal Values

Increased	Decreased
Cardiovascular disease	Addison's disease
Chronic lung diseases	Anemias
Congenital heart defects	Bone marrow suppression
Cushing's disease	Chronic infection
Hemoconcentration	Hemodilution
Hepatic cancer	Hodgkin's disease
Polycythemia vera	Hypothyroidism
Renal cyst	Leukemia
Secondary polycythemia	Multiple myeloma
	Rheumatic fever
	Subacute bacterial endocarditis
	Systemic lupus erythematosus
	Vitamin deficiency (B_6, B_{12}, folic acid)

Contributing Factors to Abnormal Values

- Hemolysis of the sample may alter test results.
- Factors that might alter test results include: age, altitude, exercise, posture, and pregnancy.
- False low results have occurred in the presence of cold agglutinins.
- Drugs that might *increase* RBC count: gentamicin, methyldopa.
- Drugs that might *decrease* RBC count: acetaminophen, aminosalicylic acid, ampicillin, antineoplastic agents, chloramphenicol, indomethacin, isoniazid, methyldopa, phenobarbital, phenytoin, rifampin, tetracyclines, thiazide diuretics, tolbutamide, vitamin A.

Pre-Test Nursing Care

- Explain to the patient the purpose of the test and the need for a blood sample to be drawn.
- No fasting is required before the test.

Procedure

- The 7-mL blood sample is drawn in a collection tube containing EDTA.
- Gloves are worn throughout the procedure.

Post-Test Nursing Care

- Invert and gently mix the sample with the anticoagulant.
- Apply pressure at venipuncture site. Apply dressing, periodically assessing for continued bleeding.
- Label the specimen and transport it to the laboratory.
- Report abnormal findings to the primary care provider.
- Instruct patients diagnosed with polycythemia vera to maintain physical activity. The purpose of this activity is to prevent venous stasis with resultant venous thrombosis. This can occur because of the relative "thickness" of the blood in these patients.

• • • • • • • • • • • • • •

R

Red Blood Cell Distribution Width
(RDW)

The red blood cell distribution width (RDW) is calculated by machine from the mean corpuscular volume (MCV) and the red blood cell count. It is a quantitative measure of anisocytosis, a condition in which the red blood cells are unequal in size. This assists in distinguishing iron deficiency anemia from thalassemia. Both conditions have a low MCV; however, iron deficiency anemia has a high RDW, whereas thalassemia has a normal RDW. The RDW may become abnormal before the anemia occurs.

Normal Values

11.5%–14.5%

Possible Meanings of Abnormal Values

Increased	Decreased
Folic acid deficiency anemia	Alcohol abuse
Iron deficiency anemia	
Pernicious anemia	
Sickle cell anemia	

Contributing Factors to Abnormal Values

- Hemolysis of the sample may alter test results.

Pre-Test Nursing Care

- Explain to the patient the purpose of the test and the need for a blood sample to be drawn.
- No fasting is required before the test.

Procedure

- The 5-mL sample is drawn in a collection tube containing EDTA.
- Gloves are worn throughout the procedure.

Post-Test Nursing Care

- Invert and gently mix the sample and the anticoagulant.
- Apply pressure at venipuncture site. Apply dressing, periodically assessing for continued bleeding.
- Label the specimen and transport it to the laboratory.
- Report abnormal findings to the primary care provider.

• • • • • • • • • • • • • •

R

Red Blood Cell Indices

(Blood Indices, Mean Corpuscular Hemoglobin [MCH], Mean Corpuscular Hemoglobin Concentration [MCHC], Mean Corpuscular Volume [MCV], RBC Indices)

The red blood cell indices are the mean corpuscular hemoglobin (MCH), the mean corpuscular hemoglobin concentration (MCHC), and the mean corpuscular volume (MCV). The indices are used to determine whether the red blood cells are normal in size and whether they contain an appropriate amount of hemoglobin. The indices are calculated using three measurements of the red blood cells: hematocrit, hemoglobin, and red blood cell count.

$$\textbf{MCH} = \frac{\text{Hgb (g/100 mL)} \times 10}{\text{RBC (millions/mm}^3)}$$

$$\textbf{MCHC (in \%)} = \frac{\text{Hgb (g/100 mL)} \times 100}{\text{Hct}}$$

$$\textbf{MCV} = \frac{\text{Hct (\%)} \times 10}{\text{RBC (millions/mm}^3)}$$

Normal Values

MCH	28–33 pg/cell	(28–33 pg/cell, SI units)
MCHC	32–36 g/dL (or 32–36%)	(320–360 g/L, SI units)
MCV	86–98 mcg^3	(86–98 fL, SI units)

Possible Meanings of Abnormal Values

Mean Corpuscular Hemoglobin (MCH)

Increased	Decreased
Macrocytic anemias: aplastic, hemolytic, pernicious	Hypochromic anemia (hemoglobin deficiency)
Macrocytic cells with overabundance of hemoglobin	Lead poisoning
	Microcytic anemia: Iron deficiency anemia
	Thalassemia

Mean Corpuscular Hemoglobin Concentration (MCHC)

Increased	Decreased
	Hypochromic anemia
	Iron deficiency anemia

R

Mean Corpuscular Volume (MCV)

Increased	Decreased
Chronic alcohol abuse	Irradiation
Chronic liver disease	Lead poisoning
Folic acid deficiency	Malignancies
Hypothyroidism	Microcytic anemia: iron
Macrocytic anemia: aplastic,	deficiency
hemolytic, pernicious	Rheumatoid arthritis
Vitamin B_{12} deficiency	Thalassemia

Contributing Factors to Abnormal Values

- False elevations of MCH and MCHC may occur with high heparin blood concentration.
- False elevations of MCH may occur with hyperlipidemia.
- Drugs that may *increase* MCV: antimetabolites, estrogens, phenytoin.

Pre-Test Nursing Care

- Explain to the patient the purpose of the test and the need for a blood sample to be drawn.
- No fasting is required before the test.

Procedure

- The 7-mL sample is drawn in a collection tube containing EDTA.
- Gloves are worn throughout the procedure.

Post-Test Nursing Care

- Invert and gently mix the sample and the anticoagulant.
- Apply pressure at venipuncture site. Apply dressing, periodically assessing for continued bleeding.
- Label the specimen and transport it to the laboratory.
- Report abnormal findings to the primary care provider.

• • • • • • • • • • • • • • • • •

Red Blood Cell Survival Study
(Cr–51 [Chromium] Red Cell Survival, RBC Survival Study)

R ed blood cells normally remain in circulation until their natural death at the end of their expected lifespan. However, in hemolytic diseases, red blood cell death occurs earlier than normal. The red blood cell survival study involves labeling a sample of the patient's red blood cells with radioactive chromium. The labeled cells are reinjected into the patient and then monitored every 3 days for several weeks through blood sampling. Scanning of the precordium, liver, spleen, and sacrum is also performed at the same intervals to find where the cells are being sequestered.

R

Normal Values

Tagged Cr-51 red cell half-life: 25–35 days
Gamma camera scan: Slight radioactivity in the spleen, liver, and bone marrow

Possible Meanings of Abnormal Values

Decreased

Chronic lymphocytic leukemia
Congenital nonspherocytic hemolytic anemia
Elliptocytosis
Hemoglobin C disease
Hereditary spherocytosis
Idiopathic acquired hemolytic anemia
Paroxysmal nocturnal hemoglobinuria
Pernicious anemia
Sickle cell anemia
Sickle cell hemoglobin C disease
Uremia

Contributing Factors to Abnormal Values

- Any movement by the patient may alter quality of films taken.
- Red blood cell survival may be *decreased* by recent blood transfusion, increased red blood cell production, active bleeding, leukocytosis, and thrombocytosis.

CONTRAINDICATIONS

- Pregnant women (*Caution:* A woman in her childbearing years should undergo radiography only during her menses or 12–14 days after its onset to avoid any exposure to a fetus.)
- Patients who are lactating
- Patients who are allergic to iodine, shellfish, or contrast medium
- Patients with bleeding disorders
- Patients who are unable to cooperate because of age, mental status, pain, or other factors

Pre-Test Nursing Care

- Explain to the patient the purpose of the test. Provide any written teaching materials available on the subject. Note that the only discomfort involved with this test is owing to the venipunctures. Reassure the patient that only trace amounts of the radionuclide are involved in the test.
- The patient must remain still while the scan is being performed.
- No fasting is required before the test.

R

Procedure

- A 30-mL blood sample is drawn and mixed and with 100 microcuries of Cr-51 (sodium chromate).
- The mixture is allowed to incubate overnight, and is then returned to the patient via an intravenous injection.

- A 6-mL blood sample is drawn in a collection tube containing EDTA. This is for baseline measurement of blood and red cell volumes.
- Another 6-mL blood sample is drawn 24 hours later in a collection tube containing heparin. Additional samples are drawn at 3-day intervals for 3–4 weeks.
- At the time each sample is drawn, gamma camera scans of the precordium, liver, spleen, and sacrum are also done to assess for red blood sequestration.
- Gloves are worn during the radionuclide injection and blood sampling.

Post-Test Nursing Care

- Check the injection site for redness or swelling.
- If a woman who is lactating *must* have a nuclear scan, she should not breast feed the infant until the radionuclide has been eliminated, possibly 3 days.
- Although the amount of diagnostic radionuclide excreted in the urine is low, the urine should not be used for any laboratory tests for the time period indicated by the nuclear medicine department. Clients should be told to flush the toilet three times after voiding.
- Gloves are worn when dealing with the urine.
- Encourage fluid intake by the patient to enhance excretion of the radionuclide.
- No other radionuclide tests should be scheduled for 24–48 hours.
- Label each specimen and transport to the laboratory.
- Report abnormal findings to the primary care provider.

Renal Angiography
(Renal Arteriography)

Angiography is a general term used to indicate visualization of any blood vessels, whether they are arteries or veins. The more precise term for visualization of the arteries is *arteriography*. Arteriograms are extremely valuable for observing the blood flow to a part of the body and to detect lesions that may be amenable to surgical treatment. The purposes of renal angiography are to visualize the renal parenchyma and renal vasculature, to evaluate chronic renal disease, renal failure, and transplant donors and recipients, and to conduct post-transplant evaluation of the kidney.

Normal Values

Normal renal vasculature

Possible Meanings of Abnormal Values

Chronic pyelonephritis
Intrarenal hematoma
Renal abscess
Renal arteriovenous fistula
Renal artery aneurysms
Renal artery dysplasia
Renal artery stenosis
Renal cysts

R

Renal infarction
Renal parenchymal laceration
Renal tumors

Contributing Factors to Abnormal Values

- Any movement by the patient may alter quality of films taken.
- Bowel gas, stool, or retained barium from previous exams will hinder test results.

CONTRAINDICATIONS

- Patients who are allergic to iodine, shellfish, or contrast medium dye
- Patients with bleeding disorders
- Pregnant women (*Caution:* A woman in her childbearing years should undergo radiography only during her menses or 12–14 days after its onset to avoid any exposure to a fetus.)
- Patients who are unable to cooperate because of age, mental status, pain, or other factors
- Patients with renal failure or those susceptible to dye-induced renal failure (dehydrated patients)

Pre-Test Nursing Care

- Explain to the patient the purpose of the test. Provide any written teaching materials available on the subject. Note that discomfort involved with this test is primarily owing to lying on a hard table for an extended period of time and the needle puncture. Explain that during injection of the contrast dye, the patient may experience flushing, burning, and nausea.
- Check for allergies to iodine, shellfish, or contrast medium dye. Inform the radiologist of such possible allergy and obtain order for an antihistamine and corticosteroid to be administered before the test.
- Patients receiving metformin (Glucophage) for non–insulin dependent diabetes mellitus should discontinue the drug 2 days before elective surgery or angiographic exams. This is owing to the possible occurrence of lactic acidosis, a potentially fatal complication of biguanide therapy.
- Baseline laboratory data (CBC, PT, PTT) are obtained.
- Note any medications, such as anticoagulants or aspirin, which may prolong bleeding.
- Fasting for at least 8 hours is required before the test.
- Obtain a signed informed consent.
- Administer any pretest sedation after consent form is signed.
- Assess and document patient's peripheral pulses bilaterally before the test. Mark the location of the pulses with a marking pen.

Procedure

- The patient is assisted to a supine position on the examination table.
- A maintenance intravenous line is initiated.
- Resuscitation and suctioning equipment should be available.
- The femoral site is cleansed and then anesthetized.
- The femoral artery is punctured and a catheter is introduced and advanced to the aorta. A test bolus of contrast dye is give to determine the position of the renal arteries.
- The catheter is then replaced with a renal catheter and the contrast dye is injected through the catheter directly into the aorta near the bifurcation of the renal arteries.

R

- Radiographic films are taken.
- After films of satisfactory quality are obtained, the catheter is removed and pressure held on the puncture site for at least 15 minutes.
- Gloves are worn throughout the procedure.

Post-Test Nursing Care

Possible complications:

Allergic reaction to dye
Arterial occlusion owing to disruption of arteriosclerotic plaque or dissection of arterial lining
Bleeding at puncture site
Cardiac arrhythmias
Hypotension from a decrease in renin formation during the test
Infection at the puncture site
Renal failure

- Most allergic reactions to radiopaque dye occur within 30 minutes of administration of the contrast medium. Observe the patient closely for respiratory distress, hypotension, edema, hives, rash, tachycardia, and/or laryngeal stridor. Emergency resuscitation equipment must be readily accessible.
- A pressure dressing is applied to the puncture site. Check the dressing for bleeding and the area around the puncture site for swelling at frequent intervals.
- The patient is to remain on bedrest for 6–12 hours with the affected extremity immobilized.
- Maintain pressure on the puncture site with a sandbag.
- Monitor vital signs every 15 minutes for 1 hour, then every 30 minutes for 2 hours, then every hour for 4 hours, and then every 4 hours.
- Monitor urinary output.
- Assess the color, movement, temperature, and sensation (CMTS) and the pulse(s) of the affected extremity with each vital sign check. Compare with the other extremity.
- Encourage fluid intake to promote dye excretion.
- Renal function should be assessed before metformin is restarted.
- Report abnormal findings to the primary care provider.

Renal Biopsy
(Kidney Biopsy)

Renal biopsy, in which a sample of renal tissue is obtained for histologic study, is used to aid in the diagnosis of renal parenchymal disease. The tissue sample may be obtained by percutaneous needle biopsy through the skin, or by open biopsy through a surgical incision. This discussion will be limited to that of needle biopsy of the kidney.

Renal biopsy can be used in the diagnosis of such conditions as glomerulonephritis, pyelonephritis, and systemic lupus erythematosus. However, because of the risk of damage to the kidney tissue and the availability of alternative diagnostic tests such as ultrasonography and computed tomography (CT), the use of renal biopsy is decreasing among practitioners.

R

Normal Values

No abnormal cells or tissue present

Possible Meanings of Abnormal Values

Acute glomerulonephritis
Amyloid infiltration
Chronic glomerulonephritis
Disseminated lupus erythematosus
Pyelonephritis
Rejection of kidney transplant
Renal cell carcinoma
Renal vein thrombosis
Wilms' tumor

CONTRAINDICATIONS

- Patients with bleeding disorders
- Patients with renal tumors, hydronephrosis, perinephric abscess, or advanced renal failure with uremia
- Patients with severe hypertension
- Patients with only one kidney
- Patients unable to cooperate with the examination

Pre-Test Nursing Care

- Explain to the patient the purpose of the test and the procedure to be done. Explain to the patient that a local anesthetic will be used. Transient pain may occur as the needle enters the kidney.
- Obtain baseline chest x-ray and coagulation tests (partial thromboplastin time, platelet count, prothrombin time).
- Fasting for 8 hours is required before the test.
- Obtain a signed informed consent.
- Obtain baseline vital signs.

Procedure

- The patient is assisted to a prone position with a sandbag beneath the abdomen to shift the kidneys to a posterior position.
- The skin is cleansed with an antiseptic and draped.
- A local anesthetic is administered.
- The patient is instructed to hold his breath as the biopsy needle is inserted through the back muscles, and into the kidney capsule. The patient may then exhale.
- The specimen is obtained and the needle removed.
- Pressure is exerted on the biopsy site for 5–20 minutes, followed by application of a sterile pressure dressing.
- Gloves are worn throughout the procedure.

R

Post-Test Nursing Care

Possible complications:
> **Bleeding**
> **Infection**
> **Punctured liver, lung, bowel, aorta, or inferior vena cava**

- Send the specimen to the laboratory immediately.
- Assist the patient into a supine position. Bedrest is to be maintained for at least 12–24 hours to prevent bleeding.
- Monitor the patient's vital signs and comfort level, and check the dressing for drainage every 15 minutes for 4 hours, then every 30 minutes for 4 hours, then every hour for 4 hours, and finally, every 4 hours.
- Administer analgesics as needed.
- Encourage fluid intake. Monitor output, observing all urine for frank bleeding.
- Strenuous activity should be avoided for at least 2 weeks after the procedure.
- Observe for indications of hemorrhage: decreased blood pressure, increased pulse, pallor, backache, flank pain, shoulder pain, and lightheadedness.
- Observe for signs of punctured bowel or liver: abdominal pain or tenderness, muscle guarding and rigidity, and decreased bowel sounds.
- Report abnormal findings to the primary care provider.

• • • • • • • • • • • • • • • •

Renal Function Tests

See:
Creatinine, Blood
Creatinine Clearance
Creatinine, Urine
Osmolality, Blood
Osmolality, Urine
Urea nitrogen, Blood
Uric acid, Blood
Uric acid, Urine

• • • • • • • • • • • • • • • •

Renal Scan
(Kidney Scan)

R

The renal scan is used to study the kidneys and ureters through the scanning and recording of the dispersion, clearance, and excretion of a radionuclide. This test is used to detect renal infarction, renal arterial atherosclerosis, renal trauma, renal tumors and cysts, and primary renal disease, such as glomerulonephritis. It is also used to monitor renal transplant rejection and to detect urologic problems in patients who are unable to have intravenous pyelography owing to allergies to contrast dye.

Normal Values

Normal size, shape, and function of the kidney.

Possible Meanings of Abnormal Values

Acute tubular necrosis
Congenital abnormalities
Excretory defects
Glomerulonephritis
Nephroureteral dilation
Pyelonephritis
Renal abscess
Renal cyst
Renal infarction
Renal ischemia
Renal obstruction
Renal transplant rejection
Renal tumor
Renovascular hypertension

Contributing Factors to Abnormal Values

- Any movement by the patient may alter quality of films taken.
- Presence of contrast material from previous exams may interfere with the test.

CONTRAINDICATIONS

- Pregnant women (*Caution:* A woman in her childbearing years should undergo radiography only during her menses or 12–14 days after its onset to avoid any exposure to a fetus.)
- Patients who are lactating
- Patients who are unable to cooperate because of age, mental status, pain, or other factors

Pre-Test Nursing Care

- Explain to the patient the purpose of the test. Provide any written teaching materials available on the subject. Note that discomfort involved with this test is primarily owing to lying on a hard table for an extended period of time and the needle puncture. Reassure the patient that only trace amounts of the radionuclide are involved in the test.
- The patient must remain still while the scan is being performed.
- No fasting is required before the test. The patient needs to be well hydrated.
- Obtain a signed informed consent.

Procedure

- The radiopharmaceutical is administered by intravenous injection in a peripheral vein.
- The patient is assisted to a supine position on the examination table.
- A scintillation camera is positioned over the right upper quadrant of the patient's abdomen. This camera takes a radioactivity reading from the body. This information is transformed into a two-dimensional picture of the area.

R

- Scans are obtained to record the passing of the radionuclide through the cortex and pelvis of each kidney.
- Gloves are worn during the radionuclide injection.

Post-Test Nursing Care

- Check the injection site for redness or swelling.
- If a woman who is lactating *must* have a nuclear scan, she should not breast feed the infant until the radionuclide has been eliminated, possibly for 3 days.
- Although the amount of diagnostic radionuclide excreted in the urine is low, the urine should not be used for any laboratory tests for the time period indicated by the nuclear medicine department. Clients should be told to flush the toilet three times after voiding.
- Gloves are worn when dealing with the urine.
- Encourage fluid intake by the patient to enhance excretion of the radionuclide.
- Report abnormal findings to the primary care provider.

• • • • • • • • • • • • • • • • •

Renin Activity, Plasma
(PRA, Plasma Renal Assay)

Renin is an enzyme that is produced, stored, and released by the juxtaglomerular cells of the kidneys. It is released in response to a decrease in blood flow through the kidneys. Changes in position from recumbent to upright have also been found to increase the renin level. Sodium intake also influences renin levels: high sodium intake decreases renin levels, while sodium depletion causes increased levels of renin to be released.

Renin plays a vital role in the regulation of blood pressure and fluid and electrolyte balance via the renin-angiotensin-aldosterone system. (See "Aldosterone" for diagram of this system.)

The measurement of plasma renin activity is used in the differential diagnosis of hypertension. Hypertensive patients who have low renin activity probably have a fluid volume imbalance, whereas those with high renin activity probably are hypertensive because of the vasoconstrictive effects of angiotensin, a condition known as *renovascular hypertension*.

In addition to plasma renin activity, renal vein assays for renin may be used to diagnose renovascular hypertension. For this test, which is done in the radiology department, a catheter is placed into each renal vein via the femoral vein. A sample of blood is taken from each renal vein and the inferior vena cava. The renal venous renin ratio, which is the renin level in the renal vein compared to the level in the inferior vena cava is <1.5:1.

Normal Values

Normal Salt Intake

Recumbent 6 hours: 0.5–1.6 ng/mL/hr	(0.5–1.6 µg/L/hr, SI units)
Upright 4 hours: 1.9–3.6 ng/mL/hr	(1.9–3.6 µg/L/hr, SI units)

Low Salt Intake

Recumbent 6 hours: 2.2–4.4 ng/mL/hr	(2.2–4.4 µg/L/hr, SI units)
Upright 4 hours: 4.0–8.1 ng/mL/hr	(4.0–8.1 µg/L/hr, SI units)
Upright 4 hours, with diuretic: 6.8–15.0 ng/mL/hr	(6.8–15.0 µg/L/hr, SI units)

R

Possible Meanings of Abnormal Values

Increased	Decreased
Addison's disease	Cushing's syndrome
Bartter's syndrome (renin-producing renal tumors)	Elderly
	Essential hypertension
Chronic renal failure	High-sodium diet
Cirrhosis	Licorice ingestion
Erect posture for 4 hours	Primary hyperaldosteronism
Hemorrhage	
Hypokalemia	
Hypovolemia	
Low-sodium diet	
Malignant hypertension	
Menstruation	
Nephropathy	
Pheochromocytoma	
Pregnancy	
Renal hypertension	
Secondary hyperaldosteronism	
Transplant rejection	

Contributing Factors to Abnormal Values

- The patient's position and diet may alter test results.
- Drugs that may *increase* plasma renin activity: antihypertensives, diazoxide, estrogens, furosemide, guanethidine sulfate, hydralazine hydrochloride, minoxidil, nitroprusside, oral contraceptives, spironolactone, thiazides.
- Drugs that may *decrease* plasma renin activity: clonidine hydrochloride, desmopressin acetate, lypressin, methyldopa, propranolol hydrochloride, reserpine, sodium-retaining steroids, vasopressin.

Pre-Test Nursing Care

- Explain to the patient the purpose of the test and the need for a blood sample to be drawn.
- Unless otherwise ordered, instruct the patient to follow a 3-gram sodium diet for at least 2 weeks before the test. Explain to the patient that this is considered "normal" sodium intake.
- Fasting for 8 hours is required before the test.
- If possible, drugs that may affect test results should be withheld for at least 2 weeks before the test.

Procedure

- A 7-mL blood sample is drawn in a collection tube containing EDTA that has been chilled before use.
- Gloves are worn throughout the procedure.

R

Post-Test Nursing Care

- Apply pressure at venipuncture site. Apply dressing, periodically assessing for continued bleeding.
- The tube should be tilted several times to mix the blood with the anticoagulant.
- Label the specimen, place it on ice and transport it immediately to the laboratory. The position of the patient during the blood sampling should be included on the laboratory slip.
- Report abnormal findings to the primary care provider.

• • • • • • • • • • • • • • • • • •

Reticulocyte Count
(Retic Count)

A reticulocyte is a less mature type of red blood cell. It gets its name from the fine network, or reticulum, which becomes visible on its surface when stained. After 1 to 4 days in the bloodstream, the reticulocyte becomes a mature red blood cell. The reticulocyte count provides data regarding the rate of red blood cell production, and thus, bone marrow function. The test is used in the differential diagnosis of anemia.

Normal Values

0.5%–2.5% red cells   (0.005–0.025 red cells, SI units)
Pregnancy: Slightly increased

Possible Meanings of Abnormal Values

Increased	Decreased
Acute blood loss	Alcoholism
After iron therapy for iron deficiency anemia	Aplastic anemia
Folic acid deficiency	Chronic infection
Hemolytic anemia	Cirrhosis of the liver
Leukemia	Iron deficiency anemia
Metastatic cancer	Irradiation
Polycythemia	Myxedema
Pregnancy	Pernicious anemia
Sickle cell anemia	
Thalassemia major	
Vitamin B_{12} deficiency	

Contributing Factors to Abnormal Values

- Hemolysis of the sample may alter test results.
- Falsely decreased values may occur after blood transfusions.
- Hemodilution of the sample, owing to drawing the blood from the arm in which an IV is infusing, may alter test results.

R

Pre-Test Nursing Care
- Explain to the patient the purpose of the test and the need for a blood sample to be drawn.
- No fasting is required before the test.

Procedure
- A 7-mL blood sample is drawn in a collection tube containing EDTA.
- Do not leave the tourniquet in place more than 1 minute.
- Gloves are worn throughout the procedure.

Post-Test Nursing Care
- Invert and gently mix the sample with the anticoagulant.
- Apply pressure at venipuncture site. Apply dressing, periodically assessing for continued bleeding.
- Label the specimen and transport it to the laboratory.
- Report abnormal findings to the primary care provider.

• • • • • • • • • • • • • • • •

Retrograde Pyelography
(Pyelography)

Retrograde pyelography is used to confirm findings found via excretory urography. The test involves examination of the kidneys using a contrast dye that is injected in a retrograde fashion. During a cystoscopic examination, a catheter is advanced through the ureters and into the pelvis of the kidney. The renal pelvis is drained, and then a radiopaque iodine-based contrast medium is injected through the catheter into the kidney. The incidence of allergic reaction to the dye is reduced, since the dye is usually not absorbed when administered in this way. Radiographic films are taken throughout the procedure.

Normal Values
Normal size, shape, position of kidneys, ureters, and bladder.

Possible Meanings of Abnormal Values
Bladder tumor
Congenital abnormalities
Hydronephrosis
Polycystic kidney disease
Prostatic enlargement
Renal calculi
Renal cysts
Renal tumor
Trauma
Ureteral calculi

R

Contributing Factors to Abnormal Values

- Retained barium, gas, or stool in the intestines may result in poor quality films.
- Any movement by the patient may alter quality of films taken.

CONTRAINDICATIONS

- Patients who are allergic to iodine, shellfish, or contrast medium dye
- Pregnant women (*Caution:* A woman in her childbearing years should undergo radiography only during her menses or 12–14 days after its onset to avoid any exposure to a fetus.)
- Patients who are unable to cooperate because of age, mental status, pain, or other factors
- Patients with renal failure or those susceptible to dye-induced renal failure (dehydrated patients)

Pre-Test Nursing Care

- Explain to the patient the purpose of the test. Provide any written teaching materials available on the subject. Note that this test is uncomfortable owing to the pressure experienced during injection of the dye.
- Check for allergies to iodine, shellfish, or contrast medium dye. Inform the radiologist of such possible allergy and obtain order for an antihistamine and corticosteroid to be administered prior to the test.
- Patients receiving metformin (Glucophage) for non–insulin-dependent diabetes mellitus should discontinue the drug 2 days before elective surgery or angiographic exams. This is owing to the possible occurrence of lactic acidosis, a potentially fatal complication of biguanide therapy.
- Obtain a signed informed consent.
- Fasting for 8 hours is required before the test. The patient should be well hydrated before the beginning of the fasting period.
- A laxative the night before the test, or an enema or suppository the morning of the test may be ordered.
- Pre-procedure sedation may be ordered.
- If barium studies are also ordered, they are to be performed *after* the retrograde pyelography has been successfully completed.
- Resuscitation and suctioning equipment should be readily available.

Procedure

- The patient is placed in a dorsal lithotomy position. The test is usually performed during a cystoscopic examination in the surgical department.
- A catheter is advanced through the ureters and into the pelvis of each kidney.
- After draining the pelvis of each kidney, a radiopaque iodine-based contrast medium is injected through the catheter into each kidney.
- Radiographic films are taken throughout the procedure.
- Additional contrast dye may be instilled as the catheters are being removed from the ureters to allow for films of the ureters to be taken.
- Gloves are worn throughout the procedure.

R

Post-Test Nursing Care

Possible complications:

    Allergic reaction to dye

    Hematuria

    Perforation of ureter or bladder

    Sepsis

    Ureteral edema

    Urinary tract infection

- Most allergic reactions to radiopaque dye occur within 30 minutes of administration of the contrast medium. Observe the patient closely for: respiratory distress, hypotension, edema, hives, rash, tachycardia, and/or laryngeal stridor. Emergency resuscitation equipment must be readily accessible.
- Resume the patient's diet. Encourage fluid intake to decrease any dysuria that might be present.
- Observe for allergic reaction to the dye for 24 hours.
- Monitor vital signs at least every 4 hours for 24 hours.
- Observe for indications of infection, including elevated temperature, chills, flushing, tachycardia, and flank pain.
- Monitor urinary output for at least 24 hours. Assess for bladder distention. Observe the urine for clots or gross hematuria. Pink-tinged urine is expected immediately after the procedure.
- Assess patient for discomfort, since bladder spasms may occur. If present, they are often treated with belladonna and opium (B & O) suppositories.
- Renal function should be assessed before metformin is restarted.
- Report abnormal findings to the primary care provider.

• • • • • • • • • • • • • • • •

Rheumatoid Factor
(RF, Rheumatoid Arthritis Factor)

Rheumatoid arthritis (RA) is a chronic progressive inflammatory condition of the connective tissue which mainly affects the small, peripheral joints such as the fingers and wrists. Although the joint destruction is most often thought of when mentioning RA, it is a systemic disease that can affect other systems of the body as well. An autoimmune reaction occurs in the synovial tissue, leading to pain, swelling, warmth, erythema, and lack of function in the affected joint. During the inflammatory process, antibodies team up with corresponding antigens to form immune complexes. These complexes are deposited in the synovial tissue, triggering the inflammatory reaction that leads to the damage seen in the joints of patients with rheumatoid arthritis.

One of the diagnostic tests for rheumatoid arthritis is the rheumatoid factor (RF) test. RF, an immunoglobulin, is present in more than 80% of patients with rheumatoid arthritis; however, a positive RF test can also occur in many other diseases. The antibody, which is produced by the synovium, appears in autoimmune and connective tissue diseases, and in chronic infections.

R

Normal Values

Qualitative: Negative
Quantitative: <30 IU/mL (<30 kIU/L, SI units)
                       or titer < 1:20

Possible Meanings of Abnormal Values

Increased

Allografts (skin, kidneys)
Ankylosing spondylitis
Cancer
Cirrhosis
Cryoglobulinemia
Cytomegalovirus
Dermatomyositis
Diabetes mellitus
Hypertension
Infectious mononucleosis
Influenza
Kidney disease
Leprosy
Liver disease
Lung disease
Osteoarthritis
Periodontal disease
Pulmonary interstitial disease
Rheumatoid arthritis
Rubella
Sarcoidosis
Scleroderma
Sjögren's syndrome
Subacute bacterial endocarditis
Syphilis
Systemic lupus erythematosus
Tuberculosis
Viral infections

Contributing Factors to Abnormal Values

- *False-positive* RF results may occur in the elderly and in individuals who have received numerous vaccinations and/or blood transfusions.
- Aspirin and nonsteroidal anti-inflammatory drugs do *not* interfere with testing for rheumatoid factor.

Pre-Test Nursing Care

- Explain to the patient the purpose of the test and the need for a blood sample to be drawn.
- No fasting is required before the test.

Procedure

- A 7-mL blood sample is drawn in a collection tube containing either no additives or a silicone gel.
- Gloves are worn throughout the procedure.

Post-Test Nursing Care

- Apply pressure at venipuncture site. Apply dressing, periodically assessing for continued bleeding.
- Label the specimen and transport it to the laboratory.
- Report abnormal findings to the primary care provider.

• • • • • • • • • • • • • • • • •

Rubella Antibody Titer
(German Measles Test, Hemagglutination Inhibition [HAI or HI] Test)

Rubella, also known as the German measles or 3-day measles, is a virus that is not usually considered a serious condition. It usually causes fever and transient rash in children and adults who contract it. Rubella is serious, however, if a woman contracts the disease during the first trimester of pregnancy. It can cause miscarriage, stillbirth, and congenital defects. Thus, it is extremely important for women considering pregnancy to be tested for susceptibility or immunity to rubella.

The rubella antibody titer test measures IgG and IgM antibody formation against the rubella virus. It can be used to diagnose rubella and to determine whether the person is immune to the virus. The test is also referred to as "hemagglutination inhibition" (HAI or HI), since the resulting antibody titer is the highest dilution of serum that completely inhibits hemagglutination.

Normal Values

Susceptible to rubella:	Titer <1:8
Past rubella exposure:	Titer 1:10–1:32
Immunity to rubella:	Titer >1:32

Abnormal Values

A diagnosis of rubella is made when a fourfold increase between the acute titer and the convalescent titer occurs.

Possible Meanings of Abnormal Values

Increased	Decreased
Rubella infection	Susceptible to rubella
Immunity to rubella	

Contributing Factors to Abnormal Values

- Hemolysis due to excessive agitation of the blood sample may alter test results.

R

Pre-Test Nursing Care

- Obtain a history regarding any possible exposure to the rubella virus.
- Explain to the patient the purpose of the test and the need to draw a blood sample.
- No fasting is required before the test.

Procedure

- A 5-mL blood sample is drawn in a collection tube containing no additives.
- If the test is being done to determine presence of immunity to rubella, only one sample is needed.
- If the test is being used to diagnose rubella, one blood sample is obtained 3 days after the onset of the rash. This is called the "acute titer." A second sample, the "convalescent titer" is drawn 2–3 weeks later.
- Gloves are worn throughout the procedure.

Post-Test Nursing Care

- Apply pressure at venipuncture site. Apply dressing, periodically assessing for continued bleeding.
- Label the specimen and transport it to the laboratory.
- Report abnormal findings to the primary care provider.
- If the test results indicate susceptibility to the rubella virus, the woman should be counseled to be immunized. However, she must also be instructed that pregnancy must be avoided for 3 months after the immunization.
- If the test results indicate susceptibility to the rubella virus and the woman is already pregnant, she must be instructed to avoid exposure to the disease.

• • • • • • • • • • • • • • • • •

Schilling Test
(Vitamin B₁₂ Absorption Test)

The Schilling test is used to evaluate the ability of the small intestine to absorb vitamin B_{12}. When vitamin B_{12} is ingested, it combines with intrinsic factor from the gastric mucosa. It is then able to be absorbed in the ileum.

This test involves the oral administration of radioactive vitamin B_{12}. Nonradioactive vitamin B_{12} is then administered intramuscularly (IM) to saturate the vitamin B_{12} binding sites. A 24-hour urine specimen is collected. Normal patients will absorb and then excrete as much as 25% of the radioactive B_{12}, since they have intrinsic factor and can thus absorb the vitamin from the gastrointestinal tract. Patients who have pernicious anemia, in which intrinsic factor is lacking, absorb little of the oral dose of B_{12}, resulting in little radioactive material being excreted in the urine. If the results of the Schilling test show low absorption of the radioactive vitamin B_{12}, the test is repeated with IM intrinsic factor given to rule out intestinal malabsorption. If the urinary excretion rises to normal levels, there is a lack of intrinsic factor. If urinary excretion remains low, malabsorption is probably the cause of the patient's anemia.

S

Normal Values

Excretion of 7% or more of test dose of radioactive B_{12}

Possible Meanings of Abnormal Values

Decreased

Hypothyroidism
Intestinal malabsorption
Liver disease
Pernicious anemia

Contributing Factors to Abnormal Values

- Receipt of radioactive nuclear material within 10 days of this test may alter test results.
- Conditions that may cause *decreased* excretion: diabetes, elderly, hypothyroidism, renal insufficiency.
- Drugs that may affect test results: laxatives.

 CONTRAINDICATIONS

- Pregnant women (*Caution:* A woman in her childbearing years should undergo radiography only during her menses or 12–14 days after its onset to avoid any exposure to a fetus.)
- Patients who are lactating
- Patients who are unable to cooperate because of age, mental status, pain, or other factors

Pre-Test Nursing Care

- Explain 24-hour urine collection procedure to the patient.
- Stress the importance of saving *all* urine in the 24-hour period. Instruct the patient to avoid contaminating the urine with toilet paper or feces.
- Fasting for 12 hours is required before the test.

Procedure

- A capsule of radioactive vitamin B_{12} is administered orally.
- Next, nonradioactive B_{12} is administered IM to the patient.
- Obtain the proper container containing no preservative from the laboratory.
- Begin the testing period following the patient's first voiding, which is discarded.
- Timing of the 24-hour period begins at the time the first voiding is discarded.
- *All* urine for the next 24 hours is collected in the container, which is to be kept refrigerated or on ice.
- If any urine is accidentally discarded during the 24-hour period, the test must be discontinued and a new test begun.
- The ending time of the 24-hour collection period should be posted in the patient's room.
- Gloves are to be worn whenever dealing with the specimen collection.
- When the absorption of radioactive vitamin B_{12} is low, the test is repeated with IM intrinsic factor to rule out intestinal malabsorption. Another 24-hour urine collection is performed.

S

Post-Test Nursing Care

- Label the container and transport it on ice to the laboratory as soon as possible following the end of the 24-hour collection period.
- Report abnormal findings to the primary care provider.

• • • • • • • • • • • • • • • •

Scrotal Ultrasound
(Ultrasound of Testes)

Ultrasonography is a noninvasive method of diagnostic testing in which ultrasound waves are sent into the body with a small transducer pressed against the skin. The transducer not only sends the sound waves into the body but also receives any returning sound waves, which are deflected back as they bounce off various structures. The transducer converts the returning sound waves into electric signals that are then transformed by a computer into a visual display on a monitor.

With scrotal ultrasound, visualization of the scrotum and its contents is made possible. This test is used to assess for scrotal masses and infections, evaluate scrotal pain and trauma, locate undescended testicles, and provide monitoring of patients with previously diagnosed testicular cancer.

Normal Values

Normal size, shape, and location of testicles.

Possible Meanings of Abnormal Values

Benign testicular tumors
Epididymitis
Hematocele
Hydrocele
Malignant testicular tumors
Orchitis
Pyocele
Scrotal hernia
Spermatocele
Testicular torsion
Undescended testicle
Varicocele

Contributing Factors to Abnormal Values

- The transducer must be in good contact with the skin as it is being moved. A lubricant, such as mineral oil, glycerin, or a water-based jelly, is used to ensure good contact with the skin.

S

Pre-Test Nursing Care

- Explain to the patient the purpose of the test. Provide any written teaching materials available on the subject. Note that there is no discomfort involved with this test.
- No fasting is required before the test.

Procedure

- The patient is assisted to a supine position on the ultrasonography table.
- The scrotum is supported by a towel or held in the examiner's hand.
- A coupling agent, such as a water-based gel, is applied to the area to be evaluated.
- A transducer is placed on the skin and moved as needed to provide good visualization of the scrotal contents.
- The sound waves are transformed into a visual display on the monitor. Printed copies of this display are made.
- Gloves are worn throughout the procedure.

Post-Test Nursing Care

- Cleanse the patient's skin of remaining coupling agent.
- Report abnormal findings to the primary care provider.

• • • • • • • • • • • • • • • •

Semen Analysis
(Seminal Cytology, Sperm Count)

Semen analysis is the most common diagnostic test used in an infertility workup. The analysis includes a sperm count, determination of the percentage of normal sperm and sperm motility, semen volume, and pH. If testing indicates a low sperm count or other abnormalities, a second specimen is usually tested. Abnormal semen analysis may require additional testing.

Normal Values

Volume:	2–5 mL
pH:	7.3–7.8
Color:	Grayish white
Sperm count:	20–250 million/mL
Motility:	> 60%
Normal sperm:	> 60%

Possible Meanings of Abnormal Values

Decreased

Cryptorchidism
Hyperpyrexia
Infertility
Klinefelter's syndrome
Orchitis

S

Testicular atrophy
Testicular failure

Contributing Factors to Abnormal Values

- Drugs that may *decrease* the sperm count: antineoplastic agents, cimetidine, estrogens, keto-conazole, methyltestosterone.

Pre-Test Nursing Care

- Explain to the patient the purpose of the test and the need for a semen specimen.
- Instruct the patient to abstain from sexual intercourse and intake of alcohol for 2–3 days.

Procedure

- Provide a specimen container.
- The best specimen is one collected in the physician's office or laboratory by masturbation.
- If the patient prefers to collect the specimen at home a silastic condom with no lubricant may be used during coitus interruptus.

Post-Test Nursing Care

- The specimen needs to be labeled and delivered to the laboratory within 1 hour of collection.
- Report abnormal findings to the primary care provider.

• • • • • • • • • • • • • • • • •

Sialography

Sialography is the radiographic examination of the salivary ducts. The test is used to identify stones, tumors, strictures, or inflammatory processes of the ducts. Any of the salivary ducts may be studied, including the sublingual, submaxillary, submandibular, and parotid ducts. A baseline x-ray is first taken, followed by insertion of a catheter in the duct to be studied. Contrast dye is injected through the catheter. Films are taken from several views. The patient is then given a sour-tasting drink to stimulate salivation, and additional films are taken.

Normal Values

Normal salivary ducts.

Possible Meanings of Abnormal Values

Calculi
Inflammatory disease
Strictures
Tumors

CONTRAINDICATIONS

- Patients with mouth infections
- Patients with allergies to iodine, shellfish, or contrast media dye

S

Pre-Test Nursing Care

- Explain to the patient the purpose of the test and procedure to be followed. Inform the patient that some discomfort may be felt with insertion of the catheter into the duct.
- Check for allergies to iodine, shellfish, or contrast medium dye. Inform the radiologist of such possible allergy and obtain order for an antihistamine and corticosteroid to be administered prior to the test.
- Patients receiving metformin (Glucophage) for non–insulin-dependent diabetes mellitus should discontinue the drug 2 days before elective surgery or angiographic exams. This is owing to the possible occurrence of lactic acidosis, a potentially fatal complication of biguanide therapy.
- Obtain a signed informed consent.
- No fasting is required before the test.
- Instruct the patient to brush the teeth and rinse the mouth with mouthwash before the test to reduce bacterial flora.

Procedure

- The patient is assist into a supine position on the radiology table.
- A baseline x-ray is taken to assess for presence of a ductal stone, which could prevent dye from entering the duct.
- A catheter is inserted into the duct.
- Contrast dye is injected through the catheter, and x-rays are taken.
- The patient is then given a sour-tasting solution to drink to stimulate salivation.
- Additional x-rays are taken.
- Gloves are worn throughout the procedure.

Post-Test Nursing Care

Possible complication: Allergic reaction to the dye

- Most allergic reactions to radiopaque dye occur within 30 minutes of administration of the contrast medium. Observe the patient closely for respiratory distress, hypotension, edema, hives, rash, tachycardia, and/or laryngeal stridor. Emergency resuscitation equipment must be readily accessible.
- Monitor vital signs until stable.
- Encourage fluid intake to help eliminate dye.
- A mild analgesic may be needed for pain and swelling at the site of the procedure.
- Renal function should be assessed before metformin is restarted.
- Report abnormal findings to the primary care provider.

S

Sickle Cell Test
(Hemoglobin S Test)

S ickle cells are severely deformed erythrocytes, which are sickle or crescent shaped. Sickling of the red blood cells (RBCs) results from a genetic defect in which hemoglobin S (Hgb S) is present on the RBCs rather than hemoglobin A. Individuals who are heterozygous for this gene are considered as having *sickle cell trait*. These individuals have normal red blood cells that can be easily changed to sickled forms by reducing their available oxygen supply, such as occurs at high altitudes. Individuals with *sickle cell disease (sickle cell anemia)* are homozygous for hemoglobin S. These people have spontaneously sickled red blood cells. The abnormally shaped cells are unable to pass through the capillaries and cause plugging of these vessels. This can result in a stoppage of blood supply to certain organs.

In this test, a deoxygenating agent is added to the patient's blood. The red blood cells are then observed to see if sickling occurs, and, if so, how quickly the sickling takes place. If at least 25% of the patient's hemoglobin is Hgb S, the cells will sickle, resulting in a positive test. The test is considered negative when no sickling occurs. The sickle cell test is a screening test only. To diagnose sickle cell anemia, hemoglobin electrophoresis must be done in order to quantify the amount of hemoglobin S that might be present.

Normal Values

Negative; no sickled RBCs present.

Possible Meanings of Abnormal Values

Increased

Sickle cell anemia
Sickle cell trait

Contributing Factors to Abnormal Values

- Hemolysis of the blood sample will alter test results.
- *False-positive* results may be caused by polycythemia or high blood protein levels.
- *False-negative* results may result from having received blood transfusions within the previous 4 months or from phenothiazine therapy.

Pre-Test Nursing Care

- Explain to the patient the purpose of the test and the need for a blood sample to be drawn.
- No fasting is required before the test.

Procedure

- A 7-mL blood sample is drawn in a collection tube containing EDTA.
- Gloves are worn throughout the procedure.

Post-Test Nursing Care

- Apply pressure at venipuncture site. Apply dressing, periodically assessing for continued bleeding.

S

- Label the specimen and transport it to the laboratory.
- Report abnormal findings to the primary care provider.
- Individuals found to have sickle cell disease should be instructed to avoid hypoxic situations, including high altitudes, strenuous activity, extreme cold, and traveling in unpressurized aircraft.

• • • • • • • • • • • • • • •

Sims-Huhner Test
(Cervical Mucus Sperm Penetration Test, Cervical Mucus Test, Fern Test, Postcoital Test)

The Sims-Huhner test is an assessment of the number and motility of the sperm found in the cervical mucus of a woman after intercourse. The test is best performed 1–2 days before ovulation. At that time, two changes occur in the cervical mucus that enhance sperm survival. The elasticity of the cervical mucus, known as *spinnbarkheit (SBK)*, increases. Also, the cervical mucus contains more sodium at that time. This high sodium content can be determined by spreading the cervical mucus on a clean glass slide and allowing it to dry. A pattern of *arborization* or *ferning* occurs, which is the result of the salt and water interacting with mucus glycoproteins. Thus, the presence of excellent SBK and ferning are indications of ovulation.

The Sims-Huhner test involves the collection of an endocervical mucus sample. The total number of sperm and the number of motile sperm are reported. If the number of sperm present is adequate but they are not motile, the cervical environment is unsuitable for their survival. The test is done in conjunction with semen analysis with an infertility workup. The test is also done in suspected rape cases to document the presence of sperm.

Normal Values
Mucus tenacity:	stretches at least 10 cm
Number of motile sperm:	at least 6–20 per high-power field

Possible Meanings of Abnormal Values
Infertility
Suspected rape

Contributing Factors to Abnormal Values
- Cervical mucus specimen must be obtained 2–4 hours after intercourse. Tests results are unreliable when the specimen is collected more than 6 hours after coitus.

Pre-Test Nursing Care
- Explain to the patient the purpose of the test and the need for a cervical mucus sample to be obtained.
- Obtain a signed informed consent if procedure is being done for medicolegal purposes.
- For the test results to be most valid, lubricants are not to be used and the woman must not douche after intercourse.
- In infertility workups, the male should abstain from ejaculation for 3 days before the test.

S

- The female should remain recumbent for 15–30 minutes following intercourse and then undergo testing within 1–5 hours.

Procedure

- The patient is assisted into the lithotomy position with the legs supported in stirrups, and draped for privacy.
- An unlubricated speculum is inserted into the vagina.
- The external cervical os is visualized and wiped clear of mucus.
- The specimen is aspirated from the endocervix.
- Gloves are worn throughout the procedure.
- *Note:* If the procedure is being conducted in the investigation of rape, the specimen collection must be witnessed, and the specimen placed in a sealed plastic bag. The bag is labeled as legal evidence and must be signed by every person handling the specimen.

Post-Test Nursing Care

- Label the specimen and transport it to the laboratory immediately.
- Report abnormal findings to the primary care provider.

• • • • • • • • • • • • • • • • • •

Skeletal X-Ray
(Bone X-ray, Sella Turcica X-ray, Skeletal Radiography, Skull X-ray, Spinal X-ray, Vertebral X-ray)

Radiography is the use of radiation (roentgen rays) to cause some substances to fluoresce and affect photographic plates. X-rays penetrate air easily; therefore, areas filled with air, such as the lungs, appear very dark on the film. Conversely, bones appear almost white on the film because the x-rays cannot penetrate them to reach the x-ray film. Organs and tissues such as the heart appear as shades of gray because they have more mass than air but not as much as bone.

Skeletal radiography involves obtaining x-rays of any bone structure in the body. Examples include the spine or vertebral column, long bones, or the skull. The location of the x-ray may become even more precise, such as when an x-ray of the sella turcica, an area at the base of skull, is ordered.

All x-rays of the skeletal system involve the same basic purposes, preparation, and patient education. They differ in the portion of the body to be studied and the positioning of the patient. The basic principle of position is that the part of the body that needs to be studied should be next to the film.

The purpose of skeletal system radiography is to assess the bones for deformities, fractures, dislocations, tumors, and metabolic abnormalities, such as Paget's disease or osteoporosis. The bones are studied for their density, texture, and any erosion. Joint x-rays can reveal the presence of fluid, spur formation, narrowing, or changes in the joint structure. X-rays of the skull provide valuable information regarding the three groups of bones that comprise the skull (the vault, the mandible, and the facial bones) and possible abnormal contents of the skull, such as pituitary tumors.

S

Normal Values

Normal bone structure, location, and density

Possible Meanings of Abnormal Values

Abnormal growth pattern
Arthritis
Bone metastases
Bone spurring
Cerebral hemorrhage
Degenerative arthritic changes
Fractures
Hematoma
Infection
Joint destruction
Joint effusion
Kyphosis
Osteomyelitis
Pituitary tumor
Primary bone tumor
Scoliosis
Sinusitis
Spondylosis

Contributing Factors to Abnormal Values

- Under- or overexposure of the film may alter film quality.
- When patients are unable to hold still, because of pain or mental status, the quality of the film may be affected.

 CONTRAINDICATIONS

- Pregnant women (*Caution:* A woman in her childbearing years should undergo radiography only during her menses or 12–14 days after its onset to avoid any exposure to a fetus.)

Pre-Test Nursing Care

- Explain to the patient the purpose of the test and the benefits and risks associated with the test. Provide any written teaching materials available on the subject. Note that no discomfort is associated with this procedure.
- No fasting is required before the test.
- Instruct the patient to remove all objects containing metal, such as jewelry or undergarments, as these will show on the film.

Procedure

- The patient's reproductive organs should be covered with a lead apron to prevent unnecessary exposure to radiation.
- Position the patient as ordered. The area to be evaluated must remain motionless during the procedure. Head bands, foam pads, or sandbags may be needed to immobilize the patient's head or extremity being evaluated.

S

Post-Test Nursing Care

- No special physical post-test nursing care is needed.
- Report abnormal findings to the primary care provider.

• • • • • • • • • • • • • • •

Sodium, Blood

O f the electrolytes measured in the blood, sodium (Na⁺) is the highest concentration. It is the major cation in the extracellular fluid (ECF). Sodium plays an important role in acid-base balance and promotes neuromuscular functioning. It maintains an inverse relationship with the potassium level of the blood.

Sodium concentration in the blood is closely related to the fluid balance of the body; in fact, its concentration stimulates the kidneys to compensate for changes in the body's fluid balance. For example, as water in the body increases, the concentration of sodium in the blood decreases. This stimulates the kidneys to compensate through conservation of sodium and excretion of water. This is accomplished through the work of aldosterone. If water in the body decreases, the concentration of sodium in the blood will increase. Antidiuretic hormone (ADH) is then activated, leading to conservation of water.

A decreased level of sodium in the blood is known as *hyponatremia*. Signs of this imbalance include lethargy, confusion, abdominal cramping, apprehension, oliguria, rapid weak pulse, headache, decreased skin turgor, tremors, and possibly seizures and coma. *Hypernatremia* is the term given to blood sodium levels that are above normal. Signs of this imbalance include dry mucus membranes, fever, thirst, and restlessness.

Normal Values

135–145 mEq/L (135–145 mmol/L, SI units)

Possible Meanings of Abnormal Values

Increased (Hypernatremia)	Decreased (Hyponatremia)
Cushing's disease	Acute renal failure
Dehydration	Addison's disease
Diabetes insipidus	Burns (severe)
Exchange transfusion with	Chronic renal failure
stored blood	Cirrhosis
Impaired renal function	Congestive heart failure
Overuse of IV saline solutions	Diabetic acidosis
Primary aldosteronism	Diaphoresis
Tracheobronchitis	Diarrhea
	Edema
	Emphysema

S

Increased (Hypernatremia)	Decreased (Hyponatremia)
	Excessive non-electrolyte IV infusions
	Gastrointestinal suctioning
	Hyperglycemia
	Hyperproteinemia
	Inadequate sodium intake
	Malabsorption
	Overhydration
	Pyloric obstruction
	Renal tubular acidosis
	Vomiting

Contributing Factors to Abnormal Values

- Falsely low levels of sodium may be found in blood containing high levels of lipids (hyperlipidemia).
- Drugs that may *increase* the serum sodium level: androgens, antibiotics, clonidine hydrochloride, corticosteroids, corticotropin, estrogens, lactulose, laxatives, licorice, mannitol, methyldopa, oral contraceptives, phenylbutazone, rauwolfia alkaloids, reserpine, sodium bicarbonate.
- Drugs that may *decrease* the serum sodium level: acetazolamide, aminoglutethimide, amitriptyline, ammonium chloride, amphotericin B, carbamazepine, chlorpropamide, cisplatin, clofibrate, cyclophosphamide, diuretics, heparin, imipramine hydrochloride, indomethacin, lithium, miconazole nitrate, nonsteroidal anti-inflammatory drugs, spironolactone, sulfonylureas, tolbutamide, triamterene, vasopressin, vincristine sulfate.

Pre-Test Nursing Care

- Explain to the patient the purpose of the test and the need for a blood sample to be drawn.
- No fasting is required before the test.

Procedure

- A 7-mL blood sample is drawn in a collection tube containing a silicone gel.
- Gloves are worn throughout the procedure.

Post-Test Nursing Care

- Apply pressure at venipuncture site. Apply dressing, periodically assessing for continued bleeding.
- Label the specimen and transport it to the laboratory.
- Report abnormal findings to the primary care provider.

• • • • • • • • • • • • • • • • •

S

Sodium, Urine

Sodium (Na$^+$) is the major cation in the extracellular fluid (ECF) of the body. It plays an important role in acid-base balance and promotes neuromuscular functioning. Although assessment of the serum sodium level is more common, the measurement of the urine sodium level is also very important. Measuring the sodium in the urine involves the collection of the patient's urine for a 24-hour period.

Determination of the sodium level in the urine provides the health care provider with data that assists in differential diagnosis when the sodium level in the blood is found to be low, an abnormality called *hyponatremia*. If the cause of this abnormality was owing to inadequate sodium intake, the sodium level in the urine would also be low. However, if the cause was owing to renal dysfunction, such as chronic renal failure, the sodium level in the urine would be high.

The maintenance of a normal urine sodium level is influenced by several factors, including the patient's dietary intake of sodium, the kidneys' ability to excrete sodium, and the effect of aldosterone, a mineralocorticoid hormone synthesized by the adrenal glands, and antidiuretic hormone (ADH, or vasopressin), which is released from the posterior pituitary. Aldosterone causes increased reabsorption of sodium in the distal tubules of the kidneys, leading to a lower level of sodium in the urine. ADH controls the reabsorption of water in the collecting ducts of the kidney, causing its return to the bloodstream. This results in decreased water in the urine and a corresponding increase in the urine sodium level.

Normal Values

40–220 mEq/24 hrs (40–220 mmol/24 hrs, SI units)

Note: Value is diet dependent.

Possible Meanings of Abnormal Values

Increased	Decreased
Adrenal cortical insufficiency	Acute renal failure
Chronic renal failure	Congestive heart failure
Dehydration	Cushing's disease
Diabetic acidosis	Diaphoresis
Fever	Diarrhea
Head trauma	Inadequate sodium intake
Hypothyroidism	Malabsorption
Renal tubular acidosis	Primary aldosteronism
Salicylate intoxication	Pulmonary emphysema
Starvation	Pyloric obstruction
Syndrome of inappropriate ADH secretion (SIADHS)	
Toxemia of pregnancy	

S

Contributing Factors to Abnormal Values

- Drugs that may *increase* sodium levels in the urine: acetazolamide, ammonium chloride, antibiotics, caffeine, calcitonin, cisplatin, dopamine hydrochloride, heparin, laxatives, lithium, niacin, steroids, sulfates, tetracycline, thiazide diuretics, vincristine sulfate.
- Drugs that may *decrease* sodium levels in the urine: corticosteroids, diazoxide, epinephrine, levarterenol, propranolol hydrochloride.

Pre-Test Nursing Care

- Explain 24-hour urine collection procedure to the patient.
- Stress the importance of saving *all* urine in the 24-hour period. Instruct the patient to avoid contaminating the urine with toilet paper or feces.
- No fasting is required before the test.

Procedure

- Obtain the proper container from the laboratory.
- Begin the testing period in the morning following the patient's first voiding, which is discarded.
- Timing of the 24-hour period begins at the time the first voiding is discarded.
- *All* urine for the next 24 hours is collected in the container and kept on ice.
- If any urine is accidentally discarded during the 24-hour period, the test must be discontinued and a new test begun.
- The ending time of the 24-hour collection period should be posted in the patient's room.
- Gloves are worn throughout the procedure.

Post-Test Nursing Care

- Label the container and transport it on ice to the laboratory as soon as possible following the end of the 24-hour collection period.
- Report abnormal findings to the primary care provider.

• • • • • • • • • • • • • • •

Somatomedin C
(Insulin-Like Growth Hormone)

Human growth hormone stimulates the secretion of peptide hormones produced in the liver known as somatomedins. These hormones are involved in cartilage and collagen formation, increased glucose metabolism, and amino acid transport in the diaphragm and heart. Somatomedin C, also known as insulin-like growth hormone, is affected by growth hormone activity. Thus, measurement of somatomedin provides information regarding the amount of growth hormone present. This test is also useful in monitoring the patient's response to growth hormone treatment in pituitary dwarfism, and to evaluate the severity of acromegaly.

S

Normal Values

Female

Preadolescent:	60.8–724.5 ng/mL	(60.8–724.5 µg/L, SI units)
Adolescent:	112.5–450.0 ng/mL	(112.5–450.0 µg/L, SI units)
Adult:	141.8–389.3 ng/mL	(141.8–389.3 µg/L, SI units)

Male

Preadolescent:	65.5–841.5 ng/mL	(65.5–841.5 µg/L, SI units)
Adolescent:	83.3–378.0 ng/mL	(83.3–378.0 µg/L, SI units)
Adult:	54.0–328.5 ng/mL	(54.0–328.5 µg/L, SI units)

Possible Meanings of Abnormal Values

Increased	Decreased
Acromegaly	Anorexia nervosa
Diabetic retinopathy	Chronic illness
Hyperpituitarism	Cirrhosis of the liver
Obesity	Delayed puberty
Precocious puberty	Diabetes mellitus
Pregnancy	Dwarfism
Pituitary gigantism	Emotional deprivation syndrome
	Growth hormone deficiency
	Hypopituitarism
	Hypothyroidism
	Kwashiorkor
	Liver disease
	Maternal deprivation syndrome
	Nutritional deficiency
	Pituitary tumor

Contributing Factors to Abnormal Values

- Radioactive scans within 7 days before the test may falsely elevate test results.
- Drugs that may *decrease* somatomedin C levels: estrogens.

Pre-Test Nursing Care

- Explain to the patient the purpose of the test and the need for a blood sample to be drawn.
- Fasting overnight is required before the test.

Procedure

- A 5-mL blood sample is drawn in a collection tube containing a silicone gel.
- Gloves are worn throughout the procedure.

S

Post-Test Nursing Care

- Apply pressure at venipuncture site. Apply dressing, periodically assessing for continued bleeding.
- Label the specimen and transport it to the laboratory.
- Report abnormal findings to the primary care provider.

• • • • • • • • • • • • • • • • •

Sputum Culture and Sensitivity
(Sputum C & S)

Sputum cultures are often used to aid in the differential diagnosis of bacterial, fungal, and non-bacterial lower respiratory tract pneumonia. However, the results obtained from such cultures can be misleading to the clinician if the sputum specimen is contaminated with the normal flora found in upper airway secretions. To assess acceptability of a sputum sample for culture, the laboratory first performs a Gram stain. Evidence of oropharyngeal contamination makes a specimen unsuitable for culture and a repeat sputum specimen collection is needed. Culture procedures differ depending on the organism suspected, thus the requisition slip should clearly indicate the suspected causative agent. Following culture, susceptibility or sensitivity testing is performed to guide the clinician in the selection of an appropriate antimicrobial agent.

Normal Values

The presence or absence of normal respiratory flora is reported. The clinician must evaluate the significance of the types and numbers present of each microbe.

Possible Meanings of Abnormal Values

Bacterial infections (e.g., pneumonia, tuberculosis)
Fungal infections
Parasitic infections
Viral infections

Contributing Factors to Abnormal Values

- Contamination of the specimen, collection of saliva, rather than sputum, delay in specimen delivery to laboratory, and initiation of antimicrobial therapy prior to sputum collection can alter test results.

Pre-Test Nursing Care

- The sputum should be collected before antimicrobial therapy is begun.
- Explain the procedure to the patient:
  - An early morning specimen is best, since sputum is most concentrated at that time.
  - The patient should brush the teeth and rinse the mouth with water before collecting the sputum to reduce contamination of the sample with normal respiratory flora.
  - The sputum must be from the bronchial tree. The patient must understand that this is different than saliva in the mouth.

S

- Teach the patient how to expectorate sputum by taking three deep breaths and forcing a deep cough.
- The sample is collected in a sterile sputum container.
- Ask the patient to notify the nurse when the specimen is ready.
- If tuberculosis is suspected, multiple morning specimens may be ordered.
- If the sputum is very thick, it can be thinned by inhaling nebulized saline or water, or by increasing fluid intake the evening before sample collection. Postural drainage and chest physiotherapy may also prove helpful.

Procedure

- The nurse wears gloves during the procedure and when handling the specimen.
- The patient should take several deep breaths and then cough deeply to obtain the specimen. At least one teaspoon of sputum is needed.
- Other ways to collect sputum include endotracheal suctioning, transtracheal aspiration, fiberoptic bronchoscopy, and gastric lavage.
- Following collection of sputum, the sample is sent to the laboratory. The laboratory determines the suitability of the specimen for culture by performing a Gram stain and microscopic evaluation. Sputum contaminated with upper respiratory secretions will contain an increased number of epithelial cells.
- Preliminary information about the primary microorganism present is also recorded during the initial microscopic examination.
- The sputum sample is then inoculated onto appropriate culture media and incubated.
- Final reports and susceptibility testing of most bacterial agents require 48–72 hours; whereas, fungal cultures can take up to 4 weeks, and mycobacteria (i.e., tuberculous agents) cultures can take up to 6 weeks for a final report.

Post-Test Nursing Care

- Label the specimen container and send to the laboratory as soon as possible. Note the suspected microorganism and any current antimicrobial therapy on the label. Do not refrigerate the specimen.
- Begin antimicrobial therapy as ordered *after* collection of the specimen.
- When available, report results of the culture and sensitivity to the primary care provider so that modifications in drug therapy are made if needed.

• • • • • • • • • • • • • • • •

Sputum Cytology

S putum cytology is used in the diagnosis of a variety of respiratory conditions. These include malignant conditions, as well as cellular changes of a premalignant nature such inflammation and inhaled toxins. Cytologic study of the sputum also assists in the diagnose of tuberculosis, bacterial infection, parasitic infection, and viral infection.

S

Normal Values

Negative

Possible Meanings of Abnormal Values

Asbestosis
Asthma
Bacterial infection
Bronchiectasis
Cancer
Emphysema
Inflammatory disease
Lipid pneumonia
Parasitic infection
Pneumonitis
Tuberculosis
Viral infection

Contributing Factors to Abnormal Values

- Test results are inaccurate if saliva, rather than sputum, is collected.
- Delay in specimen delivery to the laboratory may alter test results.

Pre-Test Nursing Care

- Explain the procedure to the patient, stressing that:
  - An early morning specimen is best, since sputum is most concentrated at that time.
  - The patient should brush the teeth and rinse the mouth with water before collecting the sputum to reduce contamination of the sample with normal respiratory flora.
  - The sputum must be from the bronchial tree. The patient must understand that this is different than saliva in the mouth.
- Teach the patient how to expectorate sputum by taking three deep breaths and forcing a deep cough.
- If the sputum is very thick, it can be thinned by inhaling nebulized saline or water, or by increasing fluid intake the evening before sample collection. Postural drainage and chest physiotherapy may also prove helpful.

Procedure

- The patient is instructed to take several deep breaths and then cough deeply to obtain the specimen. At least one teaspoon of sputum is needed.
- Other ways to collect sputum include endotracheal suctioning and fiberoptic bronchoscopy.
- Gloves are worn when handling the specimen.

Post-Test Nursing Care

- Label the specimen and transport it to the laboratory immediately.
- Report abnormal findings to the primary care provider.

• • • • • • • • • • • • • • • •

S

Stool Culture
(Stool For Ova and Parasites)

The gastrointestinal (GI) tract contains many bacteria and fungi as its normal flora. In addition, pathogens may enter the GI tract, causing symptoms such as persistent or bloody diarrhea and fever. People may be exposed to enteric pathogens in a variety of ways. For example, exposure may occur when traveling outside of the United States or through dietary intake. It is important to identify the pathogens to assist with treatment planning and prevention of complications.

Normal Values

Normal intestinal flora
Negative for pathogens

Possible Meanings of Abnormal Values

Positive

Bacterial enterocolitis
Parasitic enterocolitis
Protozoal enterocolitis

Contributing Factors to Abnormal Values

- Drugs that may cause *false-negative* results: antibiotics, barium, bismuth, mineral oil.

Pre-Test Nursing Care

- Explain to the patient the purpose of the test and the need for collection of a stool sample.
- Instruct the patient to avoid contaminating the stool with toilet paper or urine.
- No fasting is required before the test.

Procedure

- Provide the patient with a bedpan or, if ambulatory, a plastic specimen hat for the toilet.
- Once the patient has defecated, use a wooden tongue blade to place a 1-in. diameter stool sample in a sterile container and cover.
- Gloves are worn throughout the procedure.

Post-Test Nursing Care

- Label the specimen and transport it to the laboratory immediately.
- Report abnormal findings to the primary care provider.

• • • • • • • • • • • • • • • • •

S

Stool for Occult Blood
(Hematest, Hemoccult [Guaiac])

Bleeding can occur in all portions of the gastrointestinal tract. Bleeding can occur as a result of some medications and many disease processes. For example, gastric ulcers, ulcerative colitis, and hemorrhoids produce bleeding that can often be found by testing for occult blood in the stool. Most important for detection is cancer of the gastrointestinal tract, especially colorectal cancer. Early detection of this disease is essential to provide the best possible chance of recovery. Most products available for testing of stool for occult blood are able to detect blood loss of approximately 5 to 10 mL/day.

Normal Values

Negative

Possible Meanings of Abnormal Values

Increased

Colon cancer
Diaphragmatic hernia
Diverticulitis
Gastric cancer
Gastric ulcers
Gastritis
Gastrointestinal trauma
Hemorrhoids
Ulcerative colitis

Contributing Factors to Abnormal Values

- Meats and foods with high perioxidase activity (beets, broccoli, cantaloupe, cauliflower, horseradish, parsnips, and turnips) cause *false-positive* test results.
- Drugs that may cause *false-positive* results: aspirin, boric acid, bromides, colchicine, indomethacin, iodine, iron preparation, potassium, reserpine, salicylates, steroids, thiazide diuretics.
- Drugs that may cause *false-negative* results: ascorbic acid.

Pre-Test Nursing Care

- Explain to the patient the purpose of the test and the need for a small sample of stool.
- No fasting is required before the test. Some institutions require a diet of no meats or foods with high perioxidase activity (beets, broccoli, cantaloupe, cauliflower, horseradish, parsnips, and turnips) for 24–48 hours prior to the test.
- Aspirin and nonsteroidal anti-inflammatory drugs should be avoided for 2 days before the test.

S

Procedure

- Obtain a small amount of stool. Digital exam may be needed in order to obtain the stool sample. However, use caution to avoid trauma that would lead to bleeding.
- Place a smear of stool in the designated areas of a commercially prepared card. Close the card cover.
- Apply two drops of commercially prepared developing solution to the indicated areas.
- Gloves are worn throughout the procedure.

Post-Test Nursing Care

- Results need to be read between 30 and 120 seconds. Blue color is positive for occult blood.
- Report abnormal findings to the primary care provider.

• • • • • • • • • • • • • • • • •

Sweat Test
(Sweat Electrolytes Test)

Cystic fibrosis is a hereditary disease that affects the exocrine glands of the body. The mucous glands produce very thick mucus, which is especially problematic in the lungs. There is also malfunctioning of the pancreatic exocrine gland. Sweat levels of sodium, potassium, and chloride are abnormally elevated in children with cystic fibrosis and in genetic carriers of the disease.

This test involves the stimulation of sweat production by iontophoresis, the painless delivery of a small electrical current to the skin that causes the transportation of positive pilocarpine ions into the skin from gel pads applied to the skin. Once sweating has been stimulated, preweighed filter paper is attached to the area and allowed to remain for 1 hour to collect the sweat. Sweat chloride values of greater than 60 mEq/L are indicative of cystic fibrosis.

Normal Values

Sodium:	10–40 mEq/L (10–40 mmol/L, SI units)
Chloride:	0–35 mEq/L (0–35 mmol/L, SI units)

Possible Meanings of Abnormal Values

Increased	Decreased
Addison's disease	Hypoaldosteronism
Adrenal insufficiency	Sodium depletion
Cystic fibrosis	
Diabetes insipidus	
Ectodermal dysplasia	
Fucosidosis	
Glucose–6-phosphate-dehydrogenase deficiency	
Hypothyroidism	
Malnutrition	

S

Increased	Decreased
Mucopolysaccharidosis	
Renal failure	

Contributing Factors to Abnormal Values

- Drugs that may *decrease* sweat chloride levels: mineralocorticoids.

CONTRAINDICATIONS

- Persons with dermatitis

Pre-Test Nursing Care

- Explain to the patient the purpose of the test and how the test will be conducted.
- No fasting is required before the test.

Procedure

- Wash with distilled water and dry the site to be stimulated; the right forearm or right thigh are preferred sites.
- A small amount of pilocarpine-soaked gauze is applied to the skin and attached to the positive electrode.
- A small amount of saline-soaked gauze is also applied to the skin and attached to the negative electrode.
- A 4 milliamp current is delivered in 15- to 20-second intervals for 5 minutes.
- Remove and discard the electrodes.
- Place a preweighed, dry gauze pad or filter paper on the site previously covered by the pilocarpine pad, cover it with plastic, and seal the edges with waterproof tape.
- After 30–40 minutes, remove and discard the tape and plastic.
- Remove the gauze or filter paper with forceps and place it in a weighing bottle.
- Gloves are worn throughout the procedure.

Post-Test Nursing Care

- Seal and label the bottle, and transport it to the laboratory immediately.
- Wash the iontophoresed area with soap and water, and dry thoroughly. Redness of the area will disappear within a few hours.
- Report abnormal findings to the primary care provider.

• • • • • • • • • • • • • • • •

S

Syphilis Serology
(FTA-ABS, MHA-TP, RPR, VDRL)

Syphilis is a systemic, infectious disease caused by the spirochete *Treponema pallidum*. The organism is transmitted primarily through direct sexual contact. It can also be transmitted via the placenta from mother to fetus. If untreated, infected clients can develop irreversible complications, such as chronic inflammation of the joints, cardiovascular problems such as valvular involvement, and central nervous system problems such as mental illness and paralysis.

Laboratory diagnosis of syphilis can be made through direct and indirect tests. Direct tests, such as scraping of syphilis lesions, identify the causative organism. Indirect tests, such as the syphilis serologic tests, identify antibodies of the causative agent. These antibodies do not appear in the serum until 3–4 weeks after the appearance of the syphilis chancre, an ulcer located at the site where the organism initially enters the body.

The syphilis serology includes the VDRL, RPR, FTA-ABS, and MHA-TP tests. The *VDRL (Venereal Disease Research Laboratory) test* and the *RPR (rapid plasma reagin) test* are screening tests. In both of these tests, agglutination occurs in the presence of the syphilis antigen. Both of these tests have a high false-positive rate. Conditions such as infectious mononucleosis, rheumatoid arthritis, and malaria can cause false-positive reactions. Because of the high possibility of a false-positive result, any positive, or *reactive* VDRL or RPR test must be followed with a confirmatory test, such as the FTA-ABS or MHA-TP. Both of these tests identify the antibodies that are specific against *T. pallidum*. The *FTA-ABS (fluorescent treponemal antibody absorption) test* is the most sensitive test used to diagnose syphilis following a positive VDRL or RPR test. The *MHA-TP (microhemagglutination-*Treponema pallidum*) test* is less sensitive than the FTA-ABS, but is also less costly to perform. False positive reactions can also occur with the FTA-ABS and MHA-TP tests.

Normal Values

Negative (nonreactive)

Possible Meanings of Abnormal Values

Positive

Syphilis

Contributing Factors to Abnormal Values

- Hemolysis of the blood sample, presence of lipemia, and the intake of alcohol may alter test results.
- Conditions that may cause *false-positive* VDRL or RPR results: atypical pneumonia, Hansen disease, infectious hepatitis, infectious mononucleosis, malaria, malignant tumors, pregnancy, rheumatoid arthritis, systemic lupus erythematosus.
- Conditions that may cause *false-positive* FTA-ABS results: collagen vascular disorders, drug addiction, pregnancy.
- Conditions that may cause *false-positive* MHA-TP results: Hansen disease, infectious mononucleosis, systemic lupus erythematosus.

S

Pre-Test Nursing Care

- Explain to the patient the purpose of the test and the need for a blood sample to be drawn.
- No fasting is required before the test.
- No alcohol is allowed for 24 hours before the test.

Procedure

- A 7-mL blood sample is drawn in a collection tube containing no additives.
- Gloves are worn throughout the procedure.

Post-Test Nursing Care

- Apply pressure at venipuncture site. Apply dressing, periodically assessing for continued bleeding.
- Label the specimen and transport it to the laboratory.
- Report abnormal findings to the primary care provider.
- Positive screening test results require followup confirmatory testing.
- Positive confirmatory test results should be followed with appropriate antibiotic therapy and education of the patient.

• • • • • • • • • • • • • • • •

T- and B-Cell Lymphocyte Counts
(AIDS T-Lymphocyte Cell Markers, CD4 Marker, T- and B-Cell Lymphocyte Surface Markers)

The immune system is composed of two subsystems: the humoral immune system and the cellular immune system. The primary cell of the humoral immune system is the *B-lymphocyte*, which matures in the bone marrow. B cells circulate in the blood in an inactive state. When the B cell is exposed to a specific protein or microorganism (antigen) for the first time, it produces antibodies (immunoglobulins) that bind with the antigen. This antibody production can take weeks to years, but antibodies are usually detectable in the blood within 6 months. In subsequent exposures to the same antigen, the antibodies formed against it are already present in the blood, so the response occurs almost immediately.

T-lymphocytes, which mature in the thymus gland, comprise the cellular immune system. When a T cell encounters a specific protein or microorganism to which it has been programmed to respond, it can directly attack and destroy the substance. Several types of T cells are produced. *Cytotoxic T cells* release toxic chemicals that directly destroy the antigen. *Helper T cells*, which carry the CD4 marker, stimulate the response of all other T cells. They also stimulate the humoral immune response. The *suppressor T cells*, which carry the CD8 marker, are responsible for stopping both humoral and cell-mediated immune responses, when appropriate. *Memory cells* are able to remember antigens that they have previously encountered. These cells thus provide for immediate response to the antigen when it is next encountered.

Testing of T- and B-lymphocyte counts is conducted to evaluate the status of the immune system. It is typical for the measurement of T- and B-lymphocyte counts to be included within testing for immunologic status in patients infected with the human immunodeficiency virus

T

(HIV). Lymphocyte counts decrease as immune function decreases. The number of suppressor T cells remains normal or may increase. As helper T cells (CD4) become infected by HIV, their numbers decrease. Thus, as the CD4 cell count decreases, the percentage of persons developing AIDS increases. The CD4 count normally should be greater than 1000 cells/mm^3. Antiviral therapy should be started in patients whose CD4 count is less than 500–600 cells/mm^3. Obviously, periodic determinations of CD4 counts can be extremely stressful for the individual.

Normal Values

T and B Surface Markers

T cells (CD2):	60%–88%
Helper T cells (CD4):	34%–67%
Suppressor T cells (CD8):	10%–42%
B cells (CD19):	3%–21%

Absolute Values

Lymphocytes:	0.66–4.60 thousand/µL
T cells:	644–2201 cells/µL
Helper T cells:	493–1191 cells/µL
Suppressor T cells:	182–785 cells/µL
B cells:	92–392 cells/µL

Lymphocyte Ratio

Helper T cell to Suppressor T cell ratio > 1.0

Possible Meanings of Abnormal Values

T cells

Increased	Decreased
Graves' disease	Acute viral infection
	DeGeorge's syndrome
	HIV infection
	Hodgkin's disease
	Increased risk for clinical AIDS
	Increased risk for opportunistic infections
	Malignancies
	Measles
	Nezelof's syndrome

B cells

Increased	Decreased
Chronic lymphocytic leukemia	Deficiency of IgG, IgA, IgM
Systemic lupus erythematosus	Hypogammaglobulinemia
	Lymphomas
	Multiple myeloma
	Nephrotic syndrome

T

Contributing Factors to Abnormal Values

- There is a diurnal variation in test values.

Pre-Test Nursing Care

- Explain to the patient the purpose of the test and the need for a blood sample to be drawn.
- No fasting is required before the test.

Procedure

- A 10- to 20- mL blood sample is drawn in a collection tube containing heparin.
- Gloves are worn throughout the procedure.

Post-Test Nursing Care

Possible complication: Infection at venipuncture site owing to immunocompromised state

- Apply pressure at venipuncture site. Apply dressing, periodically assessing for continued bleeding.
- Teach the patient to monitor the site and to notify the health care provider if signs or symptoms of infection occur, such as drainage, redness, warmth, edema, pain at the site, or fever.
- Provide emotional support throughout the testing process.
- Report abnormal findings to the primary care provider.
- Provide information regarding counseling and other referral sources as appropriate.

• • • • • • • • • • • • • • • •

Testosterone

This test measures testosterone levels in the blood and, when analyzed in conjunction with the levels of follicle-stimulating hormone and luteinizing hormone, assists in the evaluation of gonadal dysfunction in both sexes. In men, testosterone is the primary androgen secreted by the interstitial cells of the testes, known as Leydig cells. Testosterone promotes the growth and development of the male sex organs, contributes to the enlargement of voluntary muscles, and stimulates the growth of axillary, facial, and pubic hair. In males, testosterone levels peak in the early morning and after exercise. In women, testosterone is secreted in small amounts by the ovaries and adrenal glands.

Normal Values

Female (total):	20–90 ng/dL (0.7–3.1 nmol/L, SI units)
Male (total):	300–1100 ng/dL (10.4–38.1 nmol/L, SI units)

T

Possible Meanings of Abnormal Values

Increased (Males)	Decreased (Males)
Adrenal cancer	Cirrhosis
Adrenal hyperplasia	Delayed male puberty
Benign adrenal tumor	Klinefelter's syndrome
Hyperthyroidism	Obesity
Incipient puberty	Orchiectomy
Sexual precocity	Primary hypogonadism
Testicular tumor	Prostatic cancer
	Secondary hypogonadism
	Testicular cancer

Increased (Females)

Adrenal hyperplasia
Adrenal tumor
Hirsutism
Ovarian tumor
Stein-Leventhal's syndrome

Contributing Factors to Abnormal Values

- Hemolysis of the blood sample and radioactive scans within 1 week before the test may alter test results.
- Drugs that may *increase* testosterone levels: anticonvulsants, barbiturates, cimetidine, estrogens, oral contraceptives.
- Drugs that may *decrease* testosterone levels: androgens, dexamethasone, diethylstilbestrol, digoxin (males), digitalis, estrogens (males), ethanol, glucose, halothane, ketoconazole, metoprolol tartrate, metyrapone, phenothiazines, spironolactone, tetracycline.

Pre-Test Nursing Care

- Explain to the patient the purpose of the test and the need for a blood sample to be drawn.
- No fasting is required before the test.

Procedure

- A 7-mL blood sample is drawn in a collection tube containing a silicone gel.
- Gloves are worn throughout the procedure.

Post-Test Nursing Care

- Apply pressure at venipuncture site. Apply dressing, periodically assessing for continued bleeding.
- Label the specimen and transport it to the laboratory.
- Report abnormal findings to the primary care provider.

• • • • • • • • • • • • • • • •

T

Therapeutic Drug Monitoring

Therapeutic drug monitoring is used to manage individual patient drug therapy. Such testing is essential when the margin of safety between a therapeutic drug effect and drug toxicity is narrow. An example of a drug in which there is a narrow margin of safety is digoxin.

Another example of how therapeutic drug monitoring is used is in the use of aminoglycosides. These antimicrobials, which are used for severe infections, are nephrotoxic and ototoxic. Thus, it is important to ensure that the drug level in the blood is high enough to deal with the infection, yet low enough to avoid toxic complications. Testing in this case is often referred to as "peak and trough," which refers to the therapeutic concentrations at their highest, and therefore most toxic, point and their lowest, or satisfactory, therapeutic points. When peak and trough monitoring is conducted, exact timing of the drug administration is essential.

Normal Values

Depends on specific drug being monitored and reference laboratory used

Possible Meanings of Abnormal Values

Increased	Decreased
Toxic drug levels	Subtherapeutic drug levels

Pre-Test Nursing Care

- Explain to the patient the purpose of the test and the need for a blood sample to be drawn.
- No fasting is required before the test.

Procedure

- A 7- to 10-mL blood sample is drawn in the type of tube designated by the reference laboratory.
- Gloves are worn throughout the procedure.

Post-Test Nursing Care

- Apply pressure at venipuncture site. Apply dressing, periodically assessing for continued bleeding.
- Label the specimen and transport it to the laboratory.
- Report abnormal findings to the primary care provider.

• • • • • • • • • • • • • •

T

Thoracentesis
(Pleural Fluid Analysis, Pleural Tap)

The pleural cavity is the space between the visceral pleura, which covers the lungs, and the parietal pleura, which lines the chest cavity. In some conditions, such as inflammatory diseases of the lungs and neoplasms, a large amount of pleural fluid may accumulate in the pleural cavity, an assessment finding known as *pleural effusion*. Other substances, such as air (pneumothorax) or blood (hemothorax), may also be present in the pleural cavity.

Thoracentesis refers to the removal of fluid from the pleural cavity. This may done for a diagnostic purpose to determine the cause of the fluid production, or for therapeutic purposes to remove up to 1000 mL of fluid at any one time. The fluid analysis includes red and white blood cell counts, cytologic studies, bacterial and fungal cultures, and determination of glucose, lactic dehydrogenase, and protein levels.

The fluid is classified as either an *exudate*, which is high-protein fluid that has leaked from blood vessels with increased permeability, or a *transudate*, a low-protein fluid leaked from normal blood vessels. An exudate may be caused by blocked lymphatic drainage, infection, neoplasm, pancreatitis, pulmonary infarction, rheumatoid arthritis, systemic lupus erythematosus, trauma, and tuberculosis. Transudate is caused by ascites, cirrhosis, congestive heart failure, hypertension, nephritis, and nephrosis.

Normal Values

Gross appearance:	Clear, odorless
Amount:	<20 mL
Specific gravity:	<1.016
Bacteria:	None
Cell counts:	Red blood cells (few)
	White blood cells (few lymphocytes)
Cytology:	No malignant cells present
Fibrinogen (clot):	None
Fungi:	None
Glucose:	Equal to serum level
Lactic dehydrogenase:	Equal to serum level
Protein:	<3 g/dL

Possible Meanings of Abnormal Values

Color

Milk colored:	Chyle present
Cloudy fluid:	Inflammation
Bloody fluid:	Caused by hemothorax, traumatic tap

T

Bacteria

Increased

Ruptured pulmonary abscess
Staphylococcus aureus infection
Streptococcal infection
Tuberculosis

Fungi

Increased

Candidiasis
Coccidioidomycosis
Histoplasmosis

Glucose

Decreased

Bacterial infection
Malignancy
Metastases
Nonseptic inflammation

Lactic Dehydrogenase

Increased

Malignancy

Protein

Increased

Collagen vascular disease
Infection
Neoplasm
Pulmonary infarction
Trauma
Tuberculosis

Red Blood Cells

Increased

Chest trauma
Neoplasm

White Blood Cells

Increased

Fungal effusion
Inflammation
Tuberculosis
Viral effusion

T

Contributing Factors to Abnormal Values

- Antimicrobial therapy, if started prior to the test, may decrease the bacterial count.
- Contamination of the specimen through break in sterile technique alters white blood cell count.

 ## CONTRAINDICATIONS

- Patients with bleeding disorders

Pre-Test Nursing Care

- Explain to the patient the purpose of the test and the procedure to be done. Explain that a local anesthetic will be used, but that a pressure-like pain will occur as the needle pierces the pleura and as the fluid is being withdrawn. Explain that no movement, including deep breathing or coughing, can occur during the test.
- No fasting is required before the test.
- Obtain a signed informed consent.
- A chest x-ray or ultrasound testing is usually done before the test to locate the fluid and to avoid accidental puncture of the lung.
- Obtain baseline vital signs.
- Pulse oximetry may be ordered for use throughout the procedure.

Procedure

- Assist the patient to a sitting position leaning forward with the arms supported on an overbed table. Provide support for the arms and head with pillows. If the patient cannot tolerate this position, an alternative position is lying on the unaffected side with the head of the bed elevated 30–45 degrees.
- Monitor vital signs every 15 minutes during the procedure.
- Sterile technique is used throughout the procedure.
- The area is cleansed and draped.
- A local anesthetic is administered.
- A 20-gauge or larger needle attached to a 50-mL syringe and a three-way stopcock is inserted through the parietal pleura.
- When the pocket of fluid is reached, a 50-mL sample of the fluid is obtained.
- If additional fluid is to be drained, connect a tubing between the three-way stopcock and the collection receptacle.
- A maximum of 1000 mL is allowed to drain slowly from the site. Rapid drainage, and thus hypovolemia, can be avoided by either raising the collection receptacle to slow the draining or by clamping the tubing.
- Throughout drainage of the pleural effusion, assess for respiratory distress: weakness, dyspnea, pallor, cyanosis, tachypnea, diaphoresis, hypotension, and blood-tinged frothy mucus. Atropine may be needed for bradycardia owing to vasovagal effect.
- Patients with pleural effusions caused by malignancies may have antineoplastic drugs injected into the pleural cavity through the three-way stopcock prior to needle removal.
- When the procedure is complete, the needle is removed. A pressure dressing is applied.
- Gloves are worn throughout the procedure.

T

Post-Test Nursing Care

Possible complications:

>**Air embolism**
>**Hemothorax**
>**Pneumothorax**
>**Pulmonary edema**
>**Reaction to antineoplastic drugs**
>**Shock and hypovolemia**

- Turn the patient on the *unaffected* side for 1 hour to allow for lung expansion.
- Monitor vital signs every 30 minutes for 2 hours, then every 4 hours until stable.
- Check the dressing frequently for drainage. Assess the puncture site for bleeding and the presence of crepitus.
- Continue to observe the patient for any respiratory distress. A post-procedure chest x-ray may be ordered to assess for the presence of hemothorax, pneumothorax, tension pneumothorax, or accumulation of additional fluid.
- Label the specimen and transport it to the laboratory immediately.
- Report abnormal findings to the primary care provider.

• • • • • • • • • • • • • • • •

Throat Culture and Sensitivity

A throat culture is used primarily to isolate and identify pathogens, especially group A beta-hemolytic streptococci (GABHS). This identification is important, since complications of such infections include rheumatic fever and glomerulonephritis. Although most sore throats are viral in nature, approximately 15% are caused by this particular type of streptococci. The white blood count is elevated with a bacterial infection, but not with a viral infection. Symptoms exhibited by the patient with GABHS occur abruptly and may include fever, chills, headache, sore throat, and distinctive patches on the throat. This test can be used in diagnosing glomerulonephritis, pharyngitis, scarlet fever, strep throat, and tonsillitis.

When a patient is suspected of having strep throat, a throat culture is ordered. The test involves swabbing each tonsilar area and the posterior pharynx. The throat swab should be performed prior to the beginning of antibiotic therapy. This test involves several components. First, a Gram stain of the specimen can be done and quickly reported. This provides basic information as to whether the organism is Gram positive or Gram negative. Next, the throat swab is cultured, that is, the organisms are allowed to grow in special culture media. In 48 to 72 hours, the organism is usually identified. The sensitivity portion of the test involves the testing of the organism to identify drugs to which the organism is sensitive or resistant.

Once the specimen is obtained, the patient is usually given a broad-spectrum antibiotic that is likely to be effective against strep throat, such as penicillin. After the throat culture and sensitivity results are available, the antibiotic in use should be verified as to its appropriateness according to the sensitivity report.

T

Normal Values

Negative

Possible Meanings of Abnormal Values

Positive

Bacterial pathogens, such as streptococci

Contributing Factors to Abnormal Values

- Drugs that may cause *false-negative* results: antibiotics.

Pre-Test Nursing Care

- Explain to the patient the purpose of the test and the need for a swabbing of the throat to be drawn. Warn the patient of the possibility of gagging during the procedure.
- Obtain the specimen before antibiotic therapy is begun.

Procedure

- Depress the tongue and take a swab of each tonsilar area and the posterior pharynx.
- Avoid touching the lips or tongue.
- Gloves are worn throughout the procedure.

Post-Test Nursing Care

- Place the swab in the Culturette tube and crush the distal end. This releases the culture medium that will keep the swab moist.
- Label the specimen and transport it to the laboratory immediately.
- Report abnormal findings to the primary care provider.

• • • • • • • • • • • • • • • • •

Thrombin Clotting Time
(TCT, Thrombin Time)

During the process of hemostasis, intrinsic and extrinsic pathways lead to the activation of coagulation factor X. This leads to the next step, in which prothrombin is converted to thrombin. Thrombin then stimulates the formation of fibrin from fibrinogen. This fibrin, with the addition of fibrin stabilizing factor, forms a stable fibrin clot at the site of injury. (See "Coagulation Studies" for description of the process of hemostasis.)

Thrombin clotting time (TCT) measures the time it takes for a blood sample to clot when thrombin is added to the sample. TCT is longer than normal when there is an abnormality in the conversion of fibrinogen to fibrin. The test is used to assess for bleeding disorders, such as disseminated intravascular coagulation (DIC), and for liver disease, and to monitor patients receiving fibrinolytic therapy.

T

Normal Values

14–16 seconds, or within 5 seconds of control

Possible Meanings of Abnormal Values

Increased	Decreased
Acute leukemia	Thrombocytosis
Afibrinogenemia	
Disseminated intravascular coagulation (DIC)	
Dysfibrinogenemia	
Dysproteinemias, such as multiple myeloma	
Liver disease	
Polycythemia vera	
Shock	
Stress	

Contributing Factors to Abnormal Values

- Hemolysis of the blood sample may alter test results.
- Drugs that may *increase* thrombin clotting time: asparaginase, heparin, streptokinase, tissue plasminogen activator (TPA), urokinase.

Pre-Test Nursing Care

- Explain to the patient the purpose of the test and the need for a blood sample to be drawn.
- No fasting is required before the test.
- Draw blood sample 1 hour before anticoagulant administration.

Procedure

- A 7-mL blood sample is drawn in a collection tube containing sodium citrate and citric acid.
- Gloves are worn throughout the procedure.

Post-Test Nursing Care

Possible complication: Hematoma at site owing to prolonged bleeding time.

- Apply pressure 3–5 minutes at venipuncture site. Apply dressing, periodically assessing for continued bleeding.
- Teach the patient to monitor the site. If the site begins to bleed, the patient should apply direct pressure and, if unable to control the bleeding, return to the lab or notify the nurse.
- Label the specimen, place it on ice, and transport it to the laboratory immediately.
- Report abnormal findings to the primary care provider.

• • • • • • • • • • • • • • • •

T

Thyroid Function Tests

See:
Thyroid-Stimulating Hormone
Thyroid-Stimulating Hormone Stimulation Test
Thyroid-Stimulating Immunoglobulins
Thyroxine
Thyroxine-Binding Globulin
Thyroxine, Free
Triiodothyronine
Triiodothyronine Uptake Test

• • • • • • • • • • • • • • •

Thyroid Scan

The thyroid scan involves the intravenous (IV) administration of a radioactive tracer. Scanning of the thyroid gland is then conducted in order to assess its size, shape, position, and function. Areas in which there is increased uptake of the tracer are called "hot spots." These areas are caused by hyperfunctioning thyroid nodules which are usually nonmalignant. "Cold spots," on the other hand, are nodules that do not take up the tracer. These areas have hypofunctioning tissue and are more likely to be malignant.

Normal Values

Normal size, shape, position, and function of the thyroid gland. Equal uptake of tracer throughout the thyroid gland.

Possible Meanings of Abnormal Values

Adenoma
Carcinoma
Cyst
Goiter
Graves' disease
Hashimoto's thyroidism
Hyperthyroidism
Hypothyroidism
Plummer's disease
Thyroiditis

Contributing Factors to Abnormal Values

• Any movement by the patient may alter quality of films taken.
• Recent receipt of x-ray contrast agents or ingestion of iodine-containing foods will alter test results.

T

- Drugs that may alter test results: anticoagulants, antihistamines, corticosteroids, cough medicines, iodides, multiple vitamins, oral contraceptives, phenothiazines, salicylates, thyroid drugs.

CONTRAINDICATIONS

- Pregnant women (*Caution:* A woman in her childbearing years should undergo radiography only during her menses or 12–14 days after its onset to avoid any exposure to a fetus.)
- Patients who are lactating
- Patients who are allergic to iodine, shellfish, or contrast medium
- Patients who are unable to cooperate because of age, mental status, pain, or other factors

Pre-Test Nursing Care

- Explain to the patient the purpose of the test. Provide any written teaching materials available on the subject. Note that discomfort involved with this test is primarily owing to lying on a hard table for an extended period of time and the needle puncture. Reassure the patient that only trace amounts of the radionuclide are involved in the test.
- Medications that may alter test results (see "Contributing Factors to Abnormal Values") should be withheld for 21 days before the test. Discuss this with the physician and the patient.
- The patient must remain still while the scan is being performed.
- Fasting for 8 hours is required before the test.
- Obtain a signed informed consent.

Procedure

- Oral radioactive iodine is administered 24 hours prior to the scan. If the IV route is used, administer the radioactive iodine 1/2 hour prior to the scan.
- The patient is assisted to a supine position on the examination table.
- A scintillation camera is positioned over the patient's thyroid. This camera takes a radioactivity reading from the body. This information is transformed into a two-dimensional picture of the skeleton.
- Gloves are worn during the radionuclide injection.

Post-Test Nursing Care

- Check the injection site for redness or swelling.
- If a woman who is lactating *must* have a nuclear scan, she should not breast feed the infant until the radionuclide has been eliminated, possibly for 3 days.
- Although the amount of diagnostic radionuclide excreted in the urine is low, the urine should not be used for any laboratory tests for the time period indicated by the nuclear medicine department. Clients should be told to flush the toilet three times after voiding.
- Gloves are worn when dealing with the urine.
- No other radionuclide tests should be scheduled for 24–48 hours.
- Encourage fluid intake by the patient to enhance excretion of the radionuclide.
- Report abnormal findings to the primary care provider.

• • • • • • • • • • • • • • • • • • •

T

Thyroid Sonogram
(Thyroid Ultrasound)

Ultrasonography is a noninvasive method of diagnostic testing in which ultrasound waves are sent into the body with a small transducer pressed against the skin. The transducer not only sends the sound waves into the body but also receives any returning sound waves, which are deflected back as they bounce off various structures. The transducer converts the returning sound waves into electric signals that are then transformed by a computer into a visual display on a monitor.

In thyroid ultrasonography, the size, shape, and position of the thyroid gland can be evaluated. This test is useful in distinguishing between a cyst and solid tumor of the thyroid gland. It is also used to monitor the response of the thyroid gland to suppressive therapy.

Normal Values

Normal size, shape, and position of the thyroid gland

Possible Meanings of Abnormal Values

Goiter
Thyroid cyst
Thyroid tumor

Contributing Factors to Abnormal Values

- The transducer must be in good contact with the skin as it is being moved. A lubricant, such as mineral oil, glycerin, or a water-based jelly, is used to ensure good contact with the skin.

Pre-Test Nursing Care

- Explain to the patient the purpose of the test. Provide any written teaching materials available on the subject. Note that there is no discomfort involved with this test.
- No fasting is required before the test.

Procedure

- The patient is assisted to a supine position on the ultrasonography table. A pillow is placed beneath the shoulders and the neck is hyperextended.
- A coupling agent, such as a water-based gel, is applied to the area to be evaluated.
- A transducer is placed on the skin and moved as needed to provide good visualization of the thyroid gland.
- The sound waves are transformed into a visual display on the monitor. Printed copies of this display are made.

Post-Test Nursing Care

- Cleanse the patient's skin of remaining coupling agent.
- Report abnormal findings to the primary care provider.

• • • • • • • • • • • • • • •

T

Thyroid-Stimulating Hormone
(TSH, Thyrotropin)

When thyroid hormone levels decrease in the bloodstream or the body is exposed to physiologic or psychological stress, the hypothalamus is stimulated to release thyrotropin-releasing hormone (TRH). TRH in turn stimulates the production of thyroid-stimulating hormone (TSH) by the anterior lobe of the pituitary gland. TSH then stimulates production and release of triiodothyronine (T_3) and thyroxine (T_4). As levels of T_3 and free T_4 in the blood rise, the pituitary gland is stimulated to decrease TSH production via a negative feedback mechanism.

TSH release occurs in a diurnal pattern, with peaks occurring in the late evening and troughs occurring at midmorning. Measurement of the TSH level along with free T_4, is used for differential diagnosis of primary and secondary hypothyroidism. For example, consider the patient whose thyroid gland is hypoactive, thus producing abnormally low levels of free T_4 in the blood. The anterior pituitary gland senses the low serum T_4 levels and, as a result, increases its release of TSH. This is an attempt to stimulate the thyroid gland to increase its production of T_3 and T_4. Thus, the combination of high TSH and low free T_4 levels indicate thyroid gland hypoactivity, or *hypothyroidism*. Measurement of the TSH level can also be used to monitor the effectiveness of drug therapy administered for hypothyroidism.

Correlation of TSH, free T_4, and radioactive iodine uptake (RAIU) results with the underlying cause is summarized in Table 8. "Primary" type problems, such as hypothyroidism, deal with the target organ (thyroid gland) itself, whereas "secondary" problems deal with abnormalities of the pituitary gland.

Normal Values

0.5–5.0 µU/mL (0.5–5.0 mU/L, SI units)

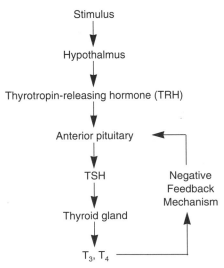

Figure 7   Thyroid hormone production.

TABLE 8
Correlation of TSH, Free T₄, and RAIU Results

Disorder	TSH	Free T4	RAIU
Hyperthyroidism			
Grave's disease	Decreased	Increased	Increased
Multinodular gland	Decreased	Increased	Increased
Autonomously functioning thyroid gland	Decreased	Increased	Increased
Subacute thyroiditis	Decreased	Increased	Decreased
Painless thyroiditis	Decreased	Increased	Decreased
Iatrogenic	Decreased	Increased	Decreased
Hypothyroidism			
Hypothyroidism	Increased	Decreased or Normal	Not Applicable

Possible Meanings of Abnormal Values

Increased	Decreased
Acute psychiatric illness	Grave's disease
Addison's disease	Hashimoto's thyroiditis
Anti-TSH antibodies	Hyperthyroidism
Euthyroid goiter	Multinodular thyroid gland
Fasting state	Organic brain syndrome
Goiter (iodine deficiency type)	Pituitary hypofunction
Hyperpituitarism	Secondary hypothyroidism
Hypothermia	
Pituitary adenoma	
Primary hypothyroidism	
Subtotal thyroidectomy	
Thyroiditis	

Contributing Factors to Abnormal Values

- Hemolysis of the blood sample may alter test results.
- Drugs that may *increase* TSH: aminodarone, aminoglutethimide, amphetamine abuse, clomiphene citrate, ethionamide, inorganic iodides, iopanoic acid, ipodate, lithium, mercaptopurine, methimazole, metoclopramide, morphine, nitroprusside sodium, phenylbutazone, propylthiouracil, radiographic dye, SSKI, sulfonamides, sulfonylureas, thyroid-releasing hormone.
- Drugs that may *decrease* TSH: dopamine hydrochloride, glucocorticoids, levodopa, phenytoin, thyroid hormones.

T

Pre-Test Nursing Care

- Explain to the patient the purpose of the test and the need for a blood sample to be drawn.
- No fasting is required before the test.
- If possible, withhold medications that may affect test results.

Procedure

- A 7-mL blood sample is drawn in a collection tube containing a silicone gel.
- Gloves are worn throughout the procedure.

Post-Test Nursing Care

- Apply pressure at venipuncture site. Apply dressing, periodically assessing for continued bleeding.
- Label the specimen and transport it to the laboratory.
- Resume medications as taken before the testing period.
- Report abnormal findings to the primary care provider.

• • • • • • • • • • • • • • • •

Thyroid-Stimulating Immunoglobulin
(TSI, TSIg, Long-Acting Thyroid Stimulator [LATS])

Thyroid-stimulating immunoglobulin (TSI), formerly called long-acting thyroid stimulator, is an autoimmune antibody which binds to or near the thyroid-stimulating hormone (TSH) receptor on thyroid cells. TSI mimics the action of TSH, stimulating the thyroid gland to release above normal levels of thyroid hormones. This test is used to assist in the diagnosis of Graves' disease, since the majority of patients with Graves' disease have positive TSI.

Normal Values

Negative

Possible Meanings of Abnormal Values

Increased

Autoimmune thyroiditis
Graves' disease
Hyperthyroidism
Malignant exophthalmos

Contributing Factors to Abnormal Values

- Radioactive iodine preparations received within 24 hours of the test may alter test results.
- Hemolysis of the sample may alter test results.

T

Pre-Test Nursing Care

- Explain to the patient the purpose of the test and the need for a blood sample to be drawn.
- No fasting is required before the test.

Procedure

- A 7-mL blood sample is drawn in a collection tube containing no additives.
- Gloves are worn throughout the procedure.

Post-Test Nursing Care

- Apply pressure at venipuncture site. Apply dressing, periodically assessing for continued bleeding.
- Label the specimen and transport it to the laboratory.
- Report abnormal findings to the primary care provider.

• • • • • • • • • • • • • • • • •

Thyroxine
(T₄, Total T₄)

When thyroid hormone levels decrease in the bloodstream or the body is exposed to physiological or psychological stress, the hypothalamus is stimulated to release thyrotropin-releasing hormone (TRH). TRH in turn stimulates the production of thyroid-stimulating hormone (TSH) by the anterior lobe of the pituitary gland. TSH then stimulates production and release of triiodothyronine (T_3) and thyroxine (T_4).

Thyroxine (T_4) is the most abundant of the thyroid hormones. There are two types of thyroxine: free thyroxine and the portion bound to plasma proteins. The total T_4 test measures both types of thyroxine. It is usually analyzed in conjunction with free thyroxine index and TSH levels to aid in the diagnosis of hyperthyroidism and hypothyroidism. It can also be used to monitor the effectiveness of drug therapy in these conditions.

Normal Values

4–12 µg/dl (51–154 nmol/L, SI units)

Possible Meanings of Abnormal Values

Increased	Decreased
Acute intermittent porphyria	Acromegaly
Acute psychiatric disorder	Cirrhosis
Excessive iodine intake	Cretinism
Goiter	Exercise
Graves' disease	Hashimoto's thyroiditis
Hyperthyroidism	Hypoproteinemia

T

Increased	Decreased
Liver disease (early)	Hypothyroidism
Lymphoma	Iodide deficiency
Newborns	Liver disease (chronic)
Obesity	Malnutrition
Pregnancy	Myxedema
Subacute thyroiditis	Nephrosis
Thyrotoxicosis	Nephrotic syndrome
	Pituitary tumor
	Simmonds' disease
	Subacute thyroiditis
	Thyroidectomy

Contributing Factors to Abnormal Values

- Hemolysis of the blood sample or having had a radionuclide scan within 1 week before the test may alter the test results.
- Drugs that may *increase* T_4 levels: amiodarone, amphetamines, clofibrate, dextrothyroxine, dinoprostone tromethamine, estrogens, 5-fluorouracil, halothane, heparin, heroin, iodothiouracil, iopanoic acid, ipodate, levarterenol, levodopa, methadone, oral contraceptives, progesterone, propranolol hydrochloride, thyroid extract, thyroid-releasing hormone, thyrotropin, thyroxine.
- Drugs that may *decrease* T_4 levels: adrenocorticoids, anabolic steroids, androgens, antithyroid drugs, asparaginase, aspirin, barbiturates, carbamazepine, chlorpromazine, corticotropin, danazol, diphenylhydantoin, ethionamide, furosemide (high doses), gold salts, iodides, isoniazid, isotretinoin, lithium carbonate, L-triiodothyronine, methimazole, penicillin, phenylbutazone, phenytoin, prednisone, propranolol hydrochloride, propylthiouracil, reserpine, salicylates, somatropin, SSKI, sulfonamides.

Pre-Test Nursing Care

- Explain to the patient the purpose of the test and the need for a blood sample to be drawn.
- No fasting is required before the test.
- If possible, thyroid medications should be withheld for one month before this test. If this is not possible, the medication being taken should be noted on the laboratory slip.

Procedure

- A 5-mL blood sample is drawn in a collection tube containing a silicone gel.
- Testing of newborns is done with a heel stick at least 3 days following birth.
- Gloves are worn throughout the procedure.

Post-Test Nursing Care

- Apply pressure at venipuncture site. Apply dressing, periodically assessing for continued bleeding.
- Label the specimen and transport it to the laboratory.
- Report abnormal findings to the primary care provider.

• • • • • • • • • • • • • • •

T

Thyroxine-Binding Globulin
(TBG)

Both of the thyroid hormones, triiodothyronine (T_3) and thyroxine (T_4) are present in the blood in two forms. These two forms are a "free" state that allows the hormone to be biologically active, and the portion bound to plasma proteins. This test measures the level of thyroxine-binding globulin (TBG), which is the primary protein carrier for both T_3 and T_4. It provides information to aid in the differential diagnosis of true thyroid disorders and those related to altered TBG levels.

Normal Values

12–18 µg/dL

Possible Meanings of Abnormal Values

Increased	Decreased
Acute intermittent porphyria	Acromegaly
Active hepatitis	Acute illness
Congenital TBG excess	Congenital TBG deficiency
Estrogen-secreting tumors	Hyperthyroidism
Hepatic disease	Hypoproteinemia
Hypothyroidism	Liver disease
Neonates	Malnutrition
Pregnancy	Nephrosis
Subacute thyroiditis	Nephrotic syndrome
	Stress
	Testosterone-producing tumors

Contributing Factors to Abnormal Values

- Hemolysis of the blood sample may alter test results.
- Drugs that may *increase* TBG levels: clofibrate, estrogens, heroin, methadone, oral contraceptives, phenothiazines.
- Drugs that may *decrease* TBG levels: androgens, corticosteroids, phenytoin, prednisone, salicylates.

Pre-Test Nursing Care

- Explain to the patient the purpose of the test and the need for a blood sample to be drawn.
- No fasting is required before the test.
- If possible, withhold drugs affecting the test for 12–24 hours before the test.

Procedure

- A 10-mL blood sample is drawn in a collection tube containing no additives.
- Gloves are worn throughout the procedure.

T

Post-Test Nursing Care

- Apply pressure at venipuncture site. Apply dressing, periodically assessing for continued bleeding.
- Label the specimen and transport it to the laboratory.
- Resume medications as taken before the test.
- Report abnormal findings to the primary care provider.

• • • • • • • • • • • • • • • • •

Thyroxine, Free
(Free T₄, FT₄)

When thyroid hormone levels decrease in the bloodstream or the body is exposed to physiologic or psychological stress, the hypothalamus is stimulated to release thyrotropin-releasing hormone (TRH). TRH in turn stimulates the production of thyroid-stimulating hormone (TSH) by the anterior lobe of the pituitary gland. TSH then stimulates production and release of triiodothyronine (T_3) and thyroxine (T_4).

Thyroxine (T_4) is the most abundant of the thyroid hormones. There are two types of thyroxine: free thyroxine and the portion bound to plasma proteins. Less than 0.05% of the total thyroxine is not bound to plasma proteins. This is known as "free thyroxine" and is the only type of thyroxine that is biologically active. This test is used to assist in diagnosing hyperthyroidism and hypothyroidism when thyroxine-binding globulin (TBG) levels are abnormal. It is a difficult test to perform because of the minute quantity of free thyroxine present in blood; thus, it is also a relatively expensive test to perform.

Normal Values

0.8–2.7 ng/dL (10–35 pmol/L, SI units)

Possible Meanings of Abnormal Values

Increased	Decreased
Acute psychiatric illness	Anorexia nervosa
Hyperthyroidism	Hypothyroidism
Nephrosis	Severe illness
Pregnancy	

Contributing Factors to Abnormal Values

- A radionuclide scan within 1 week before the test may alter test results.
- Drugs that may *increase* free thyroxine levels: amiodarone, androgens, estrogens, heparin, oral contraceptives, phenytoin, propranolol hydrochloride, radiographic dyes, thyroxine.
- Drugs that may *decrease* free thyroxine levels: carbamazepine, heparin.

T

Pre-Test Nursing Care

- Explain to the patient the purpose of the test and the need for a blood sample to be drawn.
- No fasting is required before the test.

Procedure

- A 5-mL blood sample is drawn in a collection tube containing a silicone gel.
- Gloves are worn throughout the procedure.

Post-Test Nursing Care

- Apply pressure at venipuncture site. Apply dressing, periodically assessing for continued bleeding.
- Label the specimen and transport it to the laboratory.
- Report abnormal findings to the primary care provider.

• • • • • • • • • • • • • • • •

TORCH Test

See:
Toxoplasmosis
Rubella
Cytomegalovirus
Herpes virus

The TORCH test is a screening test conducted on newborn infants to evaluate possible congenital infection to one of the following: **T**oxoplasmosis, **O**ther, **R**ubella, **C**ytomegalovirus, **H**erpes virus. "Other" tests often included are those for syphilis or hepatitis. The test may also be done on a woman during pregnancy to screen for these diseases, since they are likely to cause birth defects.

Normal Values

Negative

Possible Meanings of Abnormal Values

Increased

Presence of IgM antibodies:	Congenital infection with the indicated virus
Presence of IgG antibodies:	Transfer of antibodies from mother to newborn

Contributing Factors to Abnormal Values

- Hemolysis of the blood cells caused by excessive agitation of the sample may alter test results.

Pre-Test Nursing Care

- Explain to the mother the purpose of the test and the need for a blood sample to be drawn.
- No fasting is required before the test.

Procedure

- 3-mL of venous or umbilical cord blood is obtained from the newborn.
- Gloves are worn throughout the procedure.

Post-Test Nursing Care

- Apply pressure at venipuncture site. Apply dressing, periodically assessing for continued bleeding.
- Label the sample and transport it to the laboratory immediately, avoiding excessive agitation.
- Report abnormal findings to the primary care provider.

• • • • • • • • • • • • • • • •

Total Carbon Dioxide Content
(CO₂ Content, Carbon Dioxide Content)

Total carbon dioxide content of the blood consists of two sources. The first, accounting for more than 95% of the carbon dioxide, comes from bicarbonate (HCO_3), which is regulated by the kidneys. The other source (less than 5% of the total) is owing to the dissolved carbon dioxide and carbonic acid (H_2CO_3), which is regulated by the lungs. It is these substances that assist in maintaining the body's acid-base balance through its buffering system. Thus, measurement of the total carbon dioxide content of the blood provides a general indication of the body's buffering capacity.

Normal Values

24.0–30.9 mEq/L (24.0–30.9 mmol/L, SI units)

Possible Meanings of Abnormal Values

Increased	Decreased
Airway obstruction	Acute renal failure
Alcoholism	Dehydration
Cushing's syndrome	Diabetic acidosis
Emphysema	Diarrhea (severe)
Fat embolism	Head trauma
Hypoventilation	High fever
Metabolic alkalosis	Hyperventilation
Nasogastric suctioning	Malabsorption
Pneumonia	Metabolic acidosis
Primary aldosteronism	Renal tubular acidosis
Pyloric obstruction	Respiratory alkalosis
Respiratory acidosis	Salicylate intoxication
Vomiting	Starvation
	Uremia

T

Contributing Factors to Abnormal Values

- Use of a tourniquet or pumping of the patient's hand during acquisition of the blood sample may alter test results.
- Drugs that may *increase* total carbon dioxide content: aldosterone, antacids, barbiturates, corticotropin, cortisone acetate, ethacrynic acid, hydrocortisone, licorice, loop diuretics, mercurial diuretics, sodium bicarbonate, thiazide diuretics.
- Drugs that may *decrease* total carbon dioxide content: acetazolamide, ammonium chloride, aspirin, chlorothiazide diuretics, dimercaprol, methacillin, nitrofurantoin, paraldehyde, salicylates, tetracycline, triamterene.

Pre-Test Nursing Care

- Explain to the patient the purpose of the test and the need for a blood sample to be drawn.
- No fasting is required before the test.

Procedure

- A 7-mL blood sample is drawn. If blood sample is drawn with electrolytes, a collection tube containing a silicone gel is used. If the test is performed alone, a collection tube containing heparin is used.
- Gloves are worn throughout the procedure.

Post-Test Nursing Care

- Apply pressure at venipuncture site. Apply dressing, periodically assessing for continued bleeding.
- Label the specimen. It should be taken to the laboratory immediately. If this is not possible, it should be placed on ice.
- Report abnormal findings to the primary care provider.

· · · · · · · · · · · · · · · · · ·

Total Iron-Binding Capacity
(TIBC)

Transferrin is a plasma protein that transports iron in the blood. Approximately one-third of the transferrin available in the body actually transports iron. Total iron-binding capacity (TIBC) provides data as to the maximum amount of iron that can be bound to transferrin.

Normal Values

250–410 µg/dL (45–73 µmol/L, SI units)

T

Possible Meanings of Abnormal Values

Increased	Decreased
Acute liver damage	Blood loss
Hepatitis	Cirrhosis of the liver
Iron deficiency anemia	Hemochromatosis
Late pregnancy	Hepatitis
	Malnutrition
	Myocardial infarction
	Neoplasms
	Nephrosis
	Pernicious anemia
	Rheumatoid arthritis
	Thalassemia
	Uremia

Contributing Factors to Abnormal Values

- Hemolysis of the sample may alter test results.
- Drugs that may *increase* the total iron-binding capacity: iron salts and oral contraceptives.
- Drugs that may *decrease* the total iron-binding capacity: asparaginase, chloramphenicol, corticotropin, cortisone, dextran, steroids, testosterone.

Pre-Test Nursing Care

- Explain to the patient the purpose of the test and the need for a blood sample to be drawn.
- Fasting is required for 12 hours before the test. Water intake is allowed.
- No iron supplements are to be taken within 24–48 hours before the test.

Procedure

- Obtain the blood sample in the morning, usually after 10AM, since iron levels vary throughout the day.
- A 5-mL blood sample is obtained in a collection tube containing a silicone gel.
- Gloves are worn throughout the procedure.

Post-Test Nursing Care

- Apply pressure at venipuncture site. Apply dressing, periodically assessing for continued bleeding.
- Label the specimen and transport it to the laboratory.
- Resume medications held before the test.
- Report abnormal findings to the primary care provider.

• • • • • • • • • • • • • • •

T

Toxicology Screen
(Drug Screen)

Toxicology screening for drugs is used for determining the cause of acute drug toxicity in an unconscious person, to monitor compliance with treatment regimens for drug dependency, and to detect the presence of drugs in the body for employment or legal purposes. Blood or urine may be tested. Examples of drugs included in drug screens include amphetamines, barbiturates, benzodiazepines, cannabinoids, cocaine, ethanol, hypnotics, and narcotics.

Normal Values

Depends on drug being monitored and reference laboratory used

Possible Meanings of Abnormal Values

Increased

Intake of tested substance
Toxicity

Pre-Test Nursing Care

- Explain to the patient the purpose of the test and the need for a blood sample or a urine sample to be collected.
- No fasting is required before the test.

Procedure

- If test is to be used as legal evidence, have specimen collection witnessed.
- Follow institutional policy regarding handling of legal evidence.
- Gloves are worn throughout the procedure.

Blood Testing

- Cleanse the venipuncture site and, if needed, the top of the collection tube, with povidone-iodine solution instead of alcohol.
- A 10-mL blood sample is drawn in a collection tube containing a silicone gel.

Urine Testing

- Obtain a 50-mL random urine specimen in a clean container. Cap tightly.

Post-Test Nursing Care

- Apply pressure at venipuncture site. Apply dressing, periodically assessing for continued bleeding.
- Label the specimen and transport it to the laboratory.
- If being used as legal evidence, transport the specimen in a sealed plastic bag to the laboratory. The bag must be signed by each person handling the specimen.
- Report abnormal findings to the primary care provider.

• • • • • • • • • • • • • • • •

T

Toxoplasmosis Antibody Titer

Toxoplasmosis is a disease caused by the protozoan organism *toxoplasma gondii*. The organism can be acquired through ingestion of raw or poorly cooked meat. It is also found in the feces of cats. It is estimated that up to half of the adult population is infected with toxoplasmosis, but is asymptomatic. If symptoms do occur, they include fatigue, muscle pain, lymphadenopathy, and little or no fever.

The disease is not transmitted between humans, except through maternal–fetal transfer. If a woman is infected prior to conception, the fetus will not be affected by the organism. However, if the woman becomes infected during pregnancy, the unborn child is at risk for birth defects. Such defects include mental retardation, hydrocephalus, microcephalus, and chronic retinitis. Fetal death may occur. The Centers for Disease Control recommend testing all pregnant women for toxoplasmosis prior to the 20th week of pregnancy.

Normal Values

Titer <1:16	No previous infection

Abnormal Values

Titer 1:16–1:64	Past exposure
Titer >1:256	Recent infection
Titer >1:1024	Acute infection

Possible Meanings of Abnormal Values

Increased

Toxoplasmosis

Pre-Test Nursing Care

- Obtain a history regarding intake of raw or poorly cooked meat or contact with cats.
- Explain to the patient the purpose of the test and that it involves drawing a blood sample.
- No fasting is required before the test.

Procedure

- 5–7 mL of blood is drawn in a collection tube containing no additives.
- Gloves are worn throughout the procedure.

Post-Test Nursing Care

- Apply pressure at venipuncture site. Apply dressing, periodically assessing for continued bleeding.
- Label the specimen and transport it to the laboratory.
- Inform the patient that an additional test may be done in 7–14 days to check for rising titer levels.
- Report abnormal findings to the primary care provider.
- Teach pregnant women to avoid contact with cat litter boxes.

T

Transesophageal Echocardiography
(TEE)

Ultrasonography is a noninvasive method of diagnostic testing in which ultrasound waves are sent into the body with a small transducer pressed against the skin. The transducer not only sends the sound waves into the body but also receives any returning sound waves, which are deflected back as they bounce off various structures. The transducer converts the returning sound waves into electric signals that are then transformed by a computer into a visual display on a monitor.

In transesophageal echocardiography (TEE), a small transducer is attached to the end of a gastroscope. It is inserted into the esophagus, allowing high quality images to be taken from the posterior aspect of the heart. This allows for evaluation of thoracic, aortic, and cardiac disorders with less interference from chest wall structures.

Normal Values

No cardiac abnormalities

Possible Meanings of Abnormal Values

Aortic aneurysm
Aortic dissection
Cardiac tumors
Cardiomyopathy
Congenital heart disease
Endocarditis
Intracardiac thrombi
Myocardial ischemia
Patent ductus arteriosus
Septal defects
Valvular disease

Contributing Factors to Abnormal Values

- The transducer must be in good contact with the esophagus as it is being moved. A lubricant, such as mineral oil, glycerin, or a water-based jelly, is used to ensure good contact with the esophagus.

CONTRAINDICATIONS

- Patients with esophageal pathology, including esophageal varices or stricture, or previous esophageal surgery
- Patients with bleeding disorders
- Patients who are unable to cooperate because of age, mental status, pain, or other factors

Pre-Test Nursing Care

- Explain to the patient the purpose of the test. Provide any written teaching materials available on the subject. Note that there is minimal discomfort involved with this test.
- Obtain a signed informed consent.

T

- Fasting for 6 hours is required prior to the test.
- Have the patient remove any dentures or oral prostheses. Note any loose or capped teeth.
- Resuscitation and suctioning equipment should be available.

Procedure

- The patient is assisted to a left-lying position on the examination table.
- Cardiac monitoring, pulse oximetry, and vital sign monitoring are initiated. An IV infusion is begun, and a sedative, such as a benzodiazepine, is administered.
- The back of the patient's throat is sprayed with a topical anesthetic agent to depress the gag reflex.
- The gastroscope is introduced into the mouth and, with the patient swallowing, is advanced to the level of the right atrium of the heart.
- The sound waves are transformed into a visual display on the monitor. Printed copies of this display are made.

Post-Test Nursing Care

Possible complications:
> **Cardiac arrhythmias**
> **Esophageal bleeding**
> **Esophageal perforation**
> **Sore throat**

- Monitor the vital signs and pulse oximetry until stable.
- Keep the patient supine until the sedation is ended. A narcotic antagonist such as naloxone may be administered to reverse the sedation.
- Do not allow food or fluid intake until the gag reflex has returned.
- Report abnormal findings to the primary care provider.

• • • • • • • • • • • • • • • • •

Transferrin
(Iron-Binding Protein, Siderophilin)

Transferrin is a plasma protein that is formed in the liver and has a half-life of 7–10 days. Its primary function is to transport iron from the mucosa of the intestines to iron storage sites in the body. Transferrin is capable of binding with more than its own weight in iron. One gram of transferrin can bind with 1.43 grams of iron.

Since transferrin is a protein and has a relatively short half-life, its level decreases very quickly in cases of protein malnutrition. Because of this, measurement of transferrin is sometimes done as a way of assessing the patient's nutritional status.

Normal Values

240–480 mg/dL

T

Possible Meanings of Abnormal Values

Increased	Decreased
Estrogen therapy	Acute inflammation
Hyperestrogenism	Anemia of chronic disease
Iron deficiency anemia	Genetic defect
Pregnancy	Iron overload
	Protein deficiency owing to loss from chronic infection, chronic kidney disease, chronic liver disease, malnutrition, neoplasms, nephrosis, thermal burns

Contributing Factors to Abnormal Values

- Elevations of transferrin levels may occur in the third trimester of pregnancy and in children aged 2 1/2–10 years.
- Hemolysis of the sample may alter test results.
- Drugs that may *increase* transferrin levels: oral contraceptives.

Pre-Test Nursing Care

- Explain to the patient the purpose of the test and the need for a blood sample to be drawn.
- Fasting is required for 12 hours before the test. Water intake is allowed.
- No iron supplements are to be taken within 24–48 hours before the test.

Procedure

- Obtain the blood sample in the morning, usually after 10 AM, when serum iron levels peak.
- A 5-mL blood sample is obtained in a collection tube containing a silicone gel.
- Gloves are worn throughout the procedure.

Post-Test Nursing Care

- Apply pressure at venipuncture site. Apply dressing, periodically assessing for continued bleeding.
- Label the specimen and transport it to the laboratory.
- Report abnormal findings to the primary care provider.

• • • • • • • • • • • • • • • •

Transferrin Saturation

Transferrin saturation is a calculation that uses both the serum iron level and the total iron binding capacity (TIBC). The test is used to aid in determining the cause of abnormal iron levels and abnormal TIBC levels. The percentage of saturation is calculated as follows:

$$\frac{\text{Serum iron} \times 100}{\text{TIBC}} = \% \text{ of transferrin saturation}$$

T

Normal Values

20%–50%

Possible Meanings of Abnormal Values

Increased	Decreased
Hemochromatosis	Iron deficiency anemia
Hemosiderosis	Neoplasms
Thalassemia	Rheumatoid arthritis
	Uremia

Contributing Factors to Abnormal Values

- Any of the factors that might impact upon the serum iron levels or the total iron-binding capacity will also affect the transferrin saturation. These factors include hemolysis of the blood sample, dietary intake of iron, and receipt of blood transfusions.

Pre-Test Nursing Care

- Explain to the patient the purpose of the test and the need for a blood sample to be drawn.
- Fasting is required for 12 hours before the test. Water intake is allowed.

Procedure

- Blood should be drawn in the morning, usually after 10 AM, when serum iron levels peak.
- A 5-mL blood sample is drawn in a collection tube containing a silicone gel.
- Gloves are worn throughout the procedure.

Post-Test Nursing Care

- Apply pressure at venipuncture site. Apply dressing, periodically assessing for continued bleeding.
- Label the specimen and transport it to the laboratory.
- Report abnormal findings to the primary care provider.

• • • • • • • • • • • • • • • • •

Triglycerides

Triglycerides are synthesized in the liver from fatty acids, proteins, and glucose. They are stored in adipose tissue and can be retrieved when needed for conversion into glucose. They comprise a major part of very low-density lipoproteins and a minor part of low-density lipoproteins. Triglycerides are measured as a part of the lipid profile and are considered when analyzing an individual's risk of coronary heart disease.

T

Normal Values

40–150 mg/dL (0.45–1.69 mmol/L SI units)

Women: Slightly lower values
Elderly: Increased

Possible Meanings of Abnormal Values

Increased	Decreased
Alcoholism	Brain infarction
Diabetes mellitus	Chronic obstructive pulmonary
Glycogen storage disease	disease
Hyperlipoproteinemias	Hyperthyroidism
Hypertension	Malabsorption
Hypothyroidism	Malnutrition
Liver disease	
Nephrotic syndrome	
Pancreatic dysfunction	
Pregnancy	
Toxemia of pregnancy	

Contributing Factors to Abnormal Values

- Drugs that may *increase* triglyceride levels: alcohol, beta-adrenergic blockers, cholestyramine, corticosteroids, estrogens, oral contraceptives, thiazide diuretics.
- Drugs that may *decrease* triglyceride levels: ascorbic acid, asparaginase, colestipol hydrochloride, clofibrate, dextrothyroxine, metformin, niacin.

Pre-Test Nursing Care

- Explain to the patient the purpose of the test and the need for a blood sample to be drawn.
- Fasting for 12 hours is required before the test. Water is permitted.
- No alcohol is allowed for 24 hours before the test.

Procedure

- A 7-mL blood sample is drawn in a collection tube containing a silicone gel.
- Gloves are worn throughout the procedure.

Post-Test Nursing Care

- Apply pressure at venipuncture site. Apply dressing, periodically assessing for continued bleeding.
- Label the specimen and transport it to the laboratory.
- Report abnormal findings to the primary care provider.
- If the test results are abnormally high, counsel the patient regarding weight loss, exercise, and needed dietary changes.

• • • • • • • • • • • • • • • •

T

Triiodothyronine
(T₃, Total T₃)

When thyroid hormone levels decrease in the bloodstream or the body is exposed to physiologic or psychological stress, the hypothalamus is stimulated to release thyrotropin-releasing hormone (TRH). TRH in turn stimulates the production of thyroid-stimulating hormone (TSH) by the anterior lobe of the pituitary gland. TSH then stimulates production and release of triiodothyronine (T_3) and thyroxine (T_4).

There are two types of T_3: the free, or active, portion, and the portion bound to plasma proteins. There is significantly less T_3 in the blood than T_4. It is also bound less firmly to thyroid-binding globulin (TBG) than T_4. This test is used rather infrequently, but remains the preferred test for use in the diagnosis of T_3 thyrotoxicosis.

Normal Values
75–195 ng/dL (1.2–3.0 nmol/L, SI units)

Elderly: Decreased

Possible Meanings of Abnormal Values

Increased	Decreased
Acute psychiatric illness	Acute illness
Acute thyroiditis	Anorexia nervosa
Congenital excess of TBG	Congenital TBG deficiency
Hyperthyroidism	Goiter
Pregnancy	Hepatic cirrhosis
T_3 thyrotoxicosis	Hypothyroidism
Toxic adenoma	Myxedema
	Obesity
	Renal failure
	Starvation
	Thyroidectomy

Contributing Factors to Abnormal Values
- A radionuclide scan within 1 week before the test may alter test results.
- Hemolysis of the blood sample may alter test results.
- Drugs that may *increase* T_3 levels: antithyroid medications, clofibrate, dextrothyroxine, dinoprostone tromethamine, estrogens, heroin, L-triiodothyronine, methadone, oral contraceptives, terbutaline sulfate, thyroxine.
- Drugs that may *decrease* T_3 levels: amiodarone, anabolic steroids, androgens, antithyroid drugs, asparaginase, cimetidine, clofibrate, dexamethasone, ethionamide, heparin, iopanoic acid, ipodate, isotretinoin, lithium, methimazole, methylthiouracil, phenylbutazone, phenytoin, propranolol hydrochloride, propylthiouracil, reserpine, radiographic dyes, salicylates (large doses), steroids, sulfonamides.

T

Pre-Test Nursing Care

- Explain to the patient the purpose of the test and the need for a blood sample to be drawn.
- No fasting is required before the test.
- If possible, withhold any medications that may alter test results.

Procedure

- A 5-mL blood sample is drawn in a collection tube containing a silicone gel.
- Gloves are worn throughout the procedure.

Post-Test Nursing Care

- Apply pressure at venipuncture site. Apply dressing, periodically assessing for continued bleeding.
- Label the specimen and transport it to the laboratory.
- Resume medications as taken before the test.
- Report abnormal findings to the primary care provider.

• • • • • • • • • • • • • • •

Triiodothyronine Uptake Test
(T₃ Uptake, T₃ Resin Uptake)

This test is an indirect measurement of the amount of unsaturated thyroxine-binding globulin (TBG) based on the total quantity of TBG present and the quantity of thyroxine (T_4) bound to it. During this test, a known quantity of radioactive T_3 and a resin are added to a sample of the patient's blood. The radioactive T_3 will bind with any available TBG sites. The percentage of radioactive T_3 that remains available to become attached to the resin after all available TBG sites have been filled is determined. This percentage is inversely proportional to the percentage of TBG saturation.

Normal Values

25%–35%

Possible Meanings of Abnormal Values

Increased	Decreased
Congenital TBG deficiency	Acute hepatitis
Hyperthyroidism	Congenital TBG excess
Hypoproteinemia	Cretinism
Malnutrition	Endocrine-secreting tumors
Nephrosis	Hypothyroidism
Nephrotic syndrome	Pregnancy
Renal failure	

T

Contributing Factors to Abnormal Values

- Drugs that may *increase* T_3 uptake: androgens, barbiturates, corticosteroids, corticotropin, furosemide, glucocorticoids, heparin, penicillin, phenylbutazone, phenytoin, salicylates, thyroid extract, thyroxine.
- Drugs that may *decrease* T_3 uptake: chlorpromazine, estrogens, heroin, lithium carbonate, methadone, oral contraceptives, propylthiouracil.

Pre-Test Nursing Care

- Explain to the patient the purpose of the test and the need for a blood sample to be drawn.
- No fasting is required prior to the test.

Procedure

- A 7-mL blood sample is drawn in a collection tube containing a silicone gel.
- Gloves are worn throughout the procedure.

Post-Test Nursing Care

- Apply pressure at venipuncture site. Apply dressing, periodically assessing for continued bleeding.
- Label the specimen and transport it to the laboratory.
- Report abnormal findings to the primary care provider.

• • • • • • • • • • • • • • • •

T-Tube Cholangiography
(Postoperative Cholangiography)

When a patient undergoes a cholecystectomy with an exploration of the common bile duct, a rubber T-tube is usually inserted into the common bile duct to facilitate bile drainage. Every effort is made to find and remove any obstructions, such as stones, from within the duct. Approximately 7–10 days after surgery, the patient is taken to the radiology department for a T-tube, or postoperative, cholangiogram. This test involves the injection of contrast dye through the T-tube into the biliary ducts. The flow of the dye is observed with the fluoroscope, allowing the radiologist to verify patency of the common bile duct prior to the removal of the T-tube.

Normal Values

Even filling of the biliary ducts. No calculi, strictures, or obstructions present. Normal flow of dye into the duodenum.

Possible Meanings of Abnormal Values

Calculi
Fistulae
Neoplasms
Strictures
Surgical trauma

T

Contributing Factors to Abnormal Values

- Under- or overexposure of the film may alter film quality.
- When patients are unable to hold still, owing to pain or mental status, the quality of the film may be affected.
- Retained barium from other exams, vomiting, and diarrhea will affect test results.

 CONTRAINDICATIONS

- Pregnant women (*Caution:* A woman in her childbearing years should undergo radiography only during her menses or 12–14 days after its onset to avoid any exposure to a fetus.)
- Patients with hypersensitivity to iodine, seafood, or contrast media
- Patients who are unable to cooperate because of age, mental status, pain, or other factors

Pre-Test Nursing Care

- *Note:* If a barium swallow or an upper gastrointestinal and small-bowel series test is ordered, these should be completed *after* the T-tube cholangiography is performed. Otherwise the barium sulfate ingested during the other exams may obscure the films made of the gallbladder.
- Explain to the patient the purpose of the test and the benefits and risks associated with the test. Provide any written teaching materials available on the subject.
- Obtain a signed informed consent from the patient.
- Inform the radiologist of any potential allergy to the contrast dye and obtain order for antihistamine and steroid to be given before the procedure.
- Patients receiving metformin (Glucophage) for non–insulin-dependent diabetes mellitus should discontinue the drug 2 days before elective surgery or angiographic exams. This is owing to the possible occurrence of lactic acidosis, a potentially fatal complication of biguanide therapy.
- The patient is to be NPO for 4–6 hours before the test.
- Clamp the T-tube the day before the procedure, if ordered.
- Some physicians order a cleansing enema before the test.
- Instruct the patient to remove all objects containing metal, such as jewelry or undergarments, as these will show on the film.

Procedure

- The patient is placed in a supine position on the examination table.
- The T-tube is cleansed with povidone-iodine and approximately 5 mL of the contrast medium is injected through the tube, and a spot film is taken.
- An additional 15–20 mL of the contrast medium is injected and several films are taken in a variety of positions.
- The T-tube is then clamped, and the patient is assisted to an erect position for additional films. These films are taken to detect inadvertent injection of air through the T-tube, which can be mistaken for calculi on some films.
- Final films are taken of the contrast media emptying into the duodenum.
- Gloves are worn throughout the procedure.

Post-Test Nursing Care

Possible complications:

- **Allergic reaction to dye**
- **Sepsis**

T

- Most allergic reactions to radiopaque dye occur within 30 minutes of administration of the contrast medium. Observe the patient closely for: respiratory distress, hypotension, edema, hives, rash, tachycardia, or laryngeal stridor. Emergency resuscitation equipment must be readily accessible.
- If findings are normal, the T-tube is removed, and a dry sterile dressing is applied to the site.
- Assess the patient's vital signs until stable. Observe for signs of sepsis, such as chills and fever.
- Check the site for redness, edema, pain, and drainage often.
- If the T-tube was left in place, reconnect it to drainage.
- Resume the patient's diet and medications as taken before the test. However, renal funciton should be assessed before metformin is restarted.
- Encourage fluid intake to enhance excretion of the contrast medium.
- Report abnormal findings to the primary care provider.

• • • • • • • • • • • • • • •

Tuberculin Skin Tests
(Mantoux Test, PPD Skin Test, TB Skin Test, Tine Test)

Tuberculin skin tests are used to screen for previous infection by the tubercle bacillus. The test is unable to differentiate between active tuberculosis (TB) and dormant TB. Tuberculin skin tests are routine screening procedures for children, health care workers, individuals at high risk of being infected, and individuals who are suspected of being infected with TB. Purified protein derivative (PPD) is administered intradermally. With the Mantoux test, the PPD is administered using a tuberculin syringe and a 25- or 26-gauge needle. In multipuncture tests, such as the Tine test, there are several tines impregnated with PPD that are quickly pressed into the skin. A positive Tine test is usually confirmed with a Mantoux test. The results are read in 48–72 hours. Any area of induration (harding) is measured. Redness is not significant, and is thus not measured.

Normal Values
Negative: induration <5 mm

Possible Meanings of Abnormal Values

Positive

Active tuberculosis
Previous infection by tubercle bacilli

Contributing Factors to Abnormal Values
- Subcutaneous, rather than intradermal, injection of the PPD invalidates the test.
- Drugs that may *suppress* skin reactions when given within the past 4–6 weeks: corticosteroids, immunosuppressants, live vaccine viruses, such as measles, mumps, rubella, or polio.

CONTRAINDICATIONS
- Patients with known active tuberculosis
- Patients who have received *bacille Calmette-Guérin* (BCG), an immunization against PPD. These patients will have a positive reaction to PPD, even though they have never had the TB infection.

T

Pre-Test Nursing Care

- Explain to the patient the purpose of the test and the procedure to be performed.
- Obtain the patient's history regarding previous history of TB, previous PPD results, and previous BCG immunization.

Procedure

- The patient is placed in a sitting position, with the arm extended and supported on a flat surface.
- Cleanse the volar surface of the upper forearm with alcohol and allow to dry. Avoid moles and other areas of pigmentation for injection of the PPD.
- Inject the PPD intradermally. A wheal should appear under the skin.
- Document the site of the injection.
- Measure any area of induration in 48–72 hours.
- Gloves are worn throughout the procedure.

Post-Test Nursing Care

- Report abnormal findings to the primary care provider.

• • • • • • • • • • • • • • • • •

Tubular Reabsorption of Phosphate
(TRP, Tubular Phosphate Reabsorption [TPR])

This test is performed primarily to aid in the diagnosis of primary hyperparathyroidism. Parathyroid hormone (PTH) regulates plasma concentration and renal excretion of calcium and phosphorus. This is accomplished through stimulating reabsorption of calcium and inhibiting reabsorption of phosphate from the glomerular filtrate. By measuring the tubular reabsorption of phosphate, one gathers indirect data regarding PTH function.

Normal Values
80%–90%

Possible Meanings of Abnormal Values

Increased	Decreased
Myeloma	Primary hyperparathyroidism
Osteomalacia	
Renal tubular disease	
Uremia	

Contributing Factors to Abnormal Values

- Hemolysis of the blood sample may alter test results.
- Low phosphate intake may elevate TRP values; a high-phosphate diet may lower TRP values.

T

- Drugs that may *increase* reabsorption: furosemide, gentamicin.
- Drugs that may *decrease* reabsorption: amphotericin B, chlorothiazide diuretics.

Pre-Test Nursing Care

- Explain to the patient the purpose of the test and the need for both a blood sample and a 24-hour urine collection.
- Explain 24-hour urine collection procedure to the patient.
- Stress the importance of saving *all* urine in the 24-hour period. Instruct the patient to avoid contaminating the urine with toilet paper or feces.
- Inform the patient of the presence of a preservative in the collection bottle.
- Fasting for 8 hours is required before the test. Water is permitted.
- If possible, withhold any medications that may affect the test results.

Procedure

- A 10-mL blood sample is drawn in a collection tube containing a silicone gel.
- Begin the 24-hour urine collection, by obtaining the proper container that contains the appropriate preservative from the laboratory.
- Begin the testing period in the morning following the patient's first voiding, which is discarded.
- Timing of the 24-hour period begins at the time the first voiding is discarded.
- *All* urine for the next 24 hours is collected in the container, which is to be kept refrigerated or on ice.
- If any urine is accidentally discarded during the 24-hour period, the test must be discontinued and a new test begun.
- The ending time of the 24-hour collection period should be posted in the patient's room.
- Gloves are to be worn whenever dealing with the specimen collection.

Post-Test Nursing Care

- Apply pressure at venipuncture site. Apply dressing, periodically assessing for continued bleeding.
- Label the blood sample and transport it to the laboratory.
- Label the urine container and transport it on ice to the laboratory as soon as possible following the end of the 24-hour collection period.
- Resume any medications as taken before the test.
- Report abnormal findings to the primary care provider.

· · · · · · · · · · · · · · · ·

Tumor Markers

See:
Alpha-Fetoprotein (AFP)
CA 15-3
CA 19-9
CA-125
Carcinoembryonic Antigen (CEA)
Human Chorionic Gonadotropin (HCG)
Prostate-Specific Antigen (PSA)

T

Upper Gastrointestinal and Small-Bowel Series
(Gastric Radiography, Small Bowel Study, Stomach X-ray, Upper GI Series)

The upper gastrointestinal and small-bowel series is the fluoroscopic examination of the esophagus, stomach, and small intestine after ingestion of barium sulfate. During this procedure, a fluoroscopic screen is positioned over the structures being studied. These structures are then projected onto the fluoroscopic screen. The image remains on the monitor for continuous observation; therefore, as the patient swallows barium and it passes into the stomach, the flow of barium can be monitored on the screen. The patient's position is changed throughout the exam to allow visualization of the structures and their function, including peristalsis. This test is especially useful in the evaluation of patients experiencing dysphagia, regurgitation, burning or gnawing epigastric pain, hematemesis, melena, and weight loss. Videotapes of the fluoroscopic procedure enable the movements to be studied at a later time.

Normal Values

Normal size, shape, position, and functioning of the esophagus, stomach, and small bowel

Possible Meanings of Abnormal Values

Achalasia
Cancer of the esophagus
Chalasia
Congenital abnormalities
Duodenal cancer
Duodenal diverticula
Duodenal ulcers
Esophageal diverticula
Esophageal motility disorders, such as spasms
Esophageal ulcers
Esophageal varices
Esophagitis
External compression by pancreatic and hepatic cysts and tumors
Gastric cancer
Gastric inflammatory disease
Gastric tumors
Gastric ulcers
Gastritis
Hiatal hernia
Perforation of the esophagus, stomach, or small bowel
Polyps
Small bowel perforation
Small bowel tumors
Strictures

Contributing Factors to Abnormal Values

- Under- or overexposure of the film may alter film quality.
- When patients are unable to hold still, owing to pain or mental status, the quality of the film may be affected.

 CONTRAINDICATIONS

- Pregnant women (*Caution:* A woman in her childbearing years should undergo radiography only during her menses or 12–14 days after its onset to avoid any exposure to a fetus.)
- Patients with intestinal obstruction
- Patients with a perforated viscus (Gastrografin, a water-soluble contrast medium, would be used in place of barium.)
- Patients who are unable to cooperate because of age, mental status, pain, or other factors
- Patients with unstable vital signs

Pre-Test Nursing Care

- *Note:* If cholangiography or a barium enema test are ordered, these should be completed *before* the barium swallow is performed. Otherwise the barium sulfate ingested during the barium swallow may obscure the films made during the other exams.
- Explain to the patient the purpose of the test and the benefits and risks associated with the test. Provide any written teaching materials available on the subject. (*Note:* No discomfort is associated with this procedure. The barium, although in a milkshake-type solution, may taste chalky.)
- Fasting for 8 hours is required before the test.
- Instruct the patient to remove all objects containing metal, such as jewelry or undergarments, as these will show on the film.

Procedure

- The patient is first assisted to a supine position on the exam table. The patient is secured to the table for safety during the procedure.
- The table is tilted so that the patient is placed in an upright position for the first part of the procedure.
- The fluoroscopic screen is placed in front of the patient and the heart, lungs, and abdomen are viewed.
- The patient is instructed to take several swallows of a thick barium mixture while the video-tape is made of the pharyngeal action.
- As the patient then continues to drink the barium mixture, in addition to the fluoroscopic viewing, spot films are made of the esophageal area from a variety of angles.
- The patient drinks the barium through a straw, which allows some air to also be introduced into the abdomen. This air permits detailed examination of the gastric lining; thus, this is known as *double contrast* or *air contrast.*
- The patient is then instructed to finish drinking the barium mixture, while films are made of the filling of the stomach and the emptying of the stomach into the duodenum.
- The small intestine is observed for passage of barium, with films made at 30–60 minute intervals until the barium reaches the ileocecal valve.

Post-Test Nursing Care
Possible complication: Fecal impaction owing to retention of barium.

- Resume the patient's diet and medications as taken before the test.
- Encourage fluid intake to promote excretion of the barium.
- Instruct the patient on the need to evacuate all of the barium. Administer a cathartic as ordered. Check all stools for presence of barium, explaining to the patient that the stools will be white initially and return to normal color following passage of all of the barium.
- Notify the physician if the barium is not expelled within 2–3 days.
- Provide emotional support as the patient awaits the test results.
- Report abnormal findings to the primary care provider.

• • • • • • • • • • • • • • • • •

Urea Nitrogen, Blood
(blood urea nitrogen, BUN)

U rea is produced in the liver as a result of protein metabolism. Urea nitrogen is the nitrogen portion of urea. Urea is transported in the blood to the kidneys, where it is excreted. Since urea is cleared from the bloodstream by the kidneys, measurement of the level of urea nitrogen in the blood is an appropriate test of renal function, specifically that of glomerular function. The blood urea nitrogen (BUN) is usually determined in conjunction with the creatinine level in assessing renal function. Both of these parameters should be assessed prior to administration of any aminoglycoside to the patient. The normal ratio of BUN to creatinine ranges from 6:1 to 20:1.

Normal Values
8–25 mg/dL (2.9–8.9 mmol/L SI units)

Males:	slightly increased
Elderly:	slightly increased
Early pregnancy:	decreased (approximately 25%)
Newborn:	decreased

Possible Meanings of Abnormal Values

Increased	Decreased
Acute glomerulonephritis	Alcohol abuse
Acute myocardial infarction	Celiac disease
Congestive heart failure	Diet inadequate in protein
Diabetes mellitus	Hemodialysis
Diarrhea	Hepatitis
Gastrointestinal bleeding	Increased antidiuretic
High-protein diet	hormone (ADH)

Increased	Decreased
Mercury poisoning	Late pregnancy
Nephrotic syndrome	Malnutrition
Obstructive uropathy	Nephrosis
Severe dehydration	Overhydration
Severe infection	Severe liver failure
Shock	

Contributing Factors to Abnormal Values

- False elevation of BUN with hemolysis of blood sample.
- Drugs that may *increase* the BUN: acetohexamide, alkaline antacids, allopurinol, ammonium salts, amphotericin B, anabolic steroids, androgens, ascorbic acid, asparaginase, aspirin, bacitracin, calcium salts, captopril, chloral hydrate, chloramphenicol, chlorothiazide sodium, chlorthalidone, clonidine hydrochloride, dextran, dextrose infusions, disopyramide phosphate, doxapram, fluorides, fluphenazine, furosemide, gentamicin, guanethidine sulfate, hydroxyurea, indomethacin, kanamycin, lithium carbonate, marijuana, mercury compounds, mercurial diuretics, methicillin sodium, methotrexate, methoxyflurane, methosuximide, methyldopa, methysergide, metolazone, metoprolol tartrate, minoxidil, morphine, nalidixic acid, naproxen sodium, neomycin sulfate, nitrofurantoin, polymyxin B, probenecid, propranolol hydrochloride, rifampin, salicylates, streptokinase, sulfonamides, tetracycline, thiazide diuretics, tolmetin sodium, triamterene, vancomycin.
- Drugs that may *decrease* the BUN: chloramphenicol, streptomycin, thymol.

Pre-Test Nursing Care

- Explain to the patient the purpose of the test and the need for a blood sample to be drawn.
- No fasting is required before the test.
- Instruct the patient to avoid a diet high in red meat before the test.

Procedure

- A 7-mL blood sample is drawn in a collection tube containing a silicone gel.
- Gloves are worn throughout the procedure.

Post-Test Nursing Care

- Apply pressure at venipuncture site. Apply dressing, periodically assessing for continued bleeding.
- Label the specimen and transport it to the laboratory.
- Report abnormal findings to the primary care provider.
- If the BUN is elevated, check with the physician before administering any aminoglycoside.

• • • • • • • • • • • • • • • •

Urea Nitrogen, Urine
(Urinary Urea Nitrogen)

Testing for the level of urea nitrogen in the urine provides information regarding the nitrogen balance of the individual. This test measures the amount of urinary urea nitrogen in a 24-hour urine specimen. This finding is then compared with the amount of protein ingested during the same time period to determine the person's nitrogen balance. The nitrogen balance is determined through the following formula:

$$\text{Nitrogen balance} = \frac{\text{Protein intake (g)}}{6.25} - (24^{\circ} \text{ urinary urea nitrogen} + 4)$$

Normal Values

Urinary urea nitrogen:	6–17 g/24 hours
Nitrogen balance:	0 or greater

Possible Meanings of Abnormal Values

Decreased

Negative nitrogen balance
Impaired kidney function

Contributing Factors to Abnormal Values

- Inaccurate results may occur if any portion of the urine is disposed of, or if inaccurate intake is documented.

Pre-Test Nursing Care

- Explain 24-hour urine collection procedure to the patient.
- Stress the importance of saving *all* urine in the 24-hour period. Instruct the patient to avoid contaminating the urine with toilet paper or feces.

Procedure

- Obtain the proper container from the laboratory.
- Begin the testing period in the morning following the patient's first voiding, which is discarded.
- Timing of the 24-hour period begins at the time the first voiding is discarded.
- *All* urine for the next 24 hours is collected in the container.
- If any urine is accidentally discarded during the 24-hour period, the test must be discontinued and a new test begun.
- The ending time of the 24-hour collection period should be posted in the patient's room.
- During the 24-hour collection period, all food intake must be accurately recorded by the nurse and the protein intake determined by the dietician.
- Gloves are worn throughout the procedure.

Post-Test Nursing Care

- Label the container and transport it on ice to the laboratory as soon as possible following the end of the 24-hour collection period.
- Report abnormal findings to the primary care provider.
- If the test results indicate a negative nitrogen balance, the patient needs to be instructed on ways in which to increase the intake of protein.

• • • • • • • • • • • • • • • •

Urethral Pressure Profile

The urethral pressure profile is a manometric study that measures pressure changes along the urethra while the bladder is at rest. This study is used to diagnose urethral sphincter function abnormalities. It can also be used to evaluate the effectiveness of surgical interventions for sphincter abnormalities. Normal urethral pressures vary according to the patient's age and sex.

Normal Values

Normal maximal urethral pressures measured in cm of water:

	Female	Male
>age 64	35–75	35–105
age 45–64	40–100	40–123
age 25–44	31–115	35–113
<age 25	55–103	37–126

Possible Meanings of Abnormal Values

Urethral sphincter abnormalities

CONTRAINDICATIONS

- Patients with urinary tract infections

Pre-Test Nursing Care

- Explain to the patient the purpose of the test and how it will be performed.
- No fasting is required before the test.

Procedure

- The patient is assisted to assume a lithotomy position.
- A urinary catheterization is performed using sterile technique and proper draping. The dual-lumen catheter is connected to a transducer.
- A continuous infusion of fluids or gas are instilled through the catheter as it is withdrawn through the urethra.
- Pressures along the urethral wall are obtained as the catheter is removed.
- Gloves are worn throughout the procedure.

Post-Test Nursing Care

- Encourage the patient to increase fluid intake.
- Inform the patient that warm tub baths will provide relief from urethral discomfort that may occur after the procedure.
- Instruct the patient to report any indications of urinary tract infection: hematuria, cloudy or foul-smelling urine, inability to void, dysuria, frequency, and urgency.
- Report abnormal findings to the primary care provider.

• • • • • • • • • • • • • • • • •

Uric Acid, Blood

U ric acid is a nitrogenous compound that comes from two sources. It is the end product of the metabolism of the purines adenine and guanine during the formation and degradation of ribonucleic acid (RNA) and deoxyribonucleic acid (DNA). Uric acid is also formed as a result of the metabolism of dietary purines. Dietary sources high in purines include: anchovies, asparagus, caffeine-containing beverages, legumes, mushrooms, spinach, yeast, and organ meats, such as liver and kidneys.

Following synthesis in the liver, part of the uric acid is excreted in the urine. Excess serum uric acid can become deposited in joints and soft tissues, causing gout, an inflammatory response to the deposition of the urate crystals. Conditions in which there is rapid turnover of cells or slowing of uric acid excretion by the kidneys may cause elevated serum uric acid levels (*hyperuricemia*). Thus, this test is used to evaluate gout, kidney failure, leukemia, and toxemia of pregnancy.

Normal Values

Female:	2.3–6.6 mg/dL (137–393 umol/L SI units)
Male:	3.6–8.5 mg/dL (214–506 umol/L SI units)
Elderly:	Increased

Possible Meanings of Abnormal Values

Increased (hyperuricemia)	Decreased (hypouricemia)
Acute leukemia	Acromegaly
Acute infectious mononucleosis	Celiac disease
Alcoholism	Hodgkin's disease
Anemia	Liver disease
Congestive heart failure	Neoplasms
Dehydration	Renal tubular defects
Down syndrome	Syndrome of inappropriate
Eclampsia	ADH secretion (SIADH)
Fasting	Wilson's disease
Glomerulonephritis	Xanthinuria
Gouty arthritis	

Increased (hyperuricemia)	Decreased (hypouricemia)

Hypoparathyroidism
Hypothyroidism
Lead poisoning
Lymphomas
Malnutrition
Neoplasms
Nephritis
Pre-eclampsia
Polycythemia vera
Radiation
Renal failure
Shock
Uremia

Contributing Factors to Abnormal Values

- Drugs that may *increase* uric acid levels: acetaminophen, acetazolamide, aminophylline, ascorbic acid, asparaginase, aspirin (low dose), azathioprine, busulfan, caffeine, chlorothiazide sodium, chlorthalidone, corticosteroids, cyclophosphamide, dactinomycin, daunorubicin hydrochloride, dextran, diazoxide, epinephrine, ethacrynic acid, ethambutol hydrochloride, ethanol, fructose, furosemide, gentamicin, glucose, hydralazine hydrochloride, hydrocortisone, hydroxyurea, levodopa, mecamylamine hydrochloride, mechlorethamine, 6-mercaptopurine, methicillin sodium, methotrexate, methyldopa, metoprolol tartrate, niacin, nitrogen mustards, norepinephrine bitartrate, phenothiazines, phenytoin sodium, prednisone, probenecid, propranolol hydrochloride, propylthiouracil. pyrazinamide, quinethazone, rifampin, thiazide diuretics, 6-thioguanine, triamterene, vincristine sulfate.
- Drugs that may *decrease* uric acid levels: acetohexamide, allopurinol, anticoagulants, aspirin (high doses), azathioprine, bacitracin, chlorine, chlorpromazine, chlorprothixene, chlorthalidone, corticosteroids, corticotropin, dicumarol, ethacrynic acid, glyceryl guaiacolate, indomethacin, lithium carbonate, mannitol, marijuana, phenothiazines, phenylbutazone, piperazine, potassium oxalate, probenecid, radiographic dyes, saline infusions, sodium oxalate, sulfinpyrazone, thyroid hormone, and triamterene.

Pre-Test Nursing Care

- Explain to the patient the purpose of the test and the need for a blood sample to be drawn.
- Fasting is required for 8 hours before the test.
- Assess the patient's dietary history for intake of purine-rich foods.

Procedure

- A 7-mL blood sample is drawn in a collection tube containing a silicone gel.
- Gloves are worn throughout the procedure.

Post-Test Nursing Care

- Apply pressure at venipuncture site. Apply dressing, periodically assessing for continued bleeding.
- Label the specimen and transport it to the laboratory immediately.
- Report abnormal findings to the primary care provider.
- If the uric acid in the blood is found to be high, instruct the patient to increase the fluid intake to prevent renal stones from forming. Alcohol should be avoided in that it inhibits the excretion of urate crystals.

• • • • • • • • • • • • • • • • •

Uric Acid, Urine

Uric acid is a nitrogenous compound that comes from two sources. It is the end product of the metabolism of the purines adenine and guanine during the formation and degradation of ribonucleic acid (RNA) and deoxyribonucleic acid (DNA). Uric acid is also formed as a result of the metabolism of dietary purines. Dietary sources high in purines include: anchovies, asparagus, caffeine-containing beverages, legumes, mushrooms, spinach, yeast, and organ meats, such as liver and kidneys.

Following synthesis in the liver, part of the uric acid is excreted in the urine. Excess urinary uric acid can precipitate into urate stones in the kidneys. Thus, this test is used to evaluate gout, to determine whether there is an overexcretion of uric acid, and to determine whether renal calculi may be caused by hyperuricosuria.

Normal Values

250–650 mg/24 hours (1.48–4.43 mmol/24 hours, SI units)

Possible Meanings of Abnormal Values

Increased	Decreased
Chronic myelogenous leukemia	Alcoholism
Eclampsia	Glomerulonephritis
Gout	Lead poisoning
Infection	Urinary obstruction
Liver disease	
Polycythemia vera	
Pre-eclampsia	
Trauma	

Contributing Factors to Abnormal Values

- Drugs that may *increase* uric acid excretion: ascorbic acid, aspirin (high doses), cytotoxics, phenylbutazone (high doses), probenecid (high doses), radiographic dyes, sulfinpyrazone.

- Drugs that may *decrease* uric acid excretion: aspirin (low doses), diuretics, phenylbutazone (low doses), probenecid (low doses).

Pre-Test Nursing Care

- Explain 24-hour urine collection procedure to the patient.
- Stress the importance of saving *all* urine in the 24-hour period. Instruct the patient to avoid contaminating the urine with toilet paper or feces.
- Inform the patient of the presence of a preservative in the collection container.
- No fasting is required for this test.

Procedure

- Obtain from the laboratory, the proper container containing the alkaline preservative, sodium hydroxide.
- Begin the testing period in the morning following the patient's first voiding, which is discarded.
- Timing of the 24-hour period begins at the time the first voiding is discarded.
- *All* urine for the next 24 hours is collected in the container.
- If any urine is accidentally discarded during the 24-hour period, the test must be discontinued and a new test begun.
- The ending time of the 24-hour collection period should be posted in the patient's room.
- Gloves are worn throughout the procedure.

Post-Test Nursing Care

- Label the container and transport it on ice to the laboratory as soon as possible following the end of the 24-hour collection period.
- Report abnormal findings to the primary care provider.
- If the uric acid level in the urine is found to be high, instruct the patient on a low purine diet

• • • • • • • • • • • • • • • • • •

Urinalysis
(Routine Urinalysis, U/A)

Urinalysis includes: appearance, bilirubin, color, glucose, ketones, leukocyte esterase, nitrites, odor, pH, protein, specific gravity, urobilinogen, and microscopic exam of sediment (bacteria, casts, crystals, red blood cells, white blood cells).

The urinalysis is a routine screening test that is usually done as a part of a physical examination, during preoperative testing, and on hospital admission. It is used in the diagnosis of infections of the kidneys and urinary tract and also in the diagnosis of diseases unrelated to the urinary system.

The urinalysis consists of several components including: appearance, bilirubin, blood, color, glucose, ketones, leukocyte esterase, nitrites, odor, pH, protein, specific gravity, urobilinogen, and microscopic exam of sediment (bacteria, crystals, epithelial casts, fatty casts, granular casts, hyaline casts, red blood cells and casts, white blood cells and casts). Many of the component tests within the urinalysis are performed via dipstick method. Each of the component tests will be discussed, including a test description, normal values, possible meanings of abnormal values, and contributing factors to abnormal values.

In general, if the urine sample is left standing too long, bacteria begin to split urea into ammonia, resulting in an alkaline urine. Should this occur, test results regarding protein and the microscopic examination of casts will be inaccurate. A delay in testing may also result in falsely low glucose, ketone, bilirubin, and urobilinogen values and falsely elevated bacteria levels.

Appearance

The appearance of the urine refers to the clarity of the fluid. Deviations from the normal appearance of urine may indicate the presence of infection or hematuria.

Normal Values

Clear to slightly hazy

Possible Meanings of Abnormal Values

Cloudy urine may be caused by the presence of bacteria, fat, red blood cells, or white blood cells.
Smokey urine may be caused by the presence of blood.
Urine that *foams* on shaking may indicate the presence of bilirubin.

Contributing Factors to Abnormal Values

- If the urine sample is left standing too long, bacteria begin to split urea into ammonia, resulting in an alkaline urine. Alkaline urine (pH >7.0) results in turbid urine.
- Contamination of the sample with vaginal secretions may affect its appearance.

Bilirubin

Bilirubin, which is one of the components of bile, is formed in the liver, spleen, and bone marrow. It is also formed as a result of hemoglobin breakdown. There are three types of bilirubin: total, direct (conjugated), and indirect (unconjugated). *Total bilirubin* is composed of the direct bilirubin plus the indirect bilirubin. Normally, *direct, or conjugated, bilirubin* is excreted by the gastrointestinal (GI) tract, with only minimal amounts entering the bloodstream.

Direct bilirubin is water-soluble and is the only type of bilirubin able to cross the glomerular filter. Although it is the only type of bilirubin that could be found in the urine, it is usually not detectable in the urine, since it is converted to urobilinogen in the intestine. However, should jaundice occur because of obstruction or liver disease, the direct bilirubin is unable to reach the GI tract. It instead enters the bloodstream, where it is eventually filtered out by the kidneys and excreted in the urine. Thus, an increased level of direct bilirubin in the urine is indicative of some type of hepatic or obstructive problem.

Indirect bilirubin, also known as *free or unconjugated bilirubin,* is normally found in the blood stream. In the case of hemolytic jaundice, the breakdown of hemoglobin results in a higher level of indirect bilirubin being present in the bloodstream. *Total bilirubin* and *direct bilirubin* are measured through lab testing. The level of *indirect bilirubin* is determined by the following calculation:

$$\text{Indirect bilirubin} = \text{Total bilirubin} - \text{Direct bilirubin}$$

The test for bilirubin conducted as part of the routine urinalysis screens for the presence of direct (conjugated) bilirubin in the urine.

U

Normal Values

Negative (routine screening procedure)

No more than 0.2 mg/dL (<0.34 umol/L, SI units)

Possible Meanings of Abnormal Values

Increased

Cirrhosis of the liver
Hepatitis
Obstructive jaundice

Contributing Factors to Abnormal Values

- Drugs that may cause *false positive* results: phenazopyridine hydrochloride, phenothiazines, salicylates.
- Drug that may cause *false negative* results: ascorbic acid.
- Exposure of the specimen to light may affect test results.

Color

In general, the color of the urine should correspond to the specific gravity of the urine. For example, dilute urine with its low specific gravity is almost colorless, whereas concentrated urine, with a specific gravity, is dark yellow to amber in color. There are many factors that can affect the color of the urine, including food, drugs, and various conditions.

Normal Values

Light yellow to amber

Possible Meanings of Abnormal Values

Condition/Substance	Color of urine
Alcohol or large fluid intake	Light straw
Alkaptonuria	Black
Bacterial infections	Green
Bile	Orange
Bilirubin	Dark yellow to amber
Concentrated urine	Dark yellow to amber
Dilute urine	Very pale yellow
Excessive exercise	Red
Fever	Orange
Foods such as beets, rhubarb	Red
Foods such as carrots	Dark yellow
Melanotic tumor	Black
Porphyria	Red

Medication	Color of urine
Amitriptyline	Blue-green
Anisindione	Orange (alkaline urine)
	Pink-red-brown (acid urine)
Anthraquinones laxatives	Pink, brown
Anticoagulants	Pink, red, orange, brown
Antipyrine	Red, pink
Cascara	Brown (acid urine), yellow-pink, red (alkaline urine), black
Chloroquine hydrochloride	Brown
Deferoxamine mesylate	Red
Doxorubicin hydrochloride	Red or pink
Ferrous sulfate	Brown, black
Fluorescein sodium	Orange
Furazolidone	Brown
Ibuprofen	Red, pink
Indomethacin	Green
Levodopa	Red-brown
Methocarbamol	Dark brown, black, blue, green
Methyldopa	Red, pink brown
Methylene blue	Green-yellow, blue
Metronidazole	Dark brown
Nitrofurantoin	Brown, yellow
Oxamniquine	Red-orange
Phenazopyridine hydrochloride	Orange, red
Phenolphthalein	Pink, red, magenta (alkaline urine), orange, rust (acid urine)
Phenolsulfonphthalein	Pink, red
Phenothiazines	Pink, red, purple, orange, rust
Phensuximide	Pink, red, purple, orange, rust
Phenytoin	Pink, red, red-brown
Primaquine	Rust yellow, brown
Quinacrine hydrochloride	Dark yellow
Quinine sulfate	Brown, black
Riboflavin	Bright yellow
Rifabutin	Red-orange
Rifampin	Red-orange
Salicylates	Pink, red, brown
Senna	Red (alkaline urine), yellow-brown (acid urine)
Sulfasalazine	Orange-yellow (alkaline urine)
Sulfobromophthalein	Red
Sulfonamides	Rust, yellow, brown
Tolonium	Blue, green
Triamterene	Green, blue
Vitamins	Green

Contributing Factors to Abnormal Values

- Urine tends to darken in color on standing, thus urine specimens should be transported to the laboratory immediately after collection.

Glucose

As a part of the routine urinalysis, the urine is screened for the presence of glucose. This screening is accomplished through either the enzyme method, in which a reagent strip is dipped into the urine sample, or the reduction method, in which tablets containing cupric oxide are used. The chemical reactions result in color changes that correspond to the level of glucose in the urine. Normally, there should be no glucose present in the urine, although occasionally a trace amount will occur during pregnancy. Should glucose be found in the urine, a condition known as *glycosuria*, diabetes mellitus is suspected. However, further testing must be done to positively diagnose this condition.

Normal Values

Negative

Possible Meanings of Abnormal Values

Increased

Cushing's syndrome
Diabetes mellitus
Galactose intolerance
Hyperalimentation
Infection
Ketonuria
Lowered renal threshold for glucose (pregnancy)
Myocardial infarction
Pheochromocytoma
Stress

Contributing Factors to Abnormal Values

- Use of deteriorated reagent strips or improper technique will alter test results.
- Drugs that may cause *increased* levels of glucose in the urine: ammonium chloride, asparaginase, carbamazepine, corticosteroids, dextrothyroxine, lithium carbonate, nicotinic acid, phenothiazines, thiazide diuretics.
- Drugs that may cause *false-positive* results: aminosalicylic acid, cephalosporins, chloral hydrate, chloramphenicol, corticosteroids, indomethacin, isoniazid, nalidixic acid, nitrofurantoin, penicillin, probenecid, streptomycin, sulfonamides, tetracyclines, sugars other than glucose (lactose, fructose, galactose, pentose)
- Drugs that may cause *false-negative* results: cancer metabolites.
- Drugs that may cause *either* false-positive or false-negative results: ascorbic acid, levodopa, methyldopa, phenazopyridine hydrochloride, salicylates.

Ketones

Normally, glucose is used by the cells of the body for energy. This use of glucose as an energy source can only occur if the glucose is able to enter the cell with the assistance of insulin. When insulin is lacking, as in the patient with uncontrolled diabetes mellitus, glucose is unable to enter the cell, resulting in the need for an alternate energy source. The body then turns to the metabolism of fatty acids for energy. As fatty acids are metabolized, three ketone bodies are formed and later excreted in the urine: acetoacetic acid, acetone, and beta-hydroxybutyric acid. Thus, testing for the presence of ketones in the urine is assistive in the diagnosis of diabetes mellitus, as well as in evaluating conditions associated with ketoacidotic states, such as starvation. Testing for ketones in the urine, a situation known as *ketonuria,* can be done via use of a reagent strip or through use of test tablets. A deepening purple color is indicative of the presence of acetone.

Normal Values

Negative

Possible Meanings of Abnormal Values

Increased

Alcoholism
Anorexia
Diabetes mellitus
Diarrhea
Fasting
Fever
High protein diet
Hyperthyroidism
Post-anesthesia
Pregnancy
Starvation
Vomiting

Contributing Factors to Abnormal Values

- Diets high in fat and protein and low in carbohydrates may alter test results.
- Drugs that cause *increased* ketone levels in the urine: anesthesia using ether, isoniazid, isopropyl alcohol, and insulin (high doses).
- *False-positive* results may occur if the urine contains phenylketones (PKU) or levodopa metabolites.
- Drugs that may cause *false-positive* results: bromosulfophthalein (BSP), levodopa, phenazopyridine hydrochloride, phenothiazines, salicylates, sulfobromophthalein, phenolsulfonphthalein (PSP)

Leukocyte Esterase

Leukocyte esterase is an enzyme released from the leukocytes when pyrogenic bacteria (pyuria) are present in the urine. Testing the urine for leukocyte esterase is considered a screening test for the presence of white blood cells in the urine. A positive reaction warrants further investigation by the health care worker to determine whether a urinary tract infection truly exists. This test may be used in conjunction with a dipstick test for nitrites.

This test has been found to be very sensitive, meaning false-negative findings are extremely rare. Thus, a negative dipstick finding requires no further evaluation, unless the patient demonstrates signs and symptoms of a urinary tract infection. Any positive findings with this test should be verified by a urine culture.

Normal Values

Negative

Possible Meanings of Abnormal Values

Positive

Bacteriuria

Contributing Factors to Abnormal Values

- *False-negative* results may occur when there is ascorbic acid or protein in the urine.
- *False-positive* results may occur when there is contamination of urine sample with vaginal secretions.

Nitrites

The substance nitrate, which is derived from dietary metabolites, is normally found in the urine. When certain bacteria, such as the Gram negative bacteria associated with urinary tract infections, are present in the urine, nitrate is converted to nitrite. The presence of nitrite in the urine, then, is an indication that bacteria are also present. This test is used in conjunction with a dipstick test for leukocyte esterase to screen for the presence of bacteria during a routine urinalysis.

The conversion of nitrate to nitrite by bacteria requires the microorganism to be in contact with the nitrate for some time. Thus, the test is best conducted on the first urine specimen of the morning. A reagent strip is dipped into the urine specimen and any color change is compared with a color chart provided by the manufacturer. A negative dipstick finding requires no further evaluation, unless the patient demonstrates signs and symptoms of a urinary tract infection. Any positive findings with this test should be verified by a urine culture.

Normal Values

Negative

Possible Meanings of Abnormal Values

Positive

Bacteriuria

Contributing Factors to Abnormal Values

- *False-negative* results may occur because of:
  - Presence of yeasts or Gram positive bacteria, since there microorganisms do not convert nitrate to nitrite
  - Inadequate nitrate levels in the urine owing to diet lacking in green vegetables
  - Extremely large numbers of bacteria in urine
  - High specific gravity of urine
  - Fresh voided specimen or urine withdrawn from a urinary catheter
- *False-positive* results may occur because of:
  - Contamination of sample by Gram-negative bacteria.
- Drugs that may cause *false-negative* results: ascorbic acid (high level in the urine), antibiotics.

Odor

Another portion of the routine urinalysis, is the assessment of the urine's odor. The normal odor of urine is owing to its acidic content. Various conditions, medications, and foods may cause changes in odor of the urine.

Normal Values

Aromatic

Possible Meanings of Abnormal Values

Condition/Substance	Odor
Food (asparagus, garlic)	Musty
Ketonuria	Sweet/fruity
Maple syrup urine disease	Burnt sugar
Oathouse urine disease (methionine malabsorption)	Brewery odor
Phenylketonuria	Musty, mousey
Trimethylaminuria	Stale fish
Tyrosinemia	Fishy
Urinary tract infection	Fish/foul-smelling

Contributing Factors to Abnormal Values

- If the urine sample is left standing too long, bacteria begin to split urea into ammonia, resulting in an alkaline urine and an ammonia odor.
- Drugs that may alter urine odor: antibiotics, estrogens, paraldehyde, and vitamins.

pH

The determination of the pH of the urine provides information regarding the acid-base status of the patient. Urine is considered alkaline when the pH is greater than 7.0, and is found in such situations as the presence of urinary tract infection. When the urine pH is less than 7.0, or acidic in nature, the cause may be such problems as diarrhea or starvation. There is an inverse relationship between the pH of the urine and the ketone (acetone) level in the urine.

Normal Values

4.3–8.0 with a mean of 5.0–6.0 (diet dependent)

Possible Meanings of Abnormal Values

Increased (alkaline)	Decreased (acidic)
Bacteriuria	Alkaptonuria
Chronic renal failure	Dehydration
Fanconi's syndrome	Diabetes mellitus
Metabolic alkalosis	Diarrhea
Pyloric obstruction	Metabolic acidosis
Respiratory alkalosis	Phenylketonuria

Increased (alkaline)	Decreased (acidic)
	Pyrexia
	Renal tuberculosis
	Respiratory acidosis
	Starvation

Contributing Factors to Abnormal Values

- Foods that may *increase* the pH, making the urine more alkaline: most fruits and vegetables.
- Foods that may *decrease* the pH, making the urine more acidic: cranberry juice, eggs, meats, and pineapple juice.
- Drugs that may *increase* the pH, making the urine more alkaline: acetazolamide, amphotericin B, antibiotics, carbonic anhydrase inhibitors, potassium citrate, salicylates (high doses), sodium bicarbonate.
- Drugs that may *decrease* the pH, making the urine more acidic: ammonium chloride, ascorbic acid, diazoxide, methenamine mandelate, metolazone.

Protein

Another important component of the routine urinalysis is the testing for the presence of protein. In the individual with normal renal function, there is no protein in the urine. This is owing to the glomerular filtrate membrane of the kidney being impervious to the large protein molecules. In the case of renal dysfunction, as in glomerulonephritis, the membrane is damaged, allowing the protein to pass through and be excreted in the urine. Thus, this test is one way in which the health care provider may assess the patient for renal disease. It should be noted, however, that a small percentage of the population may have what is known as *orthostatic* or *postural proteinuria*, which is a benign condition. However, if random urine samples are consistently positive for protein, it is suggested that further testing, including the collection of a 24-hour urine sample, be conducted.

Normal Values

Negative

Possible Meanings of Abnormal Values

Increased

Diabetes mellitus
Glomerulonephritis
Malignant hypertension
Multiple myeloma
Orthostatic proteinuria
Preeclampsia
Premenstrual state
Pyelonephritis
Severe stress
Systemic lupus erythematosus

Contributing Factors to Abnormal Values

- *False-positive* results may occur if the urine is highly alkaline or highly concentrated. If the urine sample is left standing too long, bacteria begin to split urea into ammonia, resulting in an alkaline urine.
- *False-positive* results may occur after eating large amounts of protein.
- *False-negative* results may occur if the urine is highly dilute.
- Drugs that may *increase* the protein level in the urine: acetazolamide, aminoglycosides, aminosalicylic acid, amphotericin B, arsenicals, bacitracin, cephalosporins, chlorpromazine, cisplatin, dichlorphenamide, etretinate, gentamicin, gold preparations, isotretinoin, methazolamide, nafcillin sodium, penicillin (high doses), phenylbutazone, polymyxin B, promazine hydrochloride, radiopaque contrast media, sodium bicarbonate, sulfamethoxazole, sulfisoxazole, tolbutamide, tolmetin sodium, trimethadione.

Specific Gravity

The routine urinalysis also includes the determination of the specific gravity of the urine. The specific gravity is a measure of the concentration of the urine compared to the concentration of water, which is 1.000. The higher the specific gravity, the more concentrated the urine. This test value is an indication of the kidneys' ability to concentrate and excrete urine. The specific gravity is normally lower in the elderly owing to a decreased ability to concentrate urine. There is a condition, known as *fixed specific gravity,* in which the specific gravity remains at 1.010, without variance from specimen to specimen. This is usually indicative of severe renal damage.

There are two methods by which specific gravity may be determined. One method is accomplished through the use of a urinometer, or hydrometer, in which a float is placed into a test tube of urine. The higher the concentration of the urine, the higher the float rises. There are calibrations on the float to indicate the resulting specific gravity. In the second method, a drop of urine is viewed through a refractometer that, when held up to a light, provides the specific gravity reading.

Normal Values

Adult:	1.001–1.040 (Random sample usually 1.015–1.025)
Elderly:	Decreased
Infant:	1.001–1.018 (through age 2)

Possible Meanings of Abnormal Values

Increased	Decreased
Acute glomerulonephritis	ADH deficiency (diabetes insipidus)
Congestive heart failure	
Dehydration	Chronic pyelonephritis
Diabetes mellitus	Cystic fibrosis
Diarrhea	Diuretics
Excessive fluid loss	High fluid intake
Fever	Malignant hypertension
Increased secretion of ADH (owing to trauma, stress, drugs)	
Liver failure	
Low fluid intake	

Increased	Decreased
Nephrosis	
Toxemia of pregnancy	
Vomiting	

Contributing Factors to Abnormal Values

- The specific gravity may be increased when the urine sample has been contaminated with stool or toilet paper.
- Drugs that may *increase* specific gravity: albumin, dextran, glucose, radiopaque contrast media, sucrose.
- Drugs that may *decrease* specific gravity: aminoglycosides, lithium, methoxyflurane.

Urobilinogen

Bilirubin, which is one of the components of bile, is formed in the liver, spleen, and bone marrow. It is also formed as a result of hemoglobin breakdown. There are three types of bilirubin: total, direct (conjugated), and indirect (unconjugated). Conjugated bilirubin is changed into urobilinogen by intestinal bacteria in the duodenum. The majority of urobilinogen is excreted in the stool. The liver reprocesses the remaining urobilinogen into bile. A very small amount is excreted in the urine. An increase in urobilinogen is indicative of hepatic dysfunction or a hemolytic process. Urobilinogen levels are typically highest during the early to mid-afternoon. Thus, should dipstick testing for urobilinogen be positive, the collection of a 2-hour urine would be most appropriate between 1 and 3 PM

Normal Values

Negative or 0.1–1.0 Ehrlich units/dL

Possible Meanings of Abnormal Values

Increased	Decreased
Acute hepatitis	Biliary obstruction
Cirrhosis	Inflammatory disease
Cholangitis	Renal insufficiency
Hemolytic anemia	Severe diarrhea
Hemorrhage into tissues (pulmonary infarction, severe bruising)	
Severe infection	

Contributing Factors to Abnormal Values

- *False-positive* test results may occur in porphyria.
- Drugs that may *increase* urobilinogen levels: aminosalicylic acid, antipyrine, bromosulfophthalein (BSP), cascara, chlorpromazine, phenazopyridine hydrochloride, phenothiazines, sulfonamides.
- Drugs that may *decrease* urobilinogen levels: antimicrobics, chloramphenicol.

Microscopic exam of sediment

Microscopic examination of sediment in the urine includes observation of bacteria, casts, crystals, red blood cells, and white blood cells.

Bacteria

Tests for the presence of leukocyte esterase and nitrites in the urine are conducted to determine whether bacteria are present in the urine. Bacteria may also be noted via the microscopic examination of the urine. Should bacteria be found during a routine urinalysis, culture and sensitivity testing of the urine should be done to determine the organism and to provide assistance in determining appropriate antimicrobial therapy.

Normal Values

Negative

Possible Meanings of Abnormal Values

Increased

Urinary tract infection

Casts

Casts are collections of gel-like protein material which result from the agglutination of cells and cellular debris. They form in, and take the shape of, the renal tubules. Epithelial cells in the renal tubules are the components of *epithelial casts*. *Fatty casts* are formed from fat droplets. When the cellular material in epithelial cells and white blood cells breaks down, the resulting granular particles form *granular casts*. *Hyaline casts* are formed from protein, and thus indicate the presence of proteinuria.

Normal Values

Epithelial:	No casts, occasional epithelial cells
Fatty:	No casts
Granular:	No casts
Hyaline:	1–2 casts per low-power field

Possible Meanings of Abnormal Values

Type of Cast	Condition
Epithelial casts	Amyloidosis
	Eclampsia
	Glomerulonephritis
	Heavy metal poisoning
	Nephrosis
	Tubular damage
Fatty casts	Chronic renal disease
	Diabetes mellitus
	Glomerulonephritis
	Nephrotic syndrome
Granular casts	Acute renal failure

Type of Cast	Condition
	Chronic lead poisoning
	Chronic renal failure
	Glomerulonephritis
	Malignant hypertension
	Pyelonephritis
	Renal tuberculosis
	Strenuous exercise
	Toxemia of pregnancy
Hyaline casts	Acid urine
	Chronic renal failure
	Congestive heart failure
	Glomerulonephritis
	Proteinuria
	Pyelonephritis
	Strenuous exercise
	Trauma to glomerular capillary membrane

Contributing Factors to Abnormal Values

- Urine allowed to stand too long without refrigeration will become alkaline owing to bacterial conversion of urea into ammonia. Should this occur, casts may disintegrate, resulting in inaccurate test results.

Crystals

The accumulation of certain substances in the urine lead to the formation of crystals. They may also form when urine is allowed to stand at room temperature before testing or be caused by several drugs. A few crystals present in the urine have little clinical significance. However, it is problematic when numerous crystals form, resulting in the formation of renal stones. For example, numerous calcium oxalate crystals, resulting from hypercalcemia, may form calcium oxalate stones. Knowing the composition of the renal stone aids the health care provider in determining appropriate treatment modalities.

Normal Values

A few may be normally present

Possible Meanings of Abnormal Values

Increased

Renal stone formation
Urinary tract infection

Contributing Factors to Abnormal Values

- Allowing urine sample to stand at room temperature before testing may alter test results.
- Drugs that cause crystal formation in the presence of acidic urine: acetazolamide, aminosalicylic acid, ascorbic acid, nitrofurantoin, theophylline, thiazide diuretics.

Red Blood Cells and Casts

The microscopic examination of sediment also serves to determine whether any blood is present in the urine, a condition known as *hematuria*. The urine is observed for both red blood cells and red blood cell casts. When red blood cells are present in the urine, it usually indicates damage to the renal glomeruli, which would allow red blood cells to enter the urine. Since there are several interfering factors, such as trauma incurred during catheterization, which might also cause blood to be present in the urine, it is suggested that a fresh urine specimen be collected and the presence of blood be verified.

Red blood cell casts, aggregates of cells formed in the renal tubules, may also be found in the urine. Their presence usually indicates the blood is of glomerular origin, something that may occur in patients with a variety of conditions.

Normal Values

Cells:	0–2 per high-power field
Casts:	None

Possible Meanings of Abnormal Values

Increased: Red Blood Cells	Increased: Red Blood Cell Casts
Acute tubular necrosis	Acute inflammation
Benign familial hematuria	Blood dyscrasias
Benign prostatic hypertrophy	Collagen disease
Benign recurrent hematuria	Glomerulonephritis
Calculi	Goodpasture's syndrome
Foreign body	Malignant hypertension
Glomerulonephritis	Renal infarction
Hemophilia	Scurvy
Interstitial nephritis	Sickle cell anemia
Polycystic kidneys	Subacute bacterial endocarditis
Pyelonephritis	Vasculitis
Renal trauma	
Renal tuberculosis	
Renal tumor	
Subacute bacterial endocarditis	
Systemic lupus erythematosus	
Urinary tract infection	

Contributing Factors to Abnormal Values

- Hematuria may occur because of: tissue trauma from urinary catheterization, strenuous exercise, smoking, and contamination with menstrual flow.
- Drugs that may *cause hematuria:* acetylsalicylic acid, amphotericin B, bacitracin, coumarin derivatives, indomethacin, methenamine mandelate, methicillin sodium, para-aminosalicylic acid, phenylbutazone, sulfonamides.
- *False-positive* results may occur in the presence of: bromides, copper, iodides, oxidizing agents, and permanganate.

- *False-positive* results may occur after intake of certain foods, such as beets, blackberries, and rhubarb.
- *False-negative* results may occur in the presence of ascorbic acid.

White Blood Cells and Casts

A few white blood cells are normally found in the urine. If more than five white blood cells per high-power field are present, a urinary tract infection should be suspected and further testing conducted. White blood cell casts are aggregates of white blood cells that collect in the renal tubules. These casts are seen most often in patients with acute pyelonephritis.

Normal Values

Cells:	4–5 per high-power field
Casts:	None

Possible Meanings of Abnormal Values

Increased: White Blood Cells	Increased: White Blood Cell Casts
Cystitis	Acute pyelonephritis
Glomerulonephritis	Glomerulonephritis
Malignant hypertension	Lupus nephritis
Pyelonephritis	Nephrotic syndrome
	Pyogenic infection

Contributing Factors to Abnormal Values

- If the urine is contaminated with vaginal discharge, test results may be inaccurate.
- Drugs that may *increase* the number of white blood cells in the urine: allopurinol, ampicillin, aspirin, kanamycin, methicillin sodium.

Pre-Test Nursing Care

- Explain to the patient the purpose of the routine urinalysis and the need for a urine sample to be obtained.
- No fasting is required before the test.

Procedure

- Testing the first morning urine specimen, when the urine is concentrated, is preferred.
- A minimum sample of 15 ml of urine is required.
    - A clean-catch midstream technique to obtain the urine sample is recommended to prevent contamination of the specimen.
    - A clean-catch kit containing cleansing materials and a sterile specimen container is given to the patient.
    - Male patients should cleanse the urinary meatus with the materials provided or with soap and water, void a small amount of urine into the toilet, and then void directly into the specimen container.
    - Female patients should cleanse the labia minora and urinary meatus, cleansing from front to back. While keeping the labia separated, the female should void a small amount into the toilet and then void directly into the specimen container.
    - Instruct patients to avoid touching the inside of the specimen container and lid.

- For the portions of the urinalysis which involve use of dipstick testing, a reagent strip is dipped into the urine specimen. After a period of time specified by the manufacturer of the dipstick, the color of the reagent pad is compared with a color chart provided by the manufacturer.
- Gloves are worn throughout the procedure.

Post-Test Nursing Care

- Label the urine specimen and transport it to the laboratory immediately. The urine needs to be examined within 2 hours.
- If urine is collected via an indwelling urinary catheter, a syringe and needle is used. Remove the needle prior to transferring the urine to the specimen cup to avoid damage to any microscopic sediment which may be present.
- Report abnormal findings to the primary care provider.
- Obtain orders for any additional testing that may be indicated by abnormal urinalysis results.

• • • • • • • • • • • • • • • • • •

Urine Culture and Sensitivity
(Urine for C & S)

The urine is normally a sterile body fluid. Although a few bacteria reside in the urethra, in the absence of infection, bacteria should not normally be present in the urine.

When a patient is suspected of having a urinary tract infection (UTI), a urine for culture and sensitivity is ordered. The urine specimen should be obtained prior to the beginning of antibiotic therapy. This test involves several components. First a Gram stain of the specimen can be done and quickly reported. This provides basic information as to whether the organism is Gram positive or Gram negative. Next, the urine is cultured, that is, the organisms are allowed to grow in special culture media. In 48–72 hours, the organism is usually identified. The sensitivity portion of the test involves the testing of the organism to identify drugs to which the organism is sensitive or resistant.

Once the specimen is obtained, the patient is usually given a broad-spectrum antibiotic that is likely to be effective against most UTIs. After the urine culture and sensitivity results are available, the antibiotic in use should be verified as to its appropriateness according to the sensitivity report.

Normal Values

No growth

Possible Meanings of Abnormal Values

Increased

Probable sample contamination with bacterial counts < 10,000/mL
Urinary tract infection with bacterial counts > 100,000/mL

Contributing Factors to Abnormal Values

- Improper collection technique may alter test results.
- Drugs that may *decrease* bacterial counts: antibiotics.

Pre-Test Nursing Care

- Explain to the patient the purpose of the test and the need for a urine sample.
- No fasting is required before the test.

Procedure

- At least 5 ml of urine is needed for this test.
- Use of clean-catch midstream technique is recommended to prevent contamination of the specimen.
    - A clean-catch kit containing cleansing materials and a sterile specimen container is given to the patient.
    - Male patients should cleanse the urinary meatus with the materials provided or with soap and water, void a small amount of urine into the toilet, and then void directly into the specimen container.
    - Female patients should cleanse the labia minora and urinary meatus, cleansing from front to back. While keeping the labia separated, the female should void a small amount into the toilet and then void directly into the specimen container.
    - Instruct patients to avoid touching the inside of the specimen container and lid.
- Other methods for obtaining the urine specimen include catheterization of the patient solely to obtain the specimen, obtaining the sample from an indwelling urinary catheterization, or, in the case of patients with urinary diversions, obtaining the sample through the stoma. In neonates and infants, suprapubic aspiration may be necessary. A disposable pouch (U bag) is also used with infants and young children.
- Gloves are to be worn by the health care worker when dealing with the specimen.

Post-Test Nursing Care

- Label the specimen. It must be transported to the laboratory immediately or placed on ice.
- Report results of the culture and sensitivity to the primary care provider so that modifications in drug therapy are made if needed.

• • • • • • • • • • • • • • • •

Urobilinogen, Fecal

Bilirubin, which is one of the components of bile, is formed in the liver, spleen, and bone marrow. It is also formed as a result of hemoglobin breakdown. There are three types of bilirubin: total, direct (conjugated), and indirect (unconjugated).

Direct, or conjugated, bilirubin is converted to urobilinogen by intestinal bacteria in the duodenum. The majority of urobilinogen is excreted in the stool. The liver reprocesses the remaining urobilinogen into bile. A very small amount is excreted in the urine.

The fecal urobilinogen level is dependent on the amount of conjugated bilirubin excreted in the bile salts into the intestine. Fecal urobilinogen levels decrease when obstructive jaundice (as from gallstones) or hepatic jaundice occurs, since the bilirubin is unable to reach the intestines for excretion and instead enters the bloodstream for excretion by the kidneys.

There must also be adequate numbers of bacteria present in the intestine to breakdown the bilirubin into urobilinogen. With inadequate bacterial presence, as occurs following oral antibiotic therapy, the decreased urobilinogen in the feces results in a light-colored stool.

Normal Values

30–200 mg/100 g of feces (50–300 mg/24 hours)

Possible Meanings of Abnormal Values

Increased	Decreased
Hemolytic anemias	Aplastic anemia
Hemolytic jaundice	Complete biliary obstruction
	Hepatic jaundice
	Obstructive jaundice
	Oral antibiotic therapy
	Severe liver disease

Contributing Factors to Abnormal Values

- Drugs that may *increase* fecal urobilinogen levels: salicylates, sulfonamides.
- Drugs that may *decrease* fecal urobilinogen levels: broad spectrum antibiotics.

Pre-Test Nursing Care

- Explain to the patient the purpose of the test and the need for a stool sample.
- No fasting is required before the test.
- Instruct the patient to avoid contaminating the stool with toilet paper or urine.

Procedure

- Collect the stool specimen using tongue blades. Place it in a dry, clean, urine-free container.
- Gloves are worn throughout the procedure.

Post-Test Nursing Care

- Cover the specimen, label the container, and transport it to the laboratory immediately.
- Report abnormal findings to the primary care provider.

Uroflowmetry
(Urine Flow Studies, Urodynamic Studies)

Uroflowmetry is a noninvasive procedure that is used to detect dysfunctional voiding patterns. The test includes the measurement of the voiding duration, amount, and rate using a urine flowmeter, an instrument into which the patient voids. For the most accurate evaluation of urine flow patterns, recording of each voiding for 2–3 days should be performed. Uroflowmetry is usually performed in conjunction with other urinary tract testing, such as cystometry. Although the urethral pressure profile test is more often used, uroflowmetry is useful for testing patients in whom urinary catheterization is contraindicated.

Normal Values

(*Note:* Values are based on a minimum urine volume of 200 mL for adults and 100 mL for children under age 14)

	Female	Male
>age 64	10 mL/sec	9 mL/sec
age 46–64	15 mL/sec	12 mL/sec
age 14–45	18 mL/sec	21 mL/sec
age 8–13	15 mL/sec	12 mL/sec
<age 8	10 mL/sec	10 mL/sec

Possible Meanings of Abnormal Values

External sphincter dysfunction
Hypotonia of detrusor muscle
Outflow obstruction (Urethral stricture, prostatic cancer, benign prostatic hypertrophy)
Stress incontinence

Contributing Factors to Abnormal Values

- Drugs such as urinary spasmolytics and anticholinergics may alter test results.
- Contamination of the flowmeter by toilet paper or stool will alter test results.

Pre-Test Nursing Care

- Explain to the patient the purpose of the test.
- Instruct the patient to void into the urine flowmeter. No toilet paper or stool can be allowed to enter the flowmeter funnel, or the test results will be altered.
- No fasting is required before the test.

Procedure

- When the patient feels the urge to void, a normal voiding position should be assumed. Voiding should occur directly into the urine flowmeter; the bladder is to be completely empty.
- Serial recordings of each voiding over 2–3 days are usually performed.

Post-Test Nursing Care

- Uroflowmeter recordings are analyzed and displayed graphically by the instrument.
- Report abnormal findings to the primary care provider.

• • • • • • • • • • • • • • • • •

Uroporphyrinogen-I-Synthase
(Porphobilinogen Deaminase)

Uroporphyrinogen-I-synthase is an enzyme found in red blood cells that is necessary for the conversion of porphobilinogen to uroporphyrinogen during the production of heme (see "Aminolevulinic Acid" for heme synthesis pathway). This test is used to diagnose acute intermittent porphyria (AIP), during both latent and active phases. Most importantly, it can be used to detect individuals affected with AIP prior to the occurrence of any acute episodes, episodes that can be fatal.

Normal Values

Female: 8.0–16.8 nmol/sec/L
Male: 7.9–14.7 nmol/sec/L
(Values <6.0 nmol/sec/L are definitive for AIP.)

Possible Meanings of Abnormal Values

Decreased

Acute intermittent porphyria

Contributing Factors to Abnormal Values

- Hemolysis owing to rough handling of the sample
- False positive due to failure to freeze sample
- Failure to fast before the test
- Hemolytic and hepatic diseases may increase uroporphyrinogen-I-synthase levels.
- Low-carbohydrate diets, alcohol intake, infection, and certain drugs may decrease uroporphyrinogen-I-synthase levels.

Pre-Test Nursing Care

- Explain to the patient the purpose of the test and that it involves taking a blood sample.
- The patient needs to fast for 12–14 hours before the test.
- Explain to the patient that abstinence from alcohol is needed for 24 hours before the test. Intake of water is allowed.

Procedure

- A 10-mL sample of blood is drawn in a collection tube containing heparin.
- Gloves are worn throughout the procedure.

V

Post-Test Nursing Care

- Apply pressure at venipuncture site. Apply dressing, periodically assessing for continued bleeding.
- Handle blood sample gently.
- Label the specimen and transport it *on ice* to the laboratory immediately.
- Include the patient's hematocrit on the lab slip.
- Report abnormal findings to the primary care provider.
- If the patient is found to have acute intermittent porphyria, provide teaching regarding factors that have been found to precipitate acute episodes, including:
  - drugs and hormones: barbiturates, chlordiazepoxide, ergot, estrogens, glutethimide, griseofulvin, meprobamate, methyprylon, phenytoin, steroid hormones, sulfonamides
  - low-carbohydrate diets
  - alcohol consumption
  - infections

• • • • • • • • • • • • • • •

Vanillylmandelic Acid and Catecholamines
(VMA, Dopamine, Epinephrine, Norepinephrine, Metanephrine, Normetanephrine)

The major catecholamines are *dopamine,* secreted from nerve endings, and *epinephrine* and *norepinephrine,* secreted from the adrenal medulla and from nerve endings. These hormones play a vital role in the "fight or flight" response of the body that occurs with stimulation of the sympathetic nervous system. The metabolite of epinephrine, *metanephrine,* and the metabolite of norepinephrine, *normetanephrine,* may also be measured. The end-product of epinephrine and norepinephrine metabolism is *vanillylmandelic acid (VMA).*

In patients with unexplained hypertension, a catecholamine-secreting tumor of the adrenal medulla, known as *pheochromocytoma,* is suspected. By measuring 24-hour urinary levels of catecholamines, metanephrines, and VMA, the increased levels of catecholamines released by such a tumor can be found much more readily than through periodic plasma levels.

Normal Values

Vanillylmandelic acid (VMA):	1.4–6.5 mg/day (7.1–32.7 µmol/day SI units)
Catecholamines:	
Dopamine:	65–400 µ/day (424–2612 nmol/day SI units)
Epinephrine:	1.7–22.4 µ/day (9.3–122 nmol/day SI units)
Norepinephrine:	12.1–85.5 µ/day (72–505 nmol/day SI units)
Metanephrines, total:	0.0-0.9 mg/day (0.0–4.9 µmol/day SI units)

Possible Meanings of Abnormal Values

Increased	Decreased
Exercise	Anorexia nervosa
Ganglioblastoma	Familial dystonia

V

Increased	Decreased
Ganglioneuroma	Idiopathic orthostatic
Neuroblastoma	hypertension
Pheochromocytoma	
Stress	

Contributing Factors to Abnormal Values

- Drugs that may *increase* urinary catecholamine levels: alpha$_1$ blockers, ampicillin, ascorbic acid, aspirin, beta blockers, caffeine, chloral hydrate, epinephrine, erythromycin, ethanol, hydralazine hydrochloride, isoproterenol, labetalol hydrochloride, methenamine mandelate, methyldopa, nicotinic acid, quinidine, quinine sulfate, reserpine (short-term use), sympathomimetics, tetracycline, vitamin B.
- Drugs that may *decrease* urinary catecholamine levels: alpha$_2$ agonists, bromocriptine, calcium channel blockers, chlorpromazine, clonidine hydrochloride, guanethidine sulfate, methenamine mandelate, phenothiazines, reserpine (long-term use).
- Drugs that may cause *false-positive* results for urinary metanephrine levels: chlorpromazine, dopamine hydrochloride, guanethidine sulfate, hydralazine hydrochloride, hydrocortisone, imipramine hydrochloride, isoetharine, levodopa, monoamine oxidase inhibitors, nalidixic acid, phenobarbital, phenylephrine hydrochloride, tetracycline.
- Drugs that may cause *false-negative* results for urinary metanephrine levels: clonidine hydrochloride, guanethidine sulfate, levodopa, propranolol hydrochloride, radiographic contrast media, reserpine, theophylline.
- Drugs that may *increase* urinary VMA levels: aminosalicylic acid, aspirin, bromosulfophthalein, epinephrine, glyceryl guaiacolate, isoproterenol, levodopa, lithium carbonate, methocarbamol, nalidixic acid, norepinephrine bitartrate, oxytetracycline, penicillin, phenazopyridine hydrochloride, phenolsulfonphthalein, salicylates, sulfonamides.
- Drugs that may *decrease* urinary VMA levels: chlorpromazine, clofibrate, clonidine hydrochloride, disulfiram, guanethidine analogs, imipramine hydrochloride, levodopa, methyldopa, monamine oxidase inhibitors, reserpine, salicylates.
- Foods that may cause *false increases* in urinary catecholamine levels: bananas, beer, Chianti wines, cheese, coffee, walnuts.
- Foods that may cause *false increases* in urinary metanephrine levels: bananas.
- Foods that may affect urinary VMA levels: avocados, bananas, beer, cheese, Chianti wines, chocolate, citrus fruits, cocoa, coffee, fava beans, grains, tea, vanilla, walnuts.

Pre-Test Nursing Care

- Explain 24-hour urine collection procedure to the patient.
- Stress the importance of saving *all* urine in the 24-hour period. Instruct the patient to avoid contaminating the urine with toilet paper or feces.
- Inform the patient of the presence of a preservative in the collection bottle.
- Instruct the patient to avoid excessive physical activity and stress during the testing period.
- Foods known to affect test results should be avoided for 3 days before the test. The patient should otherwise consume a regular diet, since fasting will increase test results.

V

- If possible, withhold medications that may alter test results for at least 3 days. Check with laboratory regarding preferred length of time.
- Diuretics, antihypertensives, and sympathomimetics (including over-the-counter medications) should be withheld for 1–2 weeks.

Procedure

- Obtain the proper container containing the appropriate preservative from the laboratory.
- Begin the testing period in the morning following the patient's first voiding, which is discarded.
- Timing of the 24-hour period begins at the time the first voiding is discarded.
- *All* urine for the next 24 hours is collected in the container, which is to be kept refrigerated or on ice.
- If any urine is accidentally discarded during the 24-hour period, the test must be discontinued and a new test begun.
- The ending time of the 24-hour collection period should be posted in the patient's room.
- Gloves are to be worn when dealing with the specimen collection.

Post-Test Nursing Care

- Label the container and transport it on ice to the laboratory as soon as possible following the end of the 24-hour collection period.
- Resume diet and medications as taken before the testing period.
- Report abnormal findings to the primary care provider.

• • • • • • • • • • • • • • • • •

Vitamin B$_{12}$
(Cyanocobalamin, Extrinsic Factor)

Vitamin B$_{12}$ is a water-soluble vitamin obtained from dietary animal sources. It is necessary for DNA synthesis. In order for vitamin B$_{12}$ to be absorbed from the gastrointestinal tract, the intrinsic factor, a glycoprotein secreted by the parietal cells in the stomach, must be present. If the intrinsic factor is lacking, vitamin B$_{12}$ will not be absorbed, and pernicious anemia, a type of macrocytic anemia, will occur. Testing for vitamin B$_{12}$, along with testing for folic acid, is used to diagnose macrocytic anemia.

Normal Values

Normal:	205–876 pg/mL (151–646 pmol/L SI units)
Elderly:	Decreased

Abnormal Values

Borderline:	140–204 pg/mL (103–150 pmol/L SI units)
Deficient:	<140 pg/mL (<103 pmol/L, SI units)

Possible Meanings of Abnormal Values

Increased	Decreased
Chronic obstructive pulmonary disease	Alcoholic hepatitis
	Aplastic anemia
Congestive heart failure	Cancer
Diabetes	Diet deficient in folic acid
Leukemia	Hemodialysis
Leukocytosis	Hypothyroidism
Liver disease	Inflammatory bowel disease
Liver metastasis	Malabsorption
Obesity	Malnutrition
Uremia	Parasites
	Pernicious anemia
	Pregnancy
	Smoking
	Vegetarianism

Contributing Factors to Abnormal Values

- Hemolysis of the sample may interfere with test results.
- Prolonged exposure of the sample to light may alter test results.
- Patients who have received radiographic dyes within 7 days before the test may have altered test results.
- Drugs that may *increase* vitamin B$_{12}$ levels: anticonvulsants, estrogens, and ingestion of vitamin A and vitamin C.
- Drugs that may *decrease* vitamin B$_{12}$ levels: aspirin, alcohol, antibiotics, antineoplastic agents, diuretics, oral hypoglycemics, sedatives, and high doses of vitamin C.

Pre-Test Nursing Care

- Explain to the patient the purpose of the test and the need for a blood sample to be drawn.
- Fasting overnight is required before the test. Water intake is allowed.
- Testing for vitamin B$_{12}$ should be performed before the Schilling test.
- A baseline hematocrit should be obtained.

Procedure

- A 7-mL sample is drawn in a collection tube containing a silicone gel.
- Gloves are worn throughout the procedure.

Post-Test Nursing Care

- Apply pressure at venipuncture site. Apply dressing, periodically assessing for continued bleeding.
- Protect the sample from light by immediately placing the tube in a paper bag.
- Label the specimen and transport it to the laboratory immediately.
- Report abnormal findings to the primary care provider.

• • • • • • • • • • • • • • • •

White Blood Cell Count and Differential

(Basophil Count, Eosinophil Count, Leukocyte Count, Lymphocyte Count, Monocyte Count, Neutrophil Count, WBC Count, and Differential)

W

The purpose of white blood cells is to protect the body from the threat of foreign agents, such as bacteria. All blood cells, including white blood cells, originate from a common stem cell. Blood cell differentiation takes place in the bone marrow. This differentiation results in the development of the phagocytic white blood cells and the immune white blood cells.

The phagocytic white blood cells, which include granulocytes and monocytes, play an important role in the process of phagocytosis, the digestion of cellular debris. The *granulocytes* are so named because of their granular appearance. They are also called *polymorphonuclear leukocytes* (polys) because of their multilobed nucleus. The three types of granulocytes are neutrophils, eosinophils, and basophils. Monocytes, along with lymphocytes, are considered *mononuclear leukocytes,* since their nuclei are not multilobed. They have also been called *agranulocytes* since at one time it was thought they had no granules on their surfaces. However, it is now known that their surfaces do contain extremely small granules.

Neutrophils are the first white blood cells to arrive at an area of inflammation. They begin working to clear the area of cellular debris through the process of phagocytosis. Neutrophils have a lifespan of approximately 4 days. Mature neutrophils are distinguishable by their segmented appearance, thus they are often called "segs." Immature neutrophils, which are nonsegmented, are known as "bands" or "stabs." In the case of an acute infectious process, the body reacts quickly by releasing the neutrophils before they have reached maturity. When this increase in bands is found, it is known as a "shift to the left." As the infection or inflammation resolves and the immature neutrophils are replaced with mature cells, the return to normal is called a "shift to the right." This term is also used to mean that the cells have more than the usual number of nuclear segments. This may be seen in liver disease, pernicious anemia, megaloblastic anemia, and Down syndrome.

Eosinophils play an important role in the defense against parasitic infections. They also phagocytize cell debris, but to a lesser degree than neutrophils, and do so in the later stages of inflammation. They are also active in allergic reactions.

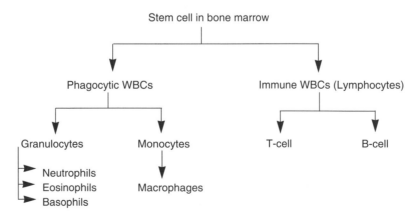

Figure 8 White Blood Cell differentiation.

Basophils release histamine, bradykinin, and serotonin when activated by injury or infection. These substances are important to the inflammatory process since they increase capillary permeability and thus increase the blood flow to the affected area. Basophils are also involved in producing allergic responses. In addition, the granules on the surface of basophils secrete the natural anticoagulating substance, heparin. This provides some balance to the clotting and coagulation pathways.

Monocytes, which live months or even years, are not considered phagocytic cells. However, after they are present in the tissues for several hours, monocytes mature into macrophages, which are phagocytic cells.

The immune white blood cells, which include the *T lymphocytes,* or T cells, and the *B lymphocytes,* or B cells, mature in lymphoid tissue (thymus and bursa) and migrate between the blood and lymph. They play an integral part in the antibody response to antigens. The lymphocytes have a lifespan of days or years, depending on their type. For an in-depth description of these cells, see "T- and B-Cell Lymphocyte Counts."

The white blood cell count and differential test, which is included in a complete blood count, includes two components. The "white blood cell count" denotes the total number of white blood cells (leukocytes) in one cubic millimeter of blood. The "differential" denotes the percentage of basophils, eosinophils, lymphocytes, monocytes, and neutrophils within a sample of 100 white blood cells. Since the differential percentages always equal 100%, an increase in the *percentage* of one type of white blood cell causes a mandatory decrease in the *percentage* of at least one other type of white blood cell. Also included are the absolute values for normal counts of each of the five types of white blood cells.

Normal Values

White blood cell count:	4,300–10,800/mm^3 or	
	4.3–10.8 × 10^9/L (SI units)	
Differential:		
Basophils	0%–2% or	0.00-0.02 (SI units)
Eosinophils	0%–7% or	0.00-0.07 (SI units)
Lymphocytes	16%–45% or	0.16-0.45 (SI units)
Monocytes	4%–10% or	0.04-0.10 (SI units)
Neutrophils:		
Segs	45%–74% or	0.45-0.74 (SI units)
Bands	0%–4% or	0.00-0.04 (SI units)
Absolute counts:		
Basophils	0–216	
Eosinophils	0–756	
Lymphocytes	688–4,860	
Monocytes	172–1,080	
Neutrophils:		
Segs	1,935–7,942	
Bands	0–432	

Possible Meanings of Abnormal Values

Increased Basophils: Basophilia

Certain skin diseases
Chicken pox

Chronic myelogenous leukemia
Chronic sinusitis
Irradiation
Measles
Myeloproliferative disorders (polycythemia vera, Hodgkin's disease)
Myxedema
Postsplenectomy
Smallpox
Ulcerative colitis

Decreased Basophils: Basopenia

Acute infection
Adrenocortical stimulation
Grave's disease (hyperthyroidism)
Irradiation
Pregnancy
Shock
Stress

Increased Eosinophils: Eosinophilia

Addison's disease
Allergic disease (bronchial asthma, hay fever, urticaria, allergic rhinitis)
Cancer of lung, stomach, ovary
Chronic myelogenous leukemia
Hodgkin's disease
Irradiation
Parasitic infections (trichinosis)
Pernicious anemia
Polycythemia
Rheumatoid arthritis
Scarlet fever
Scleroderma
Systemic lupus erythematosus
Ulcerative colitis

Decreased Eosinophils: Eosinopenia

Adrenocortical stimulation
Cushing's disease
Severe infection
Shock
Stress
Trauma

Increased Lymphocytes: Lymphocytosis

Addison's disease
Chronic lymphocytic leukemia
Crohn's disease

Cytomegalovirus
Drug hypersensitivity
Infectious mononucleosis
Pertussis
Serum sickness
Thyrotoxicosis
Toxoplasmosis
Typhoid
Ulcerative colitis
Viral disorders (mumps, rubella, rubeola, hepatitis, varicella)

Decreased Lymphocytes: Lymphocytopenia

Acute tuberculosis
Adrenocortical stimulation
AIDS
Aplastic anemia
Congestive heart failure
Hodgkin's disease
Irradiation
Lymphosarcoma
Myasthenia gravis
Obstruction of lymphatic drainage (tumor, Whipple's disease)
Renal failure
Stress
Systemic lupus erythematosus

Increased Monocytes: Monocytosis

Chronic inflammatory disorders
Chronic ulcerative colitis
Hodgkin's disease
Myeloproliferative disorders
Nonpyogenic bacterial infection (tuberculosis, subacute bacterial endocarditis, syphilis, brucel-
    losis)
Viral infections

Decreased Monocytes: Monocytopenia

Acute stress reaction
Overwhelming infection

Increased Neutrophils: Neutrophilia

Acidosis
Acute hemolysis of red blood cells
Acute pyogenic infections
Cancer of liver, gastrointestinal tract, bone marrow
Eclampsia
Emotional/physical stress (exercise, labor)
Gout

Hemorrhage
Myeloproliferative diseases
Poisoning by chemicals, drugs, venom
Rheumatic fever
Septicemia
Thyroid storm
Tissue necrosis (surgery, burns, myocardial infarction)
Uremia
Vasculitis

Decreased Neutrophils: Neutropenia

Anaphylactic shock
Anorexia nervosa
Aplastic anemia
Hypersplenism
Irradiation
Leukemia
Nonpyogenic bacterial infection
Pernicious anemia
Rheumatoid arthritis
Rickettsial infection
Septicemia
Systemic lupus erythematosus
Viral infection (infectious mononucleosis, hepatitis, measles, rubella)

Contributing Factors to Abnormal Values

- Stress, excitement, exercise, and labor may increase neutrophils.
- Eosinophil counts are lowest in the morning.
- Repeat tests should be done at the same time each time.
- Stressful conditions can decrease the eosinophil count.
- Drugs that *increase* the number of basophils: antithyroid therapy.
- Drugs that *decrease* the number of basophils: antineoplastic agents, glucocorticoids.
- Drugs that *increase* the number of eosinophils: digitalis, heparin, penicillin, propranolol hydrochloride, streptomycin, tryptophan.
- Drugs that *decrease* the number of eosinophils: corticosteroids.
- Drugs that *decrease* the number of lymphocytes: antineoplastic agents, corticosteroids.
- Drugs that *decrease* the number of monocytes: glucocorticoids, immunosuppressive agents.
- Drugs that *increase* the number of neutrophils: endotoxin, epinephrine, heparin, histamine, steroids.
- Drugs that *decrease* the number of neutrophils: analgesics, antibiotics, antineoplastic agents, antithyroid drugs, phenothiazines, sulfonamides.

Pre-Test Nursing Care

- Explain to the patient the purpose of the test and the need for a blood sample to be drawn.
- No fasting is required before the test.

Procedure

- 7-mL of blood are drawn in a collection tube containing EDTA.
- The tourniquet must not be in place longer than 60 seconds.
- Gloves are worn throughout the procedure.

Post-Test Nursing Care

- Apply pressure at venipuncture site. Apply dressing, periodically assessing for continued bleeding.
- Label the specimen and transport it to the laboratory.
- Report abnormal findings to the primary care provider.

• • • • • • • • • • • • • • • • • • •

Wound Culture and Sensitivity

When a patient is suspected of having a wound infection, a wound culture is ordered. The test involves swabbing the interior of the wound. The specimen collection should be performed before the beginning of antibiotic therapy. This test involves several components. First a Gram stain of the specimen can be done and quickly reported. This provides basic information as to whether the organism is Gram positive or Gram negative. Next, the throat swab is cultured, that is, the organisms are allowed to grow in special culture media. In 48–72 hours, the organism is usually identified. The sensitivity portion of the test involves the testing of the organism to identify drugs to which the organism is sensitive or resistant.

Once the specimen is obtained, the patient is usually given a broad-spectrum antibiotic that is likely to be effective against typical wound infections. After the wound culture and sensitivity results are available, the antibiotic in use should be verified as to its appropriateness according to the sensitivity report.

Normal Values

Negative

Possible Meanings of Abnormal Values

Positive

Wound infection

Contributing Factors to Abnormal Values

- Drugs that may cause *false-negative* results: antibiotics.

Pre-Test Nursing Care

- Explain to the patient the purpose of the test.

Procedure

- Swab the site with the cotton-tipped end of a Culturette.
- The swab needs to be of the interior of the wound itself, not of the skin surrounding the wound.
- Gloves are worn throughout the procedure.

Post-Test Nursing Care

- Place the swab in the Culturette tube and crush the distal end. This releases the culture medium that will keep the swab moist.
- Label the specimen and transport it to the laboratory immediately.
- Report abnormal findings to the primary care provider.

Drug Name Reference

Generic Name	Trade Names
acetaminophen	Tempra, Tylenol
acetazalomide	Diamox
acetohexamide	Dymelor
acetylcholine chloride	Miochol
acetylsalicylic acid	Aspirin
albumin	Albuminar, Plasbumin
albuterol	Proventil, Ventolin
allopurinol	Alloprin, Purinol, Zyloprim
alprazolam	Xanax
amiloride hydrochloride	Midamor
aminocaproic acid	Amicar
aminodarone	Cordarone
aminoglutethimide	Cytadren
aminophylline	Somophyllin, Truphylline
aminosalicylic acid	PAS, Pamisyl, Rezipas
amitriptyline	Elavil, Endep
amphotericin B	Fungizone
ampicillin	Omnipen, Polycillin, Principen
anisindione	Miradon
antipyrine	Auralgan
arginine hydrochloride	R-Gene
ascorbic acid (Vitamin C)	Ce-Vi-Sol, Vita-C, Vitamin C
asparaginase	Colaspase, Elspar
aspirin	Ascriptin, Bayer, Ecotrin
atenolol	Tenormin
atropine	Atropisol
azathioprine	Imuran
bacitracin	Bacitracin, Baci-IM
baclofen	Clofen, Lioresal
bethanecol chloride	Duvoid, Urecholine
bismuth salts	Pepto-Bismol
bromocriptine mesylate	Parlodel
bromosulfophthalein	BSP
brompheniramine maleate	Codimal-A, Dimetane
bumetanide	Bumex
busulfan	Myleran

Generic Name	Trade Names
caffeine	Caffedrine, NoDoz, Vivarin
calcitonin	Calcimar
calcium acetate	Phos-Ex, PhosLo
calcium carbonate	OsCal, Tums
calcium citrate	Citracal
calcium gluconate	Kalcinate, Titralac
captopril	Capoten
carbamazepine	Epitol, Mazepine, Tegretol
carbenicillin	Geocillin, Geopen, Pyopen
carbidopa	Lodosyn, Sinemet
carmustine	BiCNU
cascara	Cascara sagrada
cefoxitin	Mefoxin
cephalothin	Keflin
chloral hydrate	Noctec
chloramphenicol	Chloromycetin, Chloroptic
chlordiazepoxide hydrochloride	Librium, Libritabs
chloroquine hydrochloride	Aralen hydrochloride
chlorothiazide	Diuril
chlorpromazine	Promapar, Thorazine
chlorpropamide	Diabinese, Glucamide
chlorprothixene	Taractan
chlortetracycline hydrochloride	Aureomycin
chlorthalidone	Hygroton, Thalitone, Uridon
chlorzoxazone	Paraflex, Parafon Forte DSC
cholestyramine	Questran
cimetidine	Tagamet
cisplatin	CDDP Platinol
citrate	Bicritra, Polycitra
clindamycin	Cleocin
clofibrate	Atromid-S
clomiphene citrate	Clomid, Serophene
clonazepam	Klonopin
clonidine hydrochloride	Catapres

Generic Name	Trade Names	Generic Name	Trade Names
cloxacillin sodium	Cloxapen, Tegopen	droperidol	Inapsine
codeine	Codeine sulfate	epinephrine	Adrenalin chloride, Sus-Phrine
colchicine	Chochicine		
colestipol hydrochloride	Colestid	ergocalciferol	Calciferol, Deltalin, Drisdol
corticotropin	ACTH, Acthar		
cortisone acetate	Cortone	erythromycin	EES, E-Mycin
cyclophosphamide	Cytoxan, Neosar	ethacrynic acid	Edecril, Edecrin
cyclosporine	Sandimmune	ethambutol hydrochloride	Myambutol
cyproheptadine hydrochloride	Periactin		
		ethinamate	Valmid
dactinomycin	Cosmegen	ethionamide	Trecator-S.C.
danazol	Danocrine	ethosuximide	Zarontin
daunorubicin hydrochloride	Cerubidine, Daunomycin	etretinate	Tegison
		famotidine	Pepcid
deferoxamine mesylate	Desferal Mesylate	ferrous sulfate	Feosol, Mol-Iron
desmopressin acetate	DDAVP	finasteride	Proscar
dexamethasone	Decadron, Hexadrol	floxuridene	FUDR
dextran:		fludrocortisone acetate	Florinef acetate
low molecular weight	Gentran, LMD, Rheomacrodex	fluorescein sodium	Fluorescite, Funduscein-10
		fluorides	Fluoritab, Luride
high molecular weight	Dextran 75, Macrodex	fluorouracil	Adrucil, Efudex, 5-FU
dextropropoxyphene	Darvon	fluphenazine	Permitil, Prolixin
dextrothyroxine sodium	Choloxin	flurazepam hydrochloride	Dalmane
diazepam	Valium	folic acid	Folvite
diazoxide	Hyperstat, Proglycem	furazolidone	Furoxone
dichlorphenamide	Daranide	furosemide	Lasix, Myrosemide
dicumarol	Bishydroxycoumarin	gentamicin	Garamycin, Genoptic
diethylstilbestrol	DES, Stilphostrol	glucagon	Glucagon
digitoxin	Crystogidin	glutethimide	Deriglute, Doriden
digoxin	Lanoxin, Lanoxicaps	glyceryl guaiacolate	Robitussin
dimercaprol	BAL in Oil	gold salts	Myochrysine
dinoprostone	Prostaglandin E_2, Prostin E_2	gonadotropin	Glukor, Gonic
		griseofulvin	Fulvicin PG, Grisactin
diphenhydramine hydrochloride	Benadryl, Benylin	guaifenesin	Robitussin
		guanethidine sulfate	Ismelin
diphenylhydantoin	Dilantin	haloperidol	Haldol, Halperon, Peridol
dipyridamole	Persantine	halothane	Fluothane
disopyramide phosphate	Napamidc, Norpace	heparin	Heparin, Liquaemin sodium
disulfiram	Antabuse	hydralazine hydrochloride	Apresoline
dopamine hydrochloride	Dopastat, Intropin		
		hydrocortisone	Cortef, Hydrocortone
doxapram	Dopram	hydroxychloroquine hydrochloride	Plaquenil
doxepin hydrochloride	Adapin, Sinequan		
doxorubicin hydrochloride	Adriamycin, Rubex	hydroxyurea	Hydrea
		hydroxyzine hydrochloride	Atarax
doxycycline hyclate	Doxy, Vibramycin, Vibra-tabs	ibuprofen	Advil, Motrin, Nuprin

Generic Name	Trade Names	Generic Name	Trade Names
imipenem-cilastatin	Primaxin	methadone hydrochloride	Dolophine
imipramine hydrochloride	Impril, Norfranil, Tofranil	methazolamide	Meptazane
indomethacin	Indameth, Indocin, Indocin SR	methenamine mandelate	Mandelamine
insulin	Humulin	methicillin sodium	Staphcillin
iodine containing diagnostic dyes	Idotope	methimazole	Tapazole
		methocarbamol	Robaxin
iopanoic acid	Telepaque	methotrexate	Folex, Mexate, MTX, Rheumatrex
ipodate	Oragrafin		
isocarboxazid	Marplan	methoxyflurane	Penthrane
isoniazid (INH)	Laniazid, Nydrazid	methyldopa	Aldomet, Dopamet, Nu Medopa
isoproterenol	Aerolone, Isuprel, Vapo-Iso		
		methylene blue	Urolene Blue
isotretinoin	Accutane	methylphenidate	Ritalin
kanamycin	Kantrex	methyltestosterone	Android, Testred
ketoconazole	Nizoral	methyprylon	Noludar
labetalol hydrochloride	Normodyne, Trandate	methysergide	Sansert
lactulose	Cephulac, Chronulac	metoclopramide	Reglan
levarterenol	Levophed, Norepinephrine	metolazone	Zaroxolyn
levodopa	Dopar, Larodopa, L-dopa	metoprolol tartrate	Lopressor, Toprol XL
levothyroxine sodium	Synthroid, Levothroid	metronidazole	Flagyl, Metrogel, Metizol
lincomycin	Lincocin	miconazole nitrate	Nicatin, Monistat
lithium carbonate	Eskalith, Lithane, Lithobid	midazolam hydrochloride	Versed
lorazepam	Ativan	minoxidil	Loniten, Rogaine
lovastatin	Mevacor	mithramycin	Mithracin
L-tri-iodothyronine	T_3, Cytomel, Triostat	morphine sulfate	Duramorph, MS Contin, Roxanol
lypressin	Diapid		
mafenide	Sulfamylon	nafcillin sodium	Nafcil, Nallpen, Unipen
mannitol	Osmitrol	nalidixic acid	Neg-Gram
maprotiline hydrochloride	Ludiomil	naloxone hydrochloride	Narcan
		naproxen	Naprosyn
mecamylamine hydrochloride	Inversine	neomycin sulfat	Mycifradin sulfate, Myciguent
mechlorethamine	Mustargen, HN2	neostigmine	Prostigmin
meclofenamate sodium	Meclofen, Meclomen	niacin (nicotinic acid)	Nicobid, Nicolar, Nicotinex
medroxyprogesterone acetate	Depo-Provera, Provera		
		nicotine	Habitrol, Nicoderm, Nicorette
mefenamic acid	Ponstan, Ponstel	nicotinic acid (niacin)	Nicobid, Nicolar, Nicotinex
melphalan	Alkeran		
meperidine hydrochloride	Demerol hydrochloride	nifedipine	Adalat, Procardia
mephenytoin	Mesantoin	nitrazepam	Mogadon
meprobamate	Equanil, Miltown	nitrofurantoin	Furadantin, Macrodantin
mercaptopurine (6-MP)	Purinethol	nitrogen mustard	Mustargen, HN2
		nitroglycerin	Nitro-Bid, Nitro-dur, Nitrostat
metformin	Glucophage		
methacholine chloride	Provocholine	nitroprusside sodium	Nipride, Nitropress

Generic Name	Trade Names
nizatidine	Axid
norepinephrine bitartrate	Levophed
nortriptyline hydrochloride	Aventyl, Pamelor
norethindrone	Norlutin
novobiocin	Albamycin
oxacillin sodium	Bactocill, Prostaphlin
oxamniquine	Vansil
oxazepam	Serax
oxytetracyline	Terramycin, Uri-Tet
oxytocin	Pitocin, Syntocinon
papaverine hydrochloride	Carespan, Pavabid
para-aminosalicylic acid	PAS, Tubasal
paraldehyde	Paracetaldehyde, Paral
parathyroid hormone	Calderol
penicillamine	Cuprimine, Depen
pencillin	Bacillin, Pentids, Pen-Vee K, V-Cillin-K, Wycillin
pentagastrin	Papatavlon
phenazopyridine hydrochloride	Pyridium, Urodine, Urogesic
phenelzine sulfate	Nardil
phenobarbital	Luminal, Solfoton
phenolphthalein	Ex-Lax, Feen-A-Mint, Modane
phenolsulfonphthalein	PSP
phensuximide	Milontin Kapseals
phenylbutazone	Butazolidin
phenylephrine hydrochloride	Neo-synephrine
phenytoin	Dilantin, Phenytex
physostigmine	Antilirium, Isopto Eserine
phytonadione	Aquamephyton, Mephyton
piperazine	Piperazine
polymixin B sulfate	Aerosporin
potassium citrate	Citrolith, Polycitra
prednisolone	Delta Cortef, Prelone
prednisone	Deltasone, Meticorten, Orasone
primaquine	Aralen phosphate with Primaquine phosphate
primidone	Mysoline
probenecid	Benemid, Probalan
probucol	Lorelco
procainamide hydrochloride	Procan-SR, Pronestyl
prochlorperazine	Compazine

Generic Name	Trade Names
progesterone	Gesterol
promazine hydrochloride	Sparine
promethazine hydrochloride	Pentazine, Phenergan
propofol	Diprivan
propoxyphene hydrochloride	Darvon
propranolol hydrochloride	Inderal, Inderal L-A
propylthiouracil	PTU, Propyl-thyracil
pyrazinamide	Pyrazinamide
pyridostigmine bromide	Mestinon, Regonol
pyridoxine hydrochloride	Beesix
pyrimethamine	Daraprim
quinacrine hydrochloride	Atabrine hydrochloride
quinethazone	Hydromox
quinidine	Quinaglute Duratabs, Quinidex Extentabs, Quinora
quinine sulfate	Legatrin, Quinamm, Q-Vel
ranitidine	Zantac
rauwolfia serpentia	Raudixin
rescinnamine	Moderil
reserpine	Serpasil, Serpalan
rifabutin	Mycobutin
rifampin	Rifadin, Rimactane
ritodrine hydrochloride	Yutopar
secobarbital	Seconal sodium
secretin	Secretin-Ferring
senna	Senexon, Senolax
somatrem	Protropin
somatropin	Humatrope, Nutropin
spironolactone	Aldactone
SSKI	Potassium iodide
streptokinase	Streptase
streptomycin	Streptomycin
succinylcholine chloride	Anectine, Quelicin
sulfamethoxazole	Gantanol
sulfasalazine	Azulfidine, PMS Sulfasalzine
sulfinpyrazone	Anturane
sulfisoxazole	Gantrisin
tamoxifen citrate	Nolvadex
temazepam	Restoril

Generic Name	Trade Names	Generic Name	Trade Names
terbutaline sulfate	Brethaire, Brethine, Bricanyl	trimethoprim	Proloprim, Trimpex
		trimipramine maleate	Surmontil
testosterone	Delatestryl, Depo-Testosterone	troleandomycin (oleandomycin)	Tao
tetracycline	Achromycin, Sumycin	tromethamine	Tham
theophylline	Elixophyllin, Quibron, Slo-Bid, Slo-Phyllin, Theodur	trytophan	L-Trypthophan
		urea	Ureaphil
		urokinase	Abbokinase
6-thioguanine	Thioguanine	valproic acid	Depakene
thioridazine hydrochloride	Mellaril	vancomycin	Vancocin, Vancoled
		vasopressin	Pitressin
thyrotropin	Thytropar	verapamil hydrochloride	Calan, Isoptin, Verelan
thyroxine	T_4		
tolazamide	Tolinase	vincristine sulfate	Oncovin, Vincasar
tolbutamide	Orinase	vitamin A	Acon, Aquasol A
tolmetin sodium	Tolectin	vitamin C	See: ascorbic acid
t-PA (alteplase recombinant)	Activase	vitamin D	Calciferol
		vitamin E	Aquasol E, Vita-Plus E, Vitec
tranylcypromine sulfate	Parnate	warfarin sodium	Coumadin, Panwarfin, Sofarin
triamcinolone	Aristocort, Kenacort, Kenalog		
triamterene	Dyrenium		
trifluoperazine hydrochloride	Stelazine		
trimethadione	Tridione		

Drug Classification Reference

Broad Classification	Examples
adrenergic blockers	Normodyne, Regitine
aminoglycosides	Amikin, Garamycin, Kantrex, Nebcin, Streptomycin
amphetamines	Dexedrine, Desoxyn, Preludin
anabolic steroids	Depo-Testosterone, Testex
androgens	Anadrol, Cyclomen, Danocrine, Proscor, Testoderm, Ora Testryl, Testrid, Virilon
antacids	Amphojel, Gaviscon, Maalox, Mylanta, Rolaids, Tums
anticoagulants	Aspirin, Bishydroxycourmarin, Coumadin, Heparin, Levenox
anticholinergics	Atropine, Bentyl, Pro-Banthine
anticonvulsants	Depakene, Dilantin, Klonopin, Mysoline, Tegretol, Zarontin
antimalarials	Aralen, Daraprim, Lariam, Mephaquin, Plaquenil
antimicrobics	Includes anthelmintics, antibacterials, antifungals, antimarials, antiprotozoals, antivirals
antineoplastic agents	Bleomycin, Cytoxan, Elspar, Folex, 5-FU, Interferon, Platinol
antithyroid drugs	Propylthiorucail, Tapazole
antivertigo drugs.	Antivert, Compazine, Dramamine
barbiturates	Amytal, Alurate, Brevidal, Luminal, Nembutal, Pentathal, Placidyl, Seconal, Tuinal

Broad Classification	Examples
benzodiazepines	Ativan, Librium, Paxipam, Valium, Xanax
beta-blocking agents	Corgard, Inderal, Lopressor, Tenormin
calcium channel blockers	Calan, Procardia
cancer antimetabolites	Adrucil, Folex, FUDR
carbonic anhydrase inhibitors	Diamox
cephalosporins	Ceclor, Cefobid, Claforan, Duracef, Fortaz, Keflex, Kefzol, Lorabid, Rocephin
cholinergics	Antilirium, Duvoid, Mestinon, Prostigmin, Tensilon, Urecholine
corticosteroids	Aristocort, Cortef, Decadron, Deltasone, Topicort, Vanceril
coumarin derivatives	Coumadin, Miradon
cytotoxics	See: Antineoplastics
digitalis glycosides	Crystodigin, Lanoxin
diuretics	Aldactone, Bumex, Diamox, Diuril, Hydrodiuril, Lasix, Oretic, Osmitrol
estrogen blockers	Lupron
estrogens	Estrace, Estrotab, Ogen, Premarin
fibrinolytics	Abbokinase, Activase, Streptase
histamine-2 blockers	Tagamet, Pepcid, Zantac
immunosuppressive drugs	Imuran, Sandimmune
laxatives	Colace, Dialose, Dulcolax, Metamucil, Modane, Surfak

Broad Classification	Examples	Broad Classification	Examples
loop diuretics	Bumex, Edecrin, Lasix	steroids	Decadron, SoluCortef, SoluMedrol
MAO inhibitors	Marplan, Nardil, Parnate	sulfonamides	Azulfidine, Benemid, Gantanol,
nitrates	Isordil, Nitroglycerin	sulfonylureas	Diabinese, Orinase
nonsteroidal anti-inflammatory drugs (NSAIDS)	Advil, Aleve, Aspirin, Butazolidin, Clinoril, Indocin, Motrin, Naprosyn, Tolectin	sympathomimetics (adrenergics)	Adrenalin, Brethine, Dobutrex, Intropin, Isuprel, Levophed, Proventil
oral hypoglycemic agents	Glucophage	thiazide diuretics	HCTZ, Hydrochlorothiazide, Thiocyl
phenothiazines	Compazine, Phenergan, Prolixin, Tarasan, Thorazine	thyroid hormones	Euthroid, Levoid, Synthroid, Thyrolar
piperidines	Periactin, Nolahist	tricyclic antidepressants	Elavil, Pamelor, Sinequan, Tofranil
progestins	Depo Provera, Provera		
rauwolfia alkaloids	Raudixin, Serpasil		
salicylates	Aspirin, Bayer, Ascriptin, Doan's Pills, Uracel		
sedative hypnotics	Dalmane, Noctec, Restoril, Seconal		

Test Groupings

This appendix provides a quick reference for some of the more common groupings of tests.

Adrenal Function:

adrenocorticotropic hormone

adrenocorticotropic hormone stimulation test

aldosterone

cortisol, blood

cortisol, urine

dexamethasone supression test

17-hydroxycorticosteroids

17-ketosteroids

pregnanetriol

renin activity, plasma

vanillylmandelic acid and catecholamines

Anemia, Diagnosis of:

blood smear

ferritin

folic acid

free erythrocyte protoporphyrin

glucose-6-phosphate dehydrogenase

hemoglobin

iron

red blood cell distribution width

red blood cell indices

reticulocyte count

Schilling test

total iron-binding capacity

transferrin

transferrin saturation

vitamin B_{12}

Arterial Blood Gases:

base excess/deficit

bicarbonate

oxygen content

oxygen saturation

partial pressure of carbon dioxide

partial pressure of oxygen

pH, blood

Bacteria in Urine (dipstick tests):

leukocyte esterase

nitrites

Cardiac Enzymes:

asparate aminotrans-aminase (AST)

creatine kinase (CK) and isoenzymes

lactic dehydrogenase (LDH, LD) and isoenzymes

Chemistry Profiles:

(*Note:* Tests included depend on chemistry profile ordered, such as SMA 20, SMA 12, or SMA 7. Check with reference laboratory as to which of these tests is included in each.)

alanine aminotrans-ferase (ALT)

albumin (see "Protein")

alkaline phosphatase (ALP)

asparate aminotrans-ferase (AST)

bilirubin, total

calcium

chloride

cholesterol

creatine kinase (CK)

creatinine

gamma-glutamyl transferase (GGT)

glucose, blood

lactic dehydrogenase (LDH)

phosphorus

potassium, blood

protein

sodium, blood

total carbon dioxide content

triglycerides

urea nitrogen, blood

uric acid, blood

Coagulation Studies:

anti-thrombin III

bleeding time

clot retraction test

coagulation factors

D-dimer test

euglobulin lysis time

fibrin degradation products

fibrinogen

partial thromboplastin time

plasminogen

protein C

protein S

prothrombin time

thrombin clotting time

Complete Blood Count with Differential:

blood smear

hematocrit

hemoglobin

platelet count

red blood cell count

red blood cell indices (MCV, MCH, MCHC)

white blood cell count and differential

Electrolytes:

anion gap
bicarbonate
chloride (blood, urine)
potassium (blood, urine)

sodium (blood, urine)
total carbon dioxide content

Fungal Antibody Tests:

blastomycosis
coccidioidomycosis

cryptococcosis antibody
histoplasmosis

Glucose and Other Sugar Metabolism:

galactose-1-phosphate uridyl transferase
glucose, blood
glucose, postprandial

glucose tolerance tset
glycosylated hemoglobin
lactose tolerance test

Heme Biosynthesis:

aminolevulinic acid
free erythrocyte protoporphyrin

porphyrins
uroporphyrinogen-I-synthase

Iron Tests:

ferritin
iron
total iron-binding capacity

transferrin
transferrin saturation

Lipid Profile:

cholesterol
high-density lipoprotein (HDL)

low-density lipoprotein (LDL)
triglycerides

Liver Function:

alanine aminotransferase (ALT)
alkaline phosphatase (ALP)
ammonia
asparate aminotransferase (AST)

bilirubin
gamma-glutamyl transferase (GGT)
leucine aminopeptidase (LAP)
5'-nucleotidase
urobilinogen

Pancreatic Enzymes:

amylase, serum
amylase, urine

lipase

Platelet Activity:

bleeding time
capillary fragility test
platelet aggregation

platelet count
platelet, mean volume

Renal Function:

creatinine, blood
creatinine, urine
creatinine clearance
osmolality, blood

osmolality, urine
urea nitrogen, blood
uric acid, blood
uric acid, urine

TORCH Test:

toxoplasmosis antibody titer
rubella antibody titer
cytomegalovirus (CMV)

herpes simplex antibody

Tumor Markers:

acid phosphatase
CA 15-3
CA 19-9
CA 125
carcinoembryonic antigen (CEA)

human chorionic gonadotropin (HCG)
prostate-specific antigen (PSA)

Urinalysis:

appearance
bilirubin
color
glucose
ketones
leukocyte esterase
nitrites
odor
pH

protein
specific gravity
urobilinogen
microscopic exam of sediment [bacteria, casts, crystals, red blood cells, white blood cells]

White Blood Cell Count and Differential:

basophil count
eosinophil count
leukocyte count

lymphocyte count
monocyte count
neutrophil count

Bibliography

Anand, A, Bashey, B, Mir, T, et al: Epidemiology, clinical manifestations and outcome of *clostridium difficile*-associated diarrhea. American Journal of Gastroenterology 89(4): 519–521, 1994.

Anastasi, JK, Thomas, F: Dealing with HIV-related pulmonary infections. Nursing 94 24(11):60–64, 1994.

Anderson, S: ABGs: Six easy steps to interpreting blood gases. American Journal of Nursing 90(8):42–45, 1990.

Baker, W: Hypophosphatemia. American Journal of Nursing 85(9):999–1003, 1985.

Barland, P, Lipstein, E: Selection and use of laboratory tests in the rheumatic diseases. The American Journal of Medicine 100 (supp. 2A):16S–23S, 1996.

Bass, E, Curtiss, EL, Arena, VC, et al: The duration of Holter monitoring in patients with syncope: Is 24 hours enough? Archives of Internal Medicine 150(5):1073–1078, 1990.

Berkowitz, JF, Cassell, I: Diagnostic imaging: Special needs of older patients. Geriatrics 47(3):55–68.

Beutler, E, Kuhl, W, Vives-Corrons, J, et al: Molecular heterogeneity of glucose-6-phosphate-dehydrogenase. Blood 74 (7):2550–2555, 1989.

Black, JM, Matassarin-Jacobs, E: Luckmann and Sorensen's medical-surgical nursing: A psychophysiologic approach. 4 ed. Philadelphia, WB Saunders, 1993.

Bongard, FS, Sue, DY: Current Critical Care: Diagnosis & Treatment. Norwalk, CT, Appleton & Lange, 1994.

Borton, D: WBC count and differential: Reviewing the defensive roster. Nursing 96:26–31, 1996.

Bullock, BL: Pathophysiology: Adaptations and alterations in function. 4 ed. Philadelphia, JB Lippincott, 1996.

Calloway, C: When the problem involves magnesium, calcium, or phosphate. RN 50(5):30–36, 1987.

Carpenter, DR, Zielinski, DA: How do you treat and control *C. difficile* infection? American Journal of Nursing 92(9): 22–24, 1992.

Carroll, P: Analyzing the Chem 7. RN 60 (11):32–37, 1996.

Carroll, P: More arterial blood sampling tricks. RN 50(3):37, 1987.

Carroll, P: What you can learn from pulmonary function tests. RN 49:24–26, 1986.

Casciato, DA, Lowitz, BB: Manual of clinical oncology. Boston, Little, Brown, 1995.

Cheeseman, SH: Cytomegalovirus. In Gorbach, JL, Bartlett, JG, Blacklow, NR (eds): Infectious diseases. Philadelphia, WB Saunders, 1992.

Chernecky, CC, Krech, RL, Berger, BJ: Laboratory tests and diagnostic procedures. Philadelphia, WB Saunders, 1993.

Chokhavatia, S, Nguyen, L, Williams, R, et al: Sedation and analgesia for gastrointestinal endoscopy. American Journal of Gastroenterology 88(3):393–396, 1993.

Christensen, MB: The use of maternal serum alpha-fetoprotein screening to detect neural tube defects. Journal of the American Academy of Physician Assistants 7 (8):559–567, 1994.

Cohen, L, Kitzes, R: Magnesium sulfate and digitalis: Toxic arrhythmias. JAMA 249(20):2808–2810, 1983.

Coodley, EL: Coronary heart disease: Diagnostic techniques for evaluating myocardial infarction risk. Consultant 2618–2620, 2625–2626, 1996.

Cooper, C: What color is that urine specimen? American Journal of Nursing 93(8):37, 1993.

Corbett, JV: Laboratory tests & diagnostic procedures with nursing diagnoses. 4 ed. Stamford, CT, Appleton & Lange, 1996.

Corwin, EJ: Handbook of pathophysiology. Philadelphia, JB Lippincott, 1996.

Cosico, JN, Rothlauf, EB: Indications, management and patient education: Anticoagulant therapy during pregnancy. MCN American Journal of Maternal Child Health Nursing 17(3):130–135, 1992.

Cruz, C, Hricak, H, Samhouri, F, et al: Contrast media for angiography: Effect on renal function. Radiology 158(1): 109–112, 1986.

Curhan, GC, Willett, WC, Rimm, EB, et al: A prospective study of dietary calcium and other nutrients and the risk of symptomatic kidney stones. New England Journal of Medicine 328(12):833–838, 1993.

Cuzzell, JZ: the right way to culture a wound. American Journal of Nursing 93(5):48–50, 1993.

DeGroot-Kosolcharoen, J: Solving the infection puzzle with culture and sensitivity testing. Nursing 96:33–38, 1996.

Dillon, P: Ovarian cancer: Confronting the silent killer. Nursing 94 24(5):66–69, 1994.

Don, BR, Sebastian, A, Cheitlin, M, et al: Pseudohyperkalemia caused by fist clenching during phlebotomy. New England Journal of Medicine 322(18):1290–1291, 1990.

Eastwood, GL, Avunduk, C: Manual of gastroenterology. 2 ed. Boston: Little, Brown, 1994.

Ehrhardt, BS, Graham, M: Pulse oximetry: An easy way to check oxygen saturation. Nursing 90 20(3):50–54, 1990.

Englert, D, Guillory, J: For want of lactase. American Journal of Nursing 86(8):902–906, 1986.

Fenwick, JC, Cameron, J, Nalman, S, et al: Blood transfusion as a cause of leucocytosis in critically ill patients. Lancet 344:855–856, 1994.

Fischbach, F: A manual of laboratory & diagnostic tests. 4 ed. Philadelphia, JB Lippincott, 1992.

Fischbach, F: Quick reference to common laboratory and diagnostic tests. Philadelphia, JB Lippincott, 1995.

Fletcher, R: Diagnostic decision: Carcinoembryonic antigen. Annals of Internal Medicine 104(1):66–73, 1986.

Flyge, HA: Meeting the challenge of neutropenia. Nursing 93 23:61–64, 1993.

Goldstein, D, Rife, D, Derrick, K, et al: The test with a memory. Diabetes Forecast 47(5):23–25, 1994.

Goroll, AH, May, LA, Mulley, Jr, AG: Primary care medicine: Office evaluation and management of the adult patient. 3 ed. Philadelphia, JB Lippincott Company, 1995.

Graziano, FM, Bell, CL: The normal immune response and what can go wrong. Medical Clinics of North America 69(3):439–452, 1985.

Griffin, J: The bleeding patient. Nursing 86 16(6):34–40, 1986.

Gurevich, I: Hepatitis Part I: Enterically transmitted viral hepatitis: Eitiology, epidemiology, and prevention. Heart & Lung 22(4):370–372, 1993.

Gurevich, I: Hepatitis Part II: Viral hepatitis B, C, and D. Heart & Lung 22(5):450–456, 1993.

Hanson, RL, Nelson, RN, McCance, DR, et al: Comparison of screening tests for non-insulin dependent diabetes mellitus. Archives of Internal Medicine 153:2133–2140, 1993.

Harvey, RL, Roth, FJ, Yarnold, PR, et al: Deep vein thrombosis in stroke: The use of plasma D-dimer level as a screening test in the rehabilitation setting. Stroke 27 (9):1516–1520, 1996.

Hibner, CS, Moseley, MJ, Shank, TL: What is transesophageal echocardiography? American Journal of Nursing 93 (4):74–80, 1993.

Holyoake, TL, Stott, DJ, McKay, PJ, et al: Use of plasma ferritin concentration to diagnose iron dificiency in elderly patients. Journal of Clinical Pathology 46:857–860, 1993.

Holm, K, Walker, J: Osteoporosis: Treatment and prevention update. Geriatric Nursing 11(3):140–142, 1990.

Hoyer, JD: Laboratory medicine and pathology: Leukocyte differential. Mayo Clinic Proceedings 68:1027–1028, 1993.

Jordan, CD, Flood, JG, Laposata, M, et al: Normal reference laboratory values. New England Journal of Medicine 327 (10):718–724, 1992.

Kaplan, A, Jack, R, Opheim, KE, et al: Clinical chemistry: Interpretation and techniques. 4 ed. Baltimore, Williams & Wilkins, 1995.

Katzung, B, (ed): Basic and clinical pharmacology. 6 ed. Norwalk, CT, Appleton & Lange, 1995.

Kee, JL: Laboratory & diagnostic tests with nursing implications. 4 ed. Norwalk, CT, Appleton & Lange, 1995.

Keeys, MJ: Nuclear cardiology stress testing. Nursing 94 24(1): 63–64, 1994.

Kerlikowske, K, Grady, D, Rubin, SM, et al: Efficacy of screening mammography: A meta-analysis. JAMA 273(2): 149–154, 1995.

Knochel, J: The clinical status of hypophosphatemia: An update. New England Journal of Medicine 313(7):447–449, 1985.

Krall, EA, Dawson-Hughes, B: Walking is related to bone density and rates of bone loss. American Journal of Medicine 96(1):20–26, 1994.

Kramer, BS, Brown, ML, Prorok, PC, et al: Prostate cancer screening: What we know and what we need to know. Annals of Internal Medicine 119(9):914–923, 1993.

Kuper, BC, Failla, S: Shedding new light on lupus. American Journal of Nursing 94(11):26–32, 1994.

Lauver, D: Addressing infrequent cancer screening among women. Nursing Outlook 40(5):207–212, 1992.

Lavie, CJ, Milani, RV: Stable ischemic heart disease: Using stress and imaging procedures to direct therapy. Postgraduate Medicine 99 (2):63–66, 73–74, 77–81, 84, 1996.

Lawlor, GJ, Jr, Fischer, TJ, Adelman, DC: Manual of allergy and immunology. 3 ed. Boston, Little, Brown, 1995.

Lawson, T, McCarthy, D, Rogers, A: Tracking and treating acute pancreatitis. Patient Care 20(1):76–109, 1986.

Lee, HH, Chernesky, MA, Schachter, J, et al: Diagnosis of *Chlamydia trachomatis* infection in women by ligase chain reaction assay of urine. Lancet 345:213–216, 1995.

Leidy, KL: Functional performance in people with chronic obstructive pulmonary disease. Image 27(1):23–24, 1995.

Leiner, S: Recurrent urinary tract infections in otherwise healthy adult women. Nurse Practitioner 20(2):48–56, 1995.

Lewis, S: What bilirubin tests can tell you. RN 48(3):85–86, 1985.

Lieu, D: The Papanicolaou smear: Its value and limitations. The Journal of Family Practice 42(4):391–399, 1996.

Lum, G, Thiemke, W: Evaluation of a scoring system for leukocyte esterase-nitrite dipstick screening for urine culture. Laboratory Medicine 20(10).692–695, 1989.

Lutomski, DM, Bower, RH: The effect of thrombocytosis on serum potassium and phosphorus concentrations. American Journal of Medical Science 307(4):255–258, 1994.

Lyle, RM: Iron status in active women: Is there reason to be concerned? Food and Nutrition News 64(5):35–37, 1992.

Malarkey, LM, McMorrow, ME: Nurse's manual of laboratory tests and diagnostic procedures. Philadelphia, WB Saunders, 1996.

Marik, PE: The treatment of hypoalbuminemia in the critically ill patient. Heart & Lung 22(2):166–170, 1993.

Marx, J: Viral hepatitis. Nursing 93 23(1):35–41, 1993.

Mazza, JJ: Manual of clinical hematology. 2 ed. Boston, Little, Brown, 1995

McCance, KL, Huether, SE: Pathophysiology: The biologic basis for disease in adults and children. 2 ed. St. Louis, Mosby-Year Book, 1994.

McConnell, E: How to use a urinometer. Nursing 91 21(10): 28, 1991.

McLean, RM: Magnesium and its therapeutic uses: A review. American Journal of Medicine 96(1):63–76, 1994.

Mehler, E: Preparing your patient to use a fecal occult blood test. Nursing 94 24(5):32R, 1994.

Metheny, N: Why worry about IV fluids? American Journal of Nursing 90(6):50–57, 1990.

Miller, V: Diabetes: Let's stop testing urine. American Journal of Nursing 86(1):54, 1986.

Murray, S, Preuss, M, Schultz, T: How do you prep the bowel without enemas? American Journal of Nursing 92(8): 66–67, 1992.

Nettina, S: Syphilis: A new look at an old killer. American Journal of Nursing 90(4):68–70, 1990.

Niswander, KR, Evans, AT: Manual of obstetrics. 5 ed. Boston, Little, Brown, 1996.

Nugent, LS, Tamlyn-Leaman, K: The colposcopy experience: What do women know? Journal of Advanced Nursing 17: 514–520, 1992.

Olbrych, DD. Interpreting CPK and LDH results. Nursing 93 23(1):48–49, 1993.

Orebaugh, SL: Normal amylase levels in the presentation of acute pancreatitis. American Journal of Emergency Medicine 12(1):21–24, 1994.

Ostchega, Y, Culnane, M: Tumor markers. Nursing 85 15(9): 49–51, 1985.

Pagana, KD, Pagana, TJ: Mosby's diagnostic and laboratory test reference. 2 ed. St. Louis, Mosby, 1995.

Palardy, S, Havrankora, J, Leogo, R, et al: Blood glucose measurements during symptomatic episodes in patients with suspected postprandial hypoglycemia. New England Journal of Medicine 321(21):1421–1425, 1989.

Pittiglio, D, Sacher, R: Clinical Hematology and Fundamentals of Hemostasis. Philadelphia, FA Davis, 1987.

Purcell, J, Haynes, L: Using the ECG to detect MI. American Journal of Nursing 84(5):628–642, 1984.

Qureshi, N, Momin, ZA, Brandstetter, RD: Thoracentesis in clinical practice. Heart & Lung 23(5):376–383, 1994.

Raimer, F: How to identify electrolyte imbalances on your patient's ECG. Nursing 94 24(6):54–58, 1994.

Rakel, RE: Saunders manual of medical practice. Philadelphia, WB Saunders Company, 1996.

Randrup, E, Baum, N: Prostate-specific antigen testing for prostate cancer: Practical interpretation of values. Postgraduate Medicine 99(2):227–234, 1996.

Ravel R: Clinical Laboratory Medicine: Clinical Application of Laboratory Data. 6 ed. St. Louis, Mosby-Year Book, 1995.

Reece, SM: Toward the prevention of coronary heart disease: Screening of children and adolescents for high blood cholesterol. Nurse Practitioner 20(2):22–35, 1995.

Reis, GJ, Kaufman, H, Horowitz, G, et al: Usefulness of lactate dehydrogenase and lactate dehydrogenase isoenzymes for diagnosis of acute myocardial infarction. American Journal of Cardiology 61:754–758, 1988.

Richter, JM, Christensen, MR, Rustgi, AK, et al: The clinical utility of the CA 19-9 radioimmunoassay for the diagnosis of pancreatic cancer presenting as pain or weight loss: A cost-effectiveness analysis. Archives of Internal Medicine 149(10):2292–2297, 1989.

Rogers, AE, Dykstra, C: EEG: A closer look at a familiar diagnostic test. Journal of Neuroscience Nursing 21(4):227–233, 1989.

Schultz, SJ, Foley, CR, Gordon, DG: Preparing your patient for a cardiac PET scan. Nursing 91 21:63–64, 1991.

Shannon, MT, Wilson, BA, Stang, CL: Govoni & Hayes drugs and nursing implications. 8 ed. Norwalk, CT, Appleton & Lange, 1995.

Shmerling, RH: Rheumatic disease: Choosing the most useful diagnostic tests. Geriatric 51 (11):22–24, 26, 29–30, 32, 1996.

Slawson, M: Thirty-three drugs that discolor urine and/or stools. RN 43(1):490–491, 1980.

Smeltzer, SC, Bare, BG: Brunner and Suddarth's textbook of medical-surgical nursing. 8 ed. Philadelphia, JB Lippincott, 1996.

Snell, RS: Clinical anatomy for medical students. 5 ed. Boston, Little, Brown, 1995.

Souder, E, Alavi, A: A comparison of neuroimaging modalities for diagnosing dementia. Nurse Practitioner 20(1):66–74, 1995.

Springhouse Corporation: Illustrated guide to diagnostic tests: Student version. Springhouse, PA, Springhouse Corporation, 1994.

Springhouse Corporation: Nurse practitioner's drug handbook. Springhouse, PA, Springhouse Corporation, 1996.

Stoy, D: Controlling cholesterol with diet. American Journal of Nursing 89(12):1625–1627, 1989.

Stringfield, YN: Back to basics: Acidosis, alkalosis, and ABGs. American Journal of Nursing 93(11):43–44, 1993.

Surks, M, Chopra, IJ, Mariash, CN, et al: American Thyroid Association guidelines for use of laboratory tests in thyroid disorders. JAMA 263(11):1529–1532, 1985.

Swanson, JM, Dibble, SL, Chenitz, WC: Clinical features and psychosocial factors in young adults with genital herpes. Image 27(1):16–22, 1995.

Tallman, V: Effect of venipuncture on glucose, insulin and free fatty acid levels. Western Journal of Nursing Research 4(1):21–34, 1982.

Tasota, FJ, Wesmiller, SW: Assessing ABGs: Maintaining the delicate balance. Nursing 94 24(5):34–44, 1994.

Thomas, CL (ed): Taber's cyclopedic medical dictionary. 18 ed. Philadelphia, FA Davis, 1997.

Thompson, E, Detwiler, DS, Nelson, CM: Dobutamine stress echocardiography: A new, noninvasive method for detecting ischemic heart disease. Heart & Lung 25(2):87–97, 1996.

Treseler, KM: Clinical laboratory and diagnostic tests: Significance and nursing implications. Norwalk, CT, Appleton & Lange, 1995.

Varney, H: Varney's Midwifery. 3 ed. Boston, Jones and Bartlett Publishers, 1997.

Wallach, J: Interpretation of diagnostic tests: A synopsis of laboratory medicine. 5 ed. Boston, Little, Brown, 1992.

Walpert, N: Calcium metabolism disorders. Nursing 90 20 (7):60–64, 1990.

Walsh, PC: Using prostate-specific antigen to diagnose prostate cancer: Sailing in uncharted water. Annals of Internal Medicine 119(9):948–949, 1993.

Watson, J, Jaffe, MS: Nurse's manual of laboratory and diagnostic tests. 2 ed. Philadelphia, FA Davis, 1995.

Weber, MS: Thrombocytopenia. American Journal of Nursing 94(11):46, 1994.

Zaret, GL, Wackers, FJ: Nuclear cardiology. New England Journal of Medicine 329(12):855–863, 1993.

Index